Designing Bioactive Polymeric Materials for Restorative Dentistry

Designing Bioactive Polymeric Materials for Restorative Dentistry

Edited by
Mary Anne S. Melo

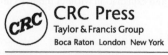

CRC Press
Taylor & Francis Group
Boca Raton London New York

CRC Press is an imprint of the
Taylor & Francis Group, an **informa** business

First edition published 2021
by CRC Press
6000 Broken Sound Parkway NW, Suite 300, Boca Raton, FL 33487-2742

and by CRC Press
2 Park Square, Milton Park, Abingdon, Oxon, OX14 4RN

© 2021 Taylor & Francis Group, LLC

CRC Press is an imprint of Taylor & Francis Group, LLC

ISBN: 978-1-4987-7886-2 (hbk)
ISBN: 978-0-429-11328-4 (ebk)

Typeset in Minion
by codeMantra

Contents

Contents

Preface

Millions of people worldwide suffer from tooth decay (dental caries disease) and its impact on their quality of life. New dental materials, currently being introduced, under development, or envisioned, are expected to be bioactive; in that, they are likely to interact with the surrounding micro-environment positively contributing to oral health. These materials will provide a wide range of functions that could benefit caries management, by inhibiting dental plaque growth, preventing tooth mineral loss, and regenerating diseased dental pulp. Additionally, because the mouth is a dynamic and harsh environment restorative material performance will change over time.

Operative dentistry is a dynamic dental discipline that has progressed and validated the development of dental materials. Operative dentistry deals with immediate placement of restorations with core functions, such as mechanical support to masticatory loads (e.g., dental crowns) and optical properties to display pleasant and natural appearance (e.g., resin composites). Historically, light-cured polymeric dental materials, well known as resin-based materials, have been a great example of an evolving material in the dental field. Over the years, Operative Dentistry has proven the success and limitations of many applied polymeric materials in restorative applications, such as sealants, resin composites, dental bondings, orthodontic adhesives, luting cement, and hybrid materials for computer-assisted design/computer-assisted manufacturing (CAD/CAM).

Advances in material design and polymer chemistry have only recently allowed us to incorporate dynamic features into dental materials. Innovative approaches range from the design of materials that hold low polymerization shrinkage, to eliminate internal stresses and stresses at the margins of the restoration, to those that have stimuli-responsive and interactive properties, where chemical or biological signals can trigger a response in dental material properties or release drugs on-demand. These developing responsive strategies result in "bioactive" materials.

Further, nanoscience and nanotechnology have opened opportunities to provide new solutions in developing dental materials by including bioactive compounds without affecting the functional-aesthetic performance and other core properties, essential for the restoration survival inside the mouth.

Dental researchers have an ongoing interest in endowing bioactivity for dental materials. Currently, limited dental materials present bioactivity. The capability of a dental material to positively affect its biological surroundings is an avenue for improving restoration longevity and clinical service inside the mouth.

Over the past decade, numerous natural or synthetic nano-to microscale agents have been screened and assessed for bioactivity, followed by formulation design and potential application of the materials in multiple clinical conditions. Data to-date clearly illustrates the increased rate of bioactive material development. Significant strides have been achieved toward the clinical application of bioactive dental materials in the last 10 years, and understanding the fundamentals of these processes unlocks future opportunities for innovative design of enhanced dental materials.

This book is organized to highlight the recent significant and exciting research that exploits the advances in dental and materials sciences in the development of dental restorative materials. We also share a forward-looking perspective on the current challenges and future directions for designing the next generation of bioactive dental materials.

In this book, experts in their fields from many countries have provided an overview of concepts for designing bioactive materials for restorative dentistry, including chapters to cover the forward-looking perspective about the current challenges for restorative dental materials, the process of designing bioactive materials, nanotechnology, and tissue engineering; chapters to focus on the different applications of bioactive materials in dentistry; and future directions for designing the next generation of bioactive dental materials.

The information presented includes practice-inspired approaches intended to provide an overview of the latest and most stimulating advances in this area. This book results from an international collaborative team with substantial scientific research publications in the preparation, characterization, and application of various emerging advanced restorative dental materials. This synopsis will give you a knowledge of multiple advances in dental materials and stimulate broad discussion and innovation among researchers and dentists.

Mary Anne S. Melo
Baltimore, MD, USA, 2020

Acknowledgments

First, I would like to show gratitude to our patients who always inspired us to investigate and discuss enhanced preventive and restorative treatment options.

I would like to thank Dr. Howard Strassler, University of Maryland Baltimore, School of Dentistry, a mentor and colleague, who shared his contagious passion for operative dentistry and inspired me to be a dental educator. Words are not adequate to express my admiration and gratitude to his wise guidance, thought-provoking daily discussion, and fostering of critical thinking.

The synopsis in this book would not be possible without the theoretical background to the practice of operative dentistry, especially in underpinning disciplines such as cariology and dental materials science. I thank our mentors, collaborators, and colleagues in these areas for their constant encouragement and contributions.

I would like to thank my undergrad dental students and MS/PhD graduate students, past and present, who have helped us so much to appreciate and enjoy the studies on bioactive restorative materials.

I am forever grateful to my family. This book would not have been possible without the unfailing support of my parents, Mary Sampaio and Anisio Melo, and my dearest husband, J. Chad Blackburn.

Editor

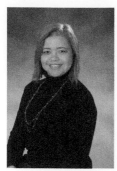

Mary Anne S. Melo, DDS, MSc, PhD FADM, is an Associate Professor and Division Director of Operative Dentistry at the School of Dentistry, University of Maryland, Baltimore, Maryland. Dr. Melo attended dental school at the University of Fortaleza, Brazil, completed a residency in operative dentistry, master's and PhD at the Federal University of Ceara, and pursued fellowship training in dental materials at the University of Maryland before joining the operative faculty.

Dr. Melo is a clinician, researcher, and educator. In her teaching work, she directs and participates in restorative dentistry predoctoral and postgraduate courses and mentors students in master's and PhD research projects. Her main areas of research focus primarily on (1) oral biofilm control with nanotechnologies by investigating anti-biofilm nanotechnologies for the oral healthcare field, (2) biofilm modeling with the development of new in vitro caries/biofilm models, (3) evaluation of the antimicrobial properties of biomaterials, and (4) translational research for the development of clinically relevant therapeutic strategies for the control of dental caries.

She has written over 100 peer-review scientific articles and serves as an ad hoc reviewer and participates in the editorial board of several scientific journals in dentistry, medicine, and biomaterials. Dr. Melo is a fellow of the Academy of Dental Materials and a member of the Academy of Operative Dentistry, the International Association for Dental Research, the Society for Color and Appearance in Dentistry, and the American Academy of Cosmetic Dentistry. Dr. Melo's unique qualifications as a researcher with clinical and materials science perspectives have successfully aligned her role for advances to the dental field.

Contributors

Abdulrahman A. Balhaddad
Dental Biomedical Science PhD
  Program
University of Maryland School of
  Dentistry
Baltimore, Maryland
and
Department of Restorative Dental
  Sciences
Imam Abdulrahman Bin Faisal
  University
Dammam, Saudi Arabia

Maximiliano Sérgio Cenci
Graduate Program in Dentistry
Federal University of Pelotas
Pelotas, Brazil

Lei Cheng
Department of Cariology and
  Endodonics West China
  Hospital of Stomatology
Sichuan University
Chengdu, China

Fabrício Mezzomo Collares
Dental Materials Laboratory
Federal University of Rio Grande
  do Sul
Porto Alegre, Brazil

Joy P. Dunkers
Biomaterials and Biosystems
  Division
National Institute of Standards and
  Technology
Gaithersburg, Maryland

Yoav Finer
George Zarb/Nobel Biocare Chair
  in Prosthodontics, Faculty of
  Dentistry
Institute of Biomaterials
  and Biomedical
  Engineering (IBBME)
University of Toronto
Toronto, Ontario, Canada

Fernando L. Esteban Florez
Department of Restorative
  Sciences Division of Dental
  Biomaterials
University of Oklahoma
Norman, Oklahoma

Isadora Martini Garcia
Dental Materials Laboratory
Federal University of Rio Grande
  do Sul
Porto Alegre, Brazil

Libang He
Department of Cariology and
  Endodonics West China
  Hospital of Stomatology
Sichuan University
Chengdu, China

Maria S. Ibrahim
Dental Biomedical Science PhD
  Program
University of Maryland School of
  Dentistry
Baltimore, Maryland
and
Department of Preventive Dental
  Sciences
Imam Abdulrahman Bin Faisal
  University
Dammam, Saudi Arabia

Sharukh S. Khajotia
Department of Restorative Sciences
  Division of Dental Biomaterials
University of Oklahoma
Norman, Oklahoma

Marlise I. Klein
Department of Dental Materials
  and Prosthodontics
São Paulo State University
São Paulo, Brazil

Jiyao Li
Department of Cariology and
  Endodonics West China
  Hospital of Stomatology
Sichuan University
Chengdu, China

Nancy J. Lin
Biomaterials and Biosystems
  Division
National Institute of Standards and
  Technology
Gaithersburg, Maryland

Sheng Lin-Gibson
Biomaterials and Biosystems
  Division
National Institute of Standards and
  Technology
Gaithersburg, Maryland

Yuan Liu
Department of Orthodontics
University of Pennsylvania
Philadelphia, Pennsylvania

Tamires Timm Maske
Graduate Program in Dentistry
Federal University of Pelotas
Pelotas, Brazil

Kimberly Ngai
George Zarb/Nobel Biocare Chair
  in Prosthodontics, Faculty of
  Dentistry
Institute of Biomaterials and
  Biomedical Engineering
  (IBBME)
University of Toronto
Toronto, Ontario, Canada

Anna Nikikova
Eastman Institute for
  Oral Health
University of Rochester
Rochester, New York

Ashley Reid
University of Maryland School of
   Dentistry
Baltimore, Maryland

Yanfang Ren
Eastman Institute for Oral Health
University of Rochester
Rochester, New York

Jirun Sun
American Dental Association
   Foundation
National Institute of Standards and
   Technology
Gaithersburg, Maryland

Françoise Hélène van de Sande
Graduate Program in Dentistry
Federal University of Pelotas
Pelotas, Brazil

Haohao Wang
Department of Cariology and
   Endodonics West China
   Hospital of Stomatology
University of Maryland School of
   Dentistry
Baltimore, Maryland
and
Department of Cariology and
   Endodonics West China
   Hospital of Stomatology
Sichuan University
Chengdu, China

Suping Wang
Department of Cariology and
   Endodonics West China
   Hospital of Stomatology
University of Maryland School of
   Dentistry
Baltimore, Maryland
and
Department of Cariology and
   Endodonics West China
   Hospital of Stomatology
Sichuan University
Chengdu, China

Michael D. Weir
Dental Biomedical Science PhD
   Program
University of Maryland School of
   Dentistry
Baltimore, Maryland
and
Department of Advanced Oral
   Sciences and Therapeutics
University of Maryland School of
   Dentistry
Baltimore, Maryland

Jin Xiao
Eastman Institute for Oral Health
University of Rochester Medical
   Center
Rochester, New York

Hockin H.K. Xu
Dental Biomedical Science PhD
  Program
Department of Advanced Oral
  Sciences and Therapeutics
University of Maryland School of
  Dentistry
Baltimore, Maryland

Xuedong Zhou
Department of Cariology and
  Endodonics West China
  Hospital of Stomatology
Sichuan University
Chengdu, China

1

An Introduction to Bioactivity via Restorative Dental Materials

Mary Anne S. Melo and Ashley Reid
University of Maryland School of Dentistry

Abdulrahman A. Balhaddad
University of Maryland School of Dentistry
Imam Abdulrahman Bin Faisal University

Contents

1.1 What Does It Mean "Bioactivity" in the Context of Restorative Materials?

"Bioactive" material is not a new term to dentistry, but inexperienced for direct restorative materials, especially for resin-based dental composites. Over the past decade, the search for a response to clinical needs imposed by an increased rate of secondary caries around faulty restorations has led to a growing exploration of this topic. The search for impairment of bioactivity in resin-based restorative material has led to a broad perspective about how a material can be defined as bioactive (Chatzistavrou et al. 2018).

The current meaning extends well beyond the medical-based description for bioactive materials. It is known as a material that can have a biological effect or be biologically active and form a bond between the tissues and the material (Dziadek et al. 2015). Under the umbrella of biomaterials, the ability to form a surface apatite-containing material (ACM), including hydroxyapatite, in a simulated body fluid (SBF) is defined as "bioactivity" (Kokubo et al. 1990). Under a dental restorative perspective, "bioactivity" describes a dynamic, positive biological process. A bioactive restorative material would be able to restore missing tooth structure, re-establish an enhanced esthetic appearance, and additionally, stimulate specific tissue responses or modulate interactions with microbiological species, for instance (Lawson and Robles 2017).

Concerning polymeric restorative materials, here, referred to as methacrylate resin-based materials that have preventive and dental restorative applications has extended the concept of bioactivity (Pratap et al. 2019). Currently, bioactive materials generally refer to biomaterials that can induce a response to the biological system upon interacting. They could have the following bioactivities as illustrated in Figure 1.1:

1. A surface that may nucleate the formation of biological-like calcium phosphates or released components involved in the induction of the bioapatite-like material when in contact with saliva or tissue fluids.
2. The release of key ions, such as calcium ions to assist in the chemical equilibrium of the mineral net into the hard dental tissues, such as enamel and dentin.
3. The release or contact of components of agents that can modulate or suppress bacterial metabolism, consequentially reducing biofilm growth.

Figure 1.2 indicates the pathways of bioactivity toward dental caries prevention via dental restorative materials.

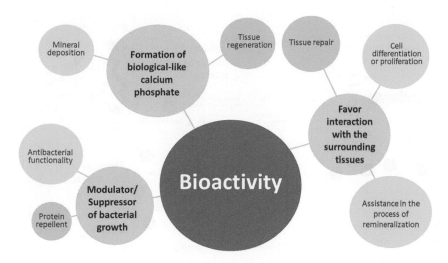

Figure 1.1 (1) A surface that may nucleate the formation of biological-like calcium phosphates or release components involved in the induction of the bioapatite-like material when in contact with saliva or tissue fluids; (2) the release of critical ions, such as calcium ions to assist in the chemical equilibrium of the mineral net into the hard dental tissues such as enamel and dentin; and (3) the release or contact of components of agents that can modulate or suppress bacterial biofilms.

1.1.1 Forecast Market for Bioactive Restorative Materials

Globally, millions of people suffer from toothache due to tooth cavities and often permanent tooth loss. Dental caries, also known as tooth decay is a biofilm-dependent infectious disease that damages teeth by loss of minerals and presents high incidence around restorative polymeric fillings (tooth-colored fillings) (Askar et al. 2020). Untreated caries results in severe pulpal pathologies, which proceeds to tooth loss because the dental enamel cannot regenerate. Also, dental caries is highly prevalent among the elderly population due to unhealthy dietary habits and poor oral hygiene. According to the World Dental Federation, approximately 3.9 billion individuals are affected by dental caries annually, which affects almost half of the world's population (Martins et al. 2017; Edelstein 2006).

The global dental fillings market size was estimated at USD 5.2 billion in 2018 and is projected to register a compound annual growth rate of 7.2% over the forecast period. The growing occurrence of secondary carious lesions, due to dental caries, is the major driving factor. Moreover, a high

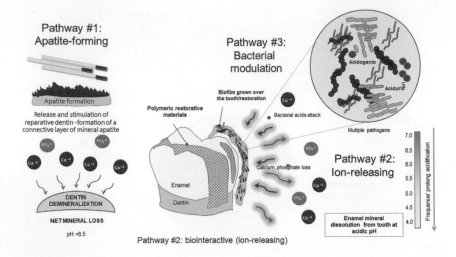

Figure 1.2   Pathways of bioactivity toward dental caries prevention via dental restorative materials can involve: Pathway #1: The use of materials that are capable of inducing bioapatite-like material, Pathway #2: Materials with remineralizing ion release, such as fluoride, calcium, and phosphate ions, to restore the minerals, and Pathway #3: Materials with contact or releasing mechanisms to modulation the dental biofilms and limit the growth of microorganisms.

prevalence of other dental conditions such as trauma, dental erosion due to unhealthy eating habits, and the growing geriatric population is expected to fuel the market ("Dental Fillings Market Size & Share | Industry Report, 2019–2026" n.d.).

The interface between dental fillings and a restored tooth is at a higher risk of pathogenic bacterial colonization. Until now, the majority of commercially available restorative polymeric filling materials present no bioactivity. The complexity of the oral biofilm and the barriers imparted for them contribute to the difficulty in developing effective novel dental materials. Nevertheless, the clinical need is pushing the market to develop new restorative products that present bioactivity.

In a similar growing trend, the bioactive materials market has been projected to exceed USD 3.29 billion in 2025. This market comprises a wide range of materials including implants, ceramics, Bioglass, and composites for medical and dental fields ("Bioactive Materials Market Analysis | Global Industry Report, 2014–2025" n.d.). The growth of the orthopedic and dental surgeries on account with these restorative treatments can offer better oral health status and quality of life, which has resulted in a rise in

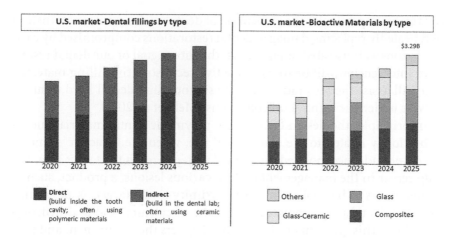

Figure 1.3 The growing trend in both dental fillings and bioactive market in the United States, according to Global Industry reports retrieved in 2019. ("Dental Fillings Market Size & Share | Industry Report, 2019–2026" n.d.; "Bioactive Materials Market Analysis | Global Industry Report, 2014–2025" n.d.)

the demand for implants. Additionally, the demand for superior properties of the bioactive materials has facilitated the rising substitution of the traditionally used implants, thereby driving growth. Figure 1.3 illustrates the growing trend in both dental fillings and bioactive market in the United States according to the Global Industry reports retrieved in 2019 ("Dental Fillings Market Size & Share | Industry Report, 2019–2026" n.d.; "Bioactive Materials Market Analysis | Global Industry Report, 2014–2025" n.d.).

Remarkably, the dental applications represented by restorative materials are the favorable demanding driver for the bioactive materials sector ("Bioactive Materials Market Analysis | Global Industry Report, 2014–2025" n.d.). The dental materials that are in high demand are pulp capping, apexification, root resorption, and root-end filling predicted over the forecast period. However, the unpredictable sizable contribution of the COVID-19 pandemic in the U.S. stock market should be considered (Baker et al. 2020).

1.1.2 Designing Bioactive Polymeric Material

Rapid advances in our understanding of cell and materials interactions provide the basis for an extensive change in the forthcoming of dental treatment, in particular the prevention of dental caries recurrence. Instead of repeatedly replacing damaged dental restorations compromised by carious lesions as illustrated in Figure 1.4, the future goal of our dental restorative intervention will be to use bioactive reconstructive filling materials that will assist the restoration and the surrounding dental hard tissue to survive under harsh intraoral conditions (Melo et al. 2013).

In principle, the design of bioactive polymeric dental materials needs to be closely related to the end clinical use, when the bioactive elements or compounds incorporated into dental material reach the target area. For pulp repair in the management of deep carious lesions, a product, such as a liner, needs to be applied in close proximity to the target tissue. In this case, the dental pulp promotes the release of calcium (Ca) and hydroxyl (OH) ions. This gradient of calcium ions triggers the recruitment and proliferation of undifferentiated cells from the pulp and activates stem cells (Gandolfi et al. 2015).

The polymer composition is the key parameter determining the bioactivity properties as the physicomechanical bulk properties of the intended polymeric restorative materials. For dental polymers, such as resin composites, the bioactive elements included in the compositions could be present in the inorganic composition or in the resin blend

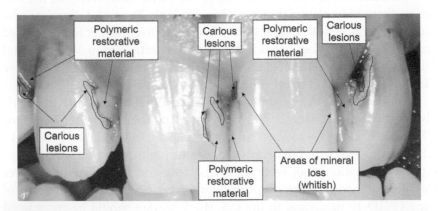

Figure 1.4 Photograph showing secondary carious lesions around polymeric restorations (resin composites). Repetitively replacing damaged dental restorations compromised by carious lesions reduces the life cycle of the teeth. Retrieved from Balhaddad, A. A., A. A. Kansara, D. Hidan, M. D. Weir, H. H. K. Xu, and M. A. S. Melo. 2019. "Toward Dental Caries: Exploring Nanoparticle-Basedplatforms and Calcium Phosphate Compounds for Dental Restorative Materials." *Bioactive Materials* 4 (1):43–55.

composition, as illustrated in Figure 1.5. Elements such as bioactive glass nanoparticles, the released profile of the ions, the nanostructures of the pores, and the surface areas will determine the bioactivity of the materials. Also, by controlling the structure, the bioactivities can be adjusted.

There are evidently other factors that influence the clinical performance of designed materials, including appropriate placement, curing, and oral hygiene. However, these secondary factors cannot overcome the simple fact that the most desirable bioactive profiling at the cost of acceptable physicomechanical or other property required for the materials' functionality will always lead to poor clinical outcomes. In this book, we discuss core additives and compositional approaches that are used to facilitate progress in polymeric restorative materials development. Specifically, we discuss the design of polymeric materials for desired physical-mechanical properties, increased bioactivity, and specific chemical interactions that favor the longevity of the restored tooth.

It seems that the complexity of living cells and their interactions with biomaterials has been a conceptual as well as a practical barrier to the use of newly developed bioactivity in biomaterials science. We will also discuss the main challenges faced by bioactive materials in the intraoral environment.

Core compositional elements for polymeric restorative materials

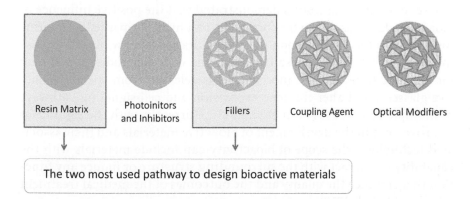

| Resin Matrix | Photoinitors and Inhibitors | Fillers | Coupling Agent | Optical Modifiers |

The two most used pathway to design bioactive materials

Figure 1.5 Basic composition of dental polymers, such as resin composites. Bioactive elements included in the compositions could be present in the inorganic composition or in the resin blend composition.

1.2 Bioactivity Concepts and Properties in Clinical Dentistry

The concept of "bioactive" was established in the late 1960s when a young professor in the Department of Materials Science and Engineering at the University of Florida, Larry Hench, invented the material we know as Bioglass. He created an entirely new paradigm for how biomaterials research viewed the interactions between synthetic materials and the human body (Greenspan 2016). The discovered Bioglass 45S5 or calcium sodium phosphosilicate material was able to replace the defective bone by the deposition of hydroxyapatite to bind the existing bone without any signs of rejection or complications (Hench et al. 1971). In the first stage of Bioglass placement, the alkali ions on the glass surface interact with the hydrogen ions from the surrounding tissue causing hydrolysis of the silica groups and an increased pH. As a result, the silanol group formation occurs and forms a silica-gel layer at the surface of the Bioglass. The calcium and phosphate ions transferred at the silica-rich layer making the structure of the Bioglass similar to the hydroxyapatite layer, which attracts the surrounding growth factors to promote the remineralization and regeneration process (Rabiee et al. 2015; Hench 2006).

Through a series of studies in the 1990s, Professor Hench and colleagues have demonstrated that not only did exposure to the Bioactive glass surface alter the cell cycle in osteoblasts but merely exposing the ionic extracts of the bioactive glass to the cells in the culture at particular ionic concentrations also led to the cell cycle effects (Zhao et al. 2011). The set of pioneering studies demonstrated that the positive influence of bioactive glass was due to the formation of a hydroxyapatite layer, forming the basis for an expansion of the exploration of how bioactive glass interacts with cells. The resulting outcome of these studies has shown for the first time that the inorganic ions released from specific bioactive glasses could alter the gene expression and cell signaling pathways of multiple cell types (Polini et al. 2013). Currently, with the significant improvement in the development of bioactive materials and their associated technology, the scope of bioactivity can include materials with the capability to interact with the surrounding structure or induce any function that enhance the quality and the outcomes of the medical treatment (Skallevold et al. 2019).

With the considerable diversity in dental applications, the concept of bioactivity may vary depending on the study field or clinical specialty. Two years ago, a clinical evaluation panel from the American Dental

Association (ADA) convened and discussed the definition of the terms for *bioactivity* and *biointeractive* ("ACE Panel Report Focuses on Bioactive Materials," n.d.). In the report, 318 practicing U.S. dentists and ADA members shared how they define bioactive materials and concerns regarding the materials. The majority of bioactive products incorporated into polymeric restorative materials are represented by liners, cements, resin composites, and dental bondings. The document also includes clinical insight gathered from literature on defining a bioactive material. This report provides some evidence-based clarity on this topic, insights on current products, and their various indications for use. Also, the report provides information about how clinicians view the essential aspects and characteristics of bioactive dental materials. Table 1.1 lists examples of the commercially available polymeric materials that claim bioactivity. According to the available research, there is still insufficient clinical evidence to support the use. Most of the available literature relies on in vitro studies (Kunert and Lukomska-Szymanska 2020). In theory, most of them that are present have the ability to release calcium, fluoride, or phosphate ions in order to assist the process of remineralization in the tooth structure surrounding the restoration.

1.2.1 Bioactivity in Restorative Dentistry

Operative or restorative dentistry is the branch of general dentistry concerned with the treatment of diseases and/or defects of the hard tissues of teeth, particularly the restoration of the form, function, and aesthetics of the hard tissues. Unfortunately, very often, the hard dental tissues undergo a bacterial acid attack causing a progressive mineral loss that may lead to the terminal stage of cavitation (Cury and Tenuta 2009). Considering this branch of Dentistry, bioactivity could be related to the ability of a material to regenerate or preserve the pulpal tissues or maintain or repair the lost minerals caused by caries and/or erosion.

The use of bioactive materials to reverse the destructive effect of demineralization can be classified into two approaches: (1) the use of bioactive materials that can deposit hydroxyapatite or fluorohydroxyapatite to remineralize demineralized surfaces and (2) the use of bioactive materials that can release molecules or interact with the attached microorganisms in order to reduce the growth and activities of caries-related pathogens, thereby inhibiting the demineralization effects caused by the pathogens. Both approaches can be used in the perspective of the conservative

TABLE 1.1　Examples of Commercially Available Bioactive Restorative Materials, Cements, and Cavity Base/Liners with Their Mechanism of Action

Name	Manufacturer	Application	Bioactive Components
Bioactive Restorative Materials			
ACTIVA™ BioACTIVE-RESTORATIVE™	(PULPDENT, Watertown, MA, USA)	Class I to V restorations, pit & fissure sealant	Calcium, phosphate, and fluoride ions release with recharging capabilities
Biodentine	(Septodont, Lancaster, PA, USA)	Temporary or permanent restorations, pulp capping, and pulpotomy. Other uses include root and furcation perforations, internal and external resorptions, apexification, and retrograde surgical filling	Tri- and di-calcium silicate that can induce remineralizing action
Doxadent	(Doxa AB, Uppsala, Sweden)	To restore posterior cavities	Calcium aluminate cement
BioCoat™	(Premier, Plymouth Meeting, PA, USA)	Pit & fissure sealant	Calcium, phosphate, and fluoride ion release
Beautifil II	(SHOFU, Japan)	Class I-V restorations	Fluoride ion release
Heliomolar	(Ivoclar Vivadent, Schaan, Principality of Liechtenstein, Liechtenstein)	Class I-V restorations	Fluoride ion release
CLEARFIL™ SE PROTECT	(Kuraray Medical Inc, Okayama, Japan)	Dental adhesive	2-Methacryloyloxy dodecyl-pyridinium bromide (MDPB) contact-killing monomer
Bioactive Cement			
ACTIVA™ BioACTIVE-Cement™	(PULPDENT, Watertown, MA, USA)	A dual-cure resin-based material to lute indirect restorations	Calcium, phosphate, and fluoride ion release

(Continued)

TABLE 1.1 (Continued) Examples of Commercially Available Bioactive Restorative Materials, Cements, and Cavity Base/Liners with Their Mechanism of Action

Name	Manufacturer	Application	Bioactive Components
Ceramir®	(Doxa AB, Uppsala, Sweden)	Implant/crown cement	Calcium aluminate/glass ionomer cement containing strontium fluoride
BioCem Universal BioActive Cement	(NuSmile, Huston, TX, USA)	Dual-cure cement	Phosphate, calcium, and fluoride ion release
TheraCem®	(BISCO, Schaumburg, IL, USA)	Dual-cure self-adhesive resin cement	Calcium and fluoride ion release
Bioactive Liners			
ACTIVA™ BioACTIVE-Base/Liner™	(PULPDENT, Watertown, MA, USA)	Base/line material	Calcium, phosphate, and fluoride ion release
Biodentine	(Septodont, Lancaster, PA, USA)	Cavity liner	Tri- and di-calcium silicate that can induce dentin bridge formation
Dycal® light cured Calcium Hydroxide	(DENTSPLY/Caulk, Milford, DE, USA)	Cavity liner	Calcium hydroxide and antibacterial action, suppress the pulp inflammation, and induce mineralization action
TheraCal LC®	(BISCO, Schaumburg, IL, USA)	Cavity liner	Calcium silicate cement with an ability to induce hydroxyapatite and secondary dentin bridge formation
Lime-Lite™	(PULPDENT, Watertown, MA, USA)	Cavity base/liner	Calcium, hydroxyl, phosphate, and fluoride ions to suppress the pulp inflammation and induce dentin bridge formation
Mineral trioxide aggregate (MTA)	(Pro Root, Tulsa Dental, Tulsa, OK, USA)	Cavity liner	Calcium hydroxide to induce pulp repair and dentin bridge formation
Calcimol LC	(Voco GmbH, Cuxhaven, Germany)	Cavity liner	Light-cured calcium hydroxide liner with calcium ion release to induce dentin bridge formation by hydroxyapatite deposition

remineralization therapy or restorative intervention that involves the removal of the carious lesions and the placement of a bioactive restoration (Balhaddad et al. 2019).

1.2.2 Bioactive Restorative Material as Sources of Deflated Ions for Mineral Content

At physiological conditions, the oral fluids (saliva, biofilm fluid) have calcium (Ca) and phosphate PO_4 in supersaturated concentrations to the mineral composition of the enamel. As a result, these ions are continually deposited onto the enamel surface or are redeposited in the enamel areas where the ions were lost. This ion-enrichment and ion-depletion effect can be considered a natural defense phenomenon promoted by saliva to preserve the mineral structure of enamel in the mouth (Naumova et al. 2019).

Therefore, remineralization can be referred to as the redeposition of minerals lost by the enamel, and this term has been used as a similar definition of enamel repair or re-hardening. Redeposition of the mineral lost by enamel can occur due to the presence of Ca, and PO_4 in the biofilm fluid or by the direct action of the salivary Ca and PO_4 soon after the biofilm is removed from the tooth surface. However, the amount of Ca and PO_4 gained is lower than what was lost, and the net result is a minute mineral loss (Nóbrega et al. 2016).

Ions released from a "biointeractive" restorative material or cement may enter the saliva, which drives the process for remineralization in surrounding tooth structure. The supersaturation by high rates of Ca and PO_4 ions released into the surrounding microenvironments under an acidic attack plays a vital role in the precipitation of crystallites. Also, it may be used to overcome the challenges associated with the limited access of ions diffused from one source of mineralizing agents, like toothpaste and mouthwashes to the areas near the materials.

Remineralization therapy involves the use of approaches to arrest early and moderate carious lesions without the need for restorative intervention. The most commonly used products in remineralization therapy are fluoride-containing products, such as fluoridated toothpastes, mouthwashes, gel, and varnish. The fluoride-containing products can provide fluoride ions in the oral environment, which then facilitate the diffusion of calcium and phosphate ions to the tooth structure (Pitts et al. 2017). Also, the deposition of fluorohydroxyapatite to the tooth structure results in higher resistance to future demineralization attack.

Likewise, the incorporation of calcium and fluoride ions into sugar-free gums and varnishes gained considerable attention in the last few years. Casein phosphopeptide-amorphous calcium phosphate (CPP-ACP) products are hypothesized to bind the enamel through casein phospho-peptide (CPP), which then can secure a considerable amount of calcium, phosphate, and fluoride ions to favor the process of remineralization. These products have the potential to keep the environments supersaturated with calcium and phosphate ions rendering the side of remineralization over demineralization (Hamba et al. 2011; Reynolds et al. 2003; Kitasako et al. 2012).

1.2.3 Bioactive Restorative Material as a Suppressor for Bacterial Growth

In operative dentistry, composite resin restorative materials represent a set of materials including bulk composite, dental adhesives, and dental primers (adhesion promoter) with a similar primary composition (Cramer et al. 2011). The bulk composite, representing the body of the restoration, does not adhere directly to the tooth requiring the application of an intermediate layer to connect the dental substrates of different resin-based materials. Dental adhesives and primers are the main reason for the bonding of the bulk composite to tooth substrates, such as enamel and dentin, and the formation of an interlocked interface.

A vast literature has shown concerns with the lifespan of these polymeric restorative materials compared to amalgam, which has mainly been attributed to their higher vulnerability to secondary caries; the foremost reason for restoration failure (Nedeljkovic et al. 2017). Many studies have focused on increasing biofilm growth observed on the composite surface as well as at the interface of the tooth/dental material (Zhang et al. 2016). The potential rationales given for this enhanced biofilm growth could be the lack of antibacterial and buffering properties of composites, the release of bacteria-stimulating compounds or the specific surface characteristics of composite materials including surface roughness, topography, charge, and hydrophobicity. Additionally, these polymeric materials undergo biodegradation in the oral cavity (Wang et al. 2018). Consequently, many researchers suggested that the degradation of composite surfaces by the bacterial acid coming from the attached biofilms can result in increased surface roughness, which will further promote bacterial accumulation leading to irregular circles with even additional impairment to the composite surface (Maktabi et al. 2018).

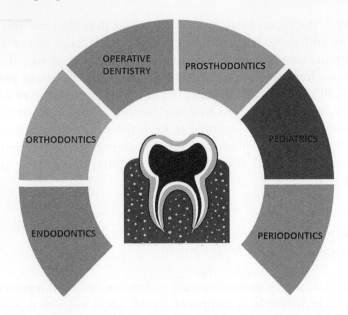

Figure 1.6   Main dental fields where the bioactivities of materials have been explored. The design and formulations are tuned to attend the clinical demands according to the material-intended applicability. The clinical applicability of the materials promotes implications to the formulation designs.

Therefore, evidence-based science materials have critically looked for the design and screen of anti-biofilm agents or compounds that can effectively minimize and modulate biofilm growth over polymeric restorative materials. In this book, many of these strategies will describe and discuss the challenges for the formulation, clinical performance-related requirements, and the material-intended applicability, according to dental disciplines and the current stages of progress toward the clinical translation (Figure 1.6).

1.2.4 Bioactivity in Other Dental Disciplines

1.2.4.1 Prosthodontics
In the large group of applied dental materials presented in this branch, the bioactive types of cement and antibacterial polymers for dentures have given the step ahead. Luting types of cement are often used to attach dental crowns and bridges in place over prepared abutment teeth. Basic mechanical, biological, and handling requirements must be met by the cement

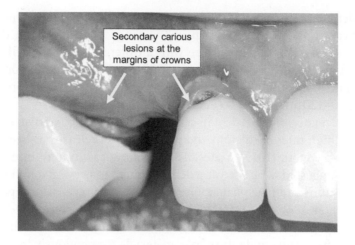

Figure 1.7 Photograph of secondary carious lesions around dental crowns. The fine line of cement between the crown margins and the tooth has been prone to bacterial accumulation and enzymatic degradation, and it is at a higher risk of secondary caries around the crowns.

such as not harming the tooth structure or tissues, allow sufficient working time to place the restoration, enough fluidity to allow complete seating of the restoration, must quickly form a hardened mass strong enough to resist functional forces, must not dissolve or wash out, and must maintain a sealed and intact restoration (Hill 2007).

The fine line of cement between the crown margins and the tooth has been prone to bacterial accumulation and enzymatic degradation, and it is at high risk of secondary caries around the crowns, as illustrated in Figure 1.7. This area is also inclined to indirect restorations not being seated correctly causing open margins. The initial target for bioactive types of cement was to overcome the formed gaps. The rationale is that bioactive types of cement would induce apatite-containing deposits at the open margin. The deposits would serve as a physical barrier occluding the cement gap at the tooth-restorative interfaces avoiding biofilm accumulation.

The preliminary findings on commercially available bioactive cements based on calcium aluminate-glass ionomer (Ceramir Crown & Bridge, Doxa Dental AB, Uppsala, Sweden) suggest the capability of surface apatite-forming. The calcium-based bioactive dental cement could seal or reseal artificial marginal gaps in simulated aqueous physiological conditions (Engstrand et al. 2012). In this study, artificial marginal gaps with dimensions of 50–120 μm appeared to be closed rapidly with apparent first-order behavior in gap closure kinetics. Yet, the single specimen with a significantly larger artificial gap in the range of 250–300 μm demonstrated a slower rate of gap closure with a different kinetic profile. Also, the calcium silicate/Portland cement-type bioactive cement demonstrated a rapid rate of closure of artificial marginal gaps with dimensions in the range of 50–120 μm (Jefferies et al. 2015).

A novel experimental dental cement containing bioactive elements capable of high rates of calcium and phosphate ion release has been investigated by Xie et al. (2019). Materials containing calcium aluminate have also been suggested to be used as a dental cement to prevent demineralization by calcium and phosphate ion release and hydroxyapatite deposition.

Another area of concentrated investigation in prosthodontics is the antibacterial polymeric denture materials. The high rates of adhesion of oral microorganisms to denture base materials tremendously impact oral health with many infections associated with the use of dentures such as oral stomatitis, candidiasis, and dental caries in teeth-supported dentures (Yitzhaki et al. 2018). Acrylic polymethyl methacrylate resin (PMMA) is considered one of the most commonly used materials as a denture base (Garcia et al. 2020). Unfortunately, PMMA is highly susceptible to microbial adhesion and infiltration (Buergers et al. 2007).

The ability to change the fungal and bacterial adhesions has influenced several investigations (Mirizadeh et al. 2018). It was found that phosphate incorporation into PMMA reduced the adhesion of *Candida albicans*. It was hypothesized that the phosphate content could decrease the contact angle and increase the hydrophilicity of the materials to reduce the fungal adhesion (Buergers et al. 2007; Dhir et al. 2007). Also, incorporating 10% of the methacrylic acidic monomer reduces *C. albicans* adhesion (Park et al. 2003). The utilization of quaternary ammonium monomers incorporated into PMMA has been promising to reduce the growth of *Streptococcus mutans* and *C. albicans* over the denture base. Another investigated avenue is the incorporation of ion-releasing metallic particles. Denture base materials that contain silver, silver zeolites, or titanium dioxide nanoparticles showed antibacterial actions against several oral species (Sivakumar et al. 2014).

1.2.4.2 Pediatrics

The polymeric restorative materials used in pediatrics overlap with the majority of restorative materials used for adult patients. Special attention has been given to convey bioactivity to a specific class of preventive materials: resin-based sealants (Monteiro et al. 2020). The purpose of using pit and fissure sealants is to act as a physical barrier against food accumulation, especially at food-stagnating areas such as occlusal pits and fissures. This class of dental materials is represented by light-curable, methacrylate-based resins formulated to present flow, strength, and adhesion to the enamel surface to act as a physical barrier, which prevents metabolic exchange between biofilm located within the fissures and oral environment (Ibrahim, Garcia et al. 2020). The class of glass ionomeric materials presents the high rates of fluoride release with rechargeability; however, the retention rate of glass ionomer sealants was found to be lower compared to resin composite sealants (Colombo and Beretta 2018). On the contrary, the retention rate of resin composite sealant is higher, but it is associated with more plaque accumulation and the lack of bioactivity making the sealant at risk of having microleakages and caries (Simonsen and Neal 2011; Simonsen 2002). Therefore, introducing bioactivity into resin-based sealants can overcome the limitations that are found in conventional resin-based sealants.

Based on the complicated pathogenesis of dental caries, the up-to-date focus of dental materials development has shifted from a single-target approach (antibacterial) to a multi-target approach (antibacterial and/or remineralizing), where several targets associated with the caries process could be affected leading to better outcomes on caries prevention. A multifunctional material intended to be used as a dental sealant with two targeting agents concurrently loaded in a researchable base resin formulation has been recently appraised (Ibrahim, Balhaddad et al. 2020).

1.2.4.3 Orthodontics

In the dental specialty, the polymeric materials are mainly proposed for the bonding of orthodontic brackets and acrylic base formulations for removable orthodontic appliances. During the orthodontic treatment, white spot lesions as incipient carious lesions are frequently observed. The accumulation of plaque around the orthodontic brackets can accelerate the demineralization process, as illustrated in Figure 1.8. Toward this problem, the use of fluoride-releasing materials was suggested to utilize the advantage of fluoride ion release to prevent the demineralization (mineral loss) (Altmann et al. 2016). The use of resin-modified glass ionomer (RMGI) adhesive and fluoride-containing mouthwash as a recharging solution is suggested to guarantee the long-term release of fluoride (Ahn et al. 2011). The development of antibacterial orthodontic adhesives may lower the incidence of white spot lesions by reducing the bacterial attachment and colonization.

An epicenter research area to deal with this problem is the development of bioactive orthodontic bonding agents that goes beyond the physical and

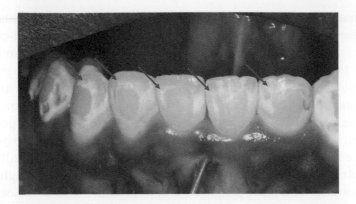

Figure 1.8 Photograph showing the areas of demineralization frequently observed during the orthodontic treatment. The pink arrows show the incipient carious lesions, known as white spot lesions. The accumulation of plaque around the orthodontic brackets can accelerate the demineralization process. Based on it, the newly developed materials should be investigated using models that resemble the actual oral disease with respect to dental anatomy and unique tissues to the oral cavity (i.e., enamel) as well as pathology (demineralization).

mechanical facet to possess bioactivity (Melo et al. 2017). The bioactive orthodontic bonding agents could stabilize/restore the mineral content and contribute to local tissue regeneration (Lim et al. 2008). In this context, orthodontic cement is in direct contact with the vulnerable enamel surface to perform their role as a carrier for remineralizing agents.

The integration of metallic nanoparticles in orthodontic adhesives shows encouraging results on the suppression of the metabolic activities of cariogenic species. The addition of nanoparticles of silver in the orthodontic adhesive is associated with less bacterial attachment and adhesion compared to conventional adhesives (Ahn et al. 2009). Similarly, zinc oxide nanoparticles were added to orthodontic adhesives and demonstrated antibacterial action against *S. mutans* (Jatania and Shivalinga 2014). Benzalkonium chloride addition to the orthodontic composite reduces the growth and adherence of *S. mutans* without affecting the mechanical properties (Othman et al. 2002). Other materials such as 1,3,5-tryacryloylhexahydro-1,3,5-triazine (TAT) and phosphate invert glass-niobium pentoxide (PIG-Nb) demonstrated antibacterial action and some amount of minerals deposition (Altmann et al. 2017).

The incorporation of quaternary ammonium nanoparticles in the orthodontic adhesives was found to reduce the growth of *S. mutans* and *Lactobacillus casei* (Sharon et al. 2018). Concerns related to bioactive agents in the orthodontic bonding agents are related to the ability of such material to maintain the bonding strength for a long time. It is also imperative that the release of such agents will not compromise the mechanical properties of the adhesive. The long-term evaluation of bioactive orthodontic adhesives is needed to confirm the benefits of these materials.

1.2.4.4 Endodontics

The use of bioactive materials in vital dental pulp therapy and root canal treatment is an essential area in dental research (Walsh et al. 2018). In clinical scenarios where pulp exposure occurs during an operative procedure for caries removal, it is the standard of care procedure that a dental material is placed directly over the exposed dental pulp to preserve its vitality. These materials are known as pulp-capping materials (Zhang and Yelick 2010). Pulp-capping materials can trigger the dental pulp to recruit odontoblasts and undifferentiated mesenchymal cells to form the reparative dentin. The main goal of this process is to preserve the pulp vitality and reduce the risk of irreversible pulpitis (Goldberg and Smith 2004).

Calcium hydroxide has been used as a gold standard for direct pulp capping procedures over the years. Because of its high alkalinity (pH 12), it is so caustic that when it is placed in contact with vital pulp tissue, the reaction produces superficial necrosis of the pulp. The irritant qualities seem to be related to its ability to stimulate the development of a calcified barrier. Several drawbacks associated with calcium hydroxide related to leakage, because of the lack of bonding with dentin, dissolution due to mist exposure, and the formation of voids (Asgary et al. 2008; Mohammadi and Dummer 2011). Mineral trioxide aggregate (MTA) has been introduced as an agent capable of promoting cell proliferation and migration, followed by differentiation to odontoblast-like cells. Human studies in primary teeth did not reveal any significant difference between calcium hydroxide and MTA (Schwendicke et al. 2016). However, human studies in permanent teeth demonstrated the ability of MTA to suppress the pulpal inflammation and form the dentin bridge more efficiently than calcium hydroxide (Li et al. 2015; Zhu et al. 2015).

Limitations reported with MTA include the delayed setting time and low handling properties (Asgary et al. 2008). As a result, a new generation of bioactive endodontic cement has been introduced as an alternative. Incorporating antibiotics into endodontic cement to induce antibacterial action and suppress the pulpal inflammation was attempted, but the pulpal healing response was less compared to MTA (AlShwaimi, Majeed et al. 2016). Besides, modifying MTA to shorten the setting time and enhance the handling characteristics were suggested using several materials including Angelus MTA, BioAggregate, EndoSequence BC RRM, and Biodentine. EndoSequence BC RRM and Biodentine revealed similar results considering pulpal healing and bridge formation compared to MTA (Komabayashi et al. 2016).

Increasing attention has been directed toward Biodentine—a bioactive tricalcium silicate cement claimed to have properties comparable to MTA (Table 1.1) (Malkondu et al. 2014). Biodentine triggers the dental pulp to produce the transforming growth factor-beta-1 (TGFβ-1), which leads to the proliferation of odontoblasts revealing the capabilities to treat dental pulp even in the most challenging cases (Laurent et al. 2012). The use of light-cured, resin-modified calcium silicate (TheraCal) was suggested in direct and indirect pulp capping. However, studies showed that Biodentine had improved repairing dentin bridge formation, less inflammatory response, and more pulpal regeneration than TheraCal (Giraud et al. 2017; Bakhtiar et al. 2017).

Another field of intense investigations on bioactive materials for endodontics is the treatment of immature tooth apex subjected to reversible pulpitis or pulpal necrosis. Traditionally, immature permanent teeth can be treated with apexification using calcium hydroxide or MTA. Unfortunately, apexification treatment cannot restore the vitality of the root canal complex in order to induce the apex formation. Therefore, the use of bioactive materials that trigger the revascularization inside the root canal system is essential to promote the apex formation and restore the vitality (Kim et al. 2018). In addition to bioactive materials, revascularization of the root canal system may include the use of stem cell therapy, pulp implantation, regenerative scaffolds, cell printing, and gene therapy (Murray et al. 2007). The stem cells could be injected into the root canal system to regenerate new pulpal tissues. The success of this technique could be improved by the presence of specific scaffolds and growth factors. In pulpal implantation, the pulpal tissue could be isolated and grown in a laboratory setting before being transferred to the pulp canal system. Also, three-dimensional cell printing has been suggested to increase the success of endodontic regeneration. The purpose of this technique is to control the position of the cells before they are transferred to the root canal system. It is suggested when performing the cell printing to keep the odontoblast cells around the peripheries and the fibroblast in the core around the nerves and blood vessels (Murray et al. 2007).

The latest technique in endodontic regeneration involves the use of gene therapy, such as remineralizing genes to induce remineralization (Nakashima and Akamine 2005). It should be mentioned that these advanced regeneration techniques are in their early stages and more in vitro and in vivo studies are needed to confirm their applicability and efficiency. The endodontic research interest should be pushed toward this direction to validate techniques that can regenerate the pulpal tissue and preserve its surrounding structure.

Another field for bioactivity in endodontics is related to the use of antibacterial root canal sealers in the root canal treatment. Root canal treatment aims to eliminate the bacterial infection, disinfect the root canal system from the bacteria and their by-products, and reduce the risk of getting recurrent infections in the future. Despite the disinfection of the root canal system, the total elimination of residual bacteria is not guaranteed and is at risk of being re-infected (Saleh et al. 2004). Therefore, the use of antibacterial canal sealers may improve the success rate of endodontic treatment. *Enterococcus faecalis* is the main endodontic pathogen that is able to invade the dentinal tubules and survive by itself in the treated canals by resisting the endodontic treatment (Sundqvist et al. 1998). The main limitation of most of the available endodontic sealers is related to the loss of their antibacterial function gradually after the setting (AlShwaimi, Bogari et al. 2016).

The formulation of an antibacterial endodontic sealer with prolonged activity has been attempted by the incorporation of antibacterial agents (Baras et al. 2019). Most of the reported studies about the antibacterial activity of endodontic sealers were performed using a mono-species model of *E. faecalis*. The need for multi-species biofilm is essential to get a better understanding of the antibacterial extent and boundaries of these sealers. The developments of a new generation of antibacterial endodontic sealers will minimize the risk of recurrent infection and root canal retreatment, and preserving the root canal system from further loss of structure due to retreatment.

1.2.4.5 Periodontics

Periodontal diseases are considered one of the leading causes of tooth loss. The destruction of the periodontal tissues involves the presence of bone resorption around the affected teeth and the formation of bone defects. Several materials are used as bone substitutes, including autografts, allografts, xenografts, and synthetic materials such as demineralized freeze-dried bone allografts (DFDBA), inorganic bovine bone, hydroxyapatite, and tricalcium phosphate (TCP). These materials can act as a scaffold that osteoblasts can deposit and form new bone. Several bioactive materials such as platelet-rich plasma (PRP), platelet-rich fibrin (PRF), enamel matrix derivative (EMD), and amnion membrane (AM) can be combined with the bone graft materials to enhance the process of bone formation and periodontal regeneration. Both PRP and PRF have multiple growth factors that induce periodontal regeneration by modulating cell proliferation, migration, and differentiation. The use of EMD is suggested to regenerate tooth cementum. The use of AM is believed to suppress the periodontal inflammation and modulate the immune system to induce angiogenesis and wound healing.

A recent systematic review investigated the efficacy of these bioactive materials to heal and generate the periodontal tissue. The use of PRF and PRP in addition to DFDBA was significantly effective to reduce the depth of periodontal pockets compared to DFDBA alone when using the pocket depth as a parameter (Zhou et al. 2018). The use of EMD and AM did not show any improvement related to the pocket depth. Also, EMD did not show any improvement in the clinical attachment gain while PRF, PRP, and AM induce attachment gain with DFDBA better than DFDBA alone. Only PRF+DFDBA showed less gingival recession compared to DFDBA alone, while the other bioactive materials did not show any improvement in the gingival recession. In addition, PRB was found to induce significant bone fill compared to DFDBA alone.

In this review, the enamel matrix derivative is the only bioactive material that did not induce any significant improvement in any of the parameters of the periodontal treatment. Another growth factors that are used in the periodontal treatment are bone morphogenetic proteins. These proteins belong to the transforming growth factor-beta (TGF-β) family that involves 20 proteins. The two most common proteins in this family are recombinant human bone morphogenetic protein-12 and recombinant human bone morphogenetic protein-2, which are used mainly in the treatment of alveolar bone defects (Wikesjö et al. 2004, 2003). Certain limitations are reported with growth factors related to their susceptibility to degradation and dilution prior to the induction of the required regeneration. Therefore, the need for scaffolds is necessary to control the delivery and release of such growth factors (Babensee et al. 2000; Anusaksathien and Giannobile 2002).

Currently, the use of guided tissue regeneration is recommended to relocate the cells to a specific site to induce the desired action of regeneration. In periodontics, combining guided tissue regeneration with grafted materials can be used to treat bone defects, furcation involvement, and gingival recession (Ramseier et al. 2012). More recently, gene delivery to the affected site may provide better stability and efficient regeneration compared to delivering such protein or growth factor. The delivery of human platelet-derived growth factor-β gene is associated with greater cementum and alveolar bone regeneration compared to the delivery of platelet-derived growth factor-β factor (Jin et al. 2004). Also, the delivery of bone morphogenetic protein genes can be used to treat significant bone defects and induce bone regeneration around dental implants (Dunn et al. 2005; Jin et al. 2003). Further research is needed to investigate the advancement of proteins and gene delivery and their interactions with surrounding tissues and oral microorganisms.

1.2.4.6 Implantology

In mplantology, the use of bioactive materials is suggested to inhibit infections caused by bacterial biofilm. Around 14% of implant failure is related to bacterial infection and contamination (Norowski and Bumgardner 2009). The planktonic microorganisms in the oral cavity can attach to the implant surface forming biofilm and causing inflammation of the soft and hard tissues leading to implant failure (Chouirfa et al. 2019). Therefore, specific approaches should be directed to prevent the attachment of oral microorganisms to preserve the implant surface from any bacterial infection. These approaches involve surface modification or coating the implant surface following chemical and physical techniques. The surface modification involves the use of methods to modify the surface of the implant, while surface coating involves the use of additional surface (Chouirfa et al. 2019).

One of the approaches to prevent bacterial attachment is to use anti-adhesion methods, such as changing the surface hydrophilicity–hydrophobicity or altering the crystalline structure of the oxide layer (Verran and Whitehead 2005; Del Curto et al. 2005). Titanium surface with strongly hydrophilic surface and oxide layer rich in crystalline anatase can reduce the bacterial adhesion (Verran and Whitehead 2005; Del Curto et al. 2005). Another approach is to coat the titanium implant surface with silver or zinc oxide particles to reduce the bacterial attachment. The released ions can target and kill the attached microorganisms without causing any cytotoxicity to the surrounding tissues (Chen et al. 2006; Petrini et al. 2006). The coating with fluoride, copper, chlorhexidine, and certain antibiotics shown antibacterial effects (Kulkarni Aranya et al. 2017).

Another constantly concerned area in implants is osseointegration, which is essential to assure the success of a dental implant. The main approaches of surface modification or coating have been implied to enhance the osseointegration around dental implants. Surface topography of the dental implant can contribute to the advantages of osseointegration. Topography changes in macro and micro levels can manipulate the growth and migration of the osteogenic cells and also the associated cytokines in bone metabolism (Smeets et al. 2016). The most significant advantages of implant topography are associated with nanoscale changes where the effect could be in cellular and protein levels, and the adhesion of the osteogenic cells could be increased (Smeets et al. 2016). Increasing the surface roughness of the dental implant can increase the surface area between the implant surface and the deposited osteogenic cells results in a great osseointegration and implant stability. Several methods for surface roughening have been discussed in the dental literature, such as blasting with ceramic particles, acid etching, plasma spraying, electrochemical anodization, and calcium phosphate coatings (Meng et al. 2016). A new approach to enhance the osseointegration involves the use of bioactive molecules and growth factors that are able to trigger the osseointegration. However, more research is needed to confirm its their beneficial effects.

1.3 Future Trends

In recent decades, bioactive polymeric materials have received an enormous amount of interest in the dental scientific community due to the recent advancement potential outcome performance in vitro and the resultant future applications in various dental fields. Bioactive materials

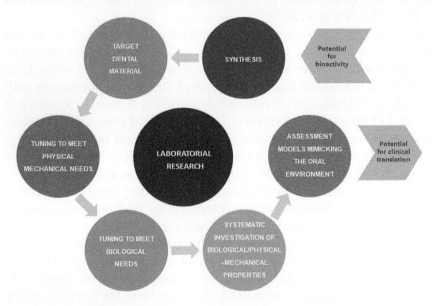

Figure 1.9 Schematic drawing for the progressing route in the development of bioactive polymeric restorative materials. Bioactive restorative materials have been developed to prevent the disease, facilitate repair, and enhance the healing of dental tissues. Although research on bioactive dental materials has made great progress in material innovation and preclinical testing, the model is in their transition from laboratorial research to clinical applications.

for restorative dentistry have evolved in a fast pace over the past three decades. This class of materials has initially presented highly biocompatible properties but low mechanical strength. Now bioactive restorative materials emerge with newly developed compositions that allows the incorporation of bioactive agents improved mechanical properties which can open the range of clinical uses in restorative dentistry.

Further developments to meet clinical survivability are anticipated in this newly emerging category of dental materials. For that, the multidisciplinary aspect of the development of bioactive materials will be critical. An integrative approach involves the study of the interactions that occur at an interface material/tooth/oral environment and is increasingly being investigated to understand, predict, and bind the occurring phenomena toward emerging applications in the dental field. This book attempts to illustrate both the current status in the use of new agents and combinatorial design strategies, as well as the promising advances in the route of progressing a bioactive restorative material from the benchtop to chairside (Figure 1.9).

This book will examine the development of biointeractive/bioactive materials in a context more closely related to restorative dentistry, with the explicit acknowledgment that much of the information has been developed in other specialty disciplines in dentistry. As such, this book will attempt to provide a better understanding of the relative position of bioactive materials in the context of the past and the present status of dental restorative materials.

References

"ACE Panel Report Focuses on Bioactive Materials." n.d. Accessed April 10, 2020. https://www.ada.org/en/publications/ada-news/2018-archive/june/ace-panel-report-focuses-on-bioactive-materials.

Ahn, S.-J., S.-J. Lee, D.-Y. Lee, and B.-S. Lim. 2011. "Effects of Different Fluoride Recharging Protocols on Fluoride Ion Release from Various Orthodontic Adhesives." *Journal of Dentistry* 39 (3): 196–201. https://doi.org/10.1016/j.jdent.2010.12.003.

Ahn, S.-J., S.-J. Lee, J.-K. Kook, and B.-S. Lim. 2009. "Experimental Antimicrobial Orthodontic Adhesives Using Nanofillers and Silver Nanoparticles." *Dental Materials* 25 (2): 206–13. https://doi.org/10.1016/j.dental.2008.06.002.

AlShwaimi, E., A. Majeed, and A. A. Ali. 2016. "Pulpal Responses to Direct Capping with Betamethasone/Gentamicin Cream and Mineral Trioxide Aggregate: Histologic and Micro-Computed Tomography Assessments." *Journal of Endodontics* 42 (1): 30–5. https://doi.org/10.1016/j.joen.2015.09.016.

AlShwaimi, E., D. Bogari, R. Ajaj, S. Al-Shahrani, K. Almas, and A. Majeed. 2016. "In Vitro Antimicrobial Effectiveness of Root Canal Sealers against Enterococcus Faecalis: A Systematic Review." *Journal of Endodontics* 42 (11): 1588–97. https://doi.org/10.1016/j.joen.2016.08.001.

Altmann, A. S. P., F. M. Collares, V. C. B. Leitune, and S. M. W. Samuel. 2016. "The Effect of Antimicrobial Agents on Bond Strength of Orthodontic Adhesives: A Meta-Analysis of In Vitro Studies." *Orthodontics & Craniofacial Research* 19 (1): 1–9. https://doi.org/10.1111/ocr.12100.

Altmann, A. S. P., F. M. Collares, V. C. B. Leitune, R. A. Arthur, A. S. Takimi, and S. M. W. Samuel. 2017. "In Vitro Antibacterial and Remineralizing Effect of Adhesive Containing Triazine and Niobium Pentoxide Phosphate Inverted Glass." *Clinical Oral Investigations* 21 (1): 93–103. https://doi.org/10.1007/s00784-016-1754-y.

Anusaksathien, O., and W. V. Giannobile. 2002. "Growth Factor Delivery to Re-Engineer Periodontal Tissues." *Current Pharmaceutical Biotechnology* 3 (2): 129–39.

Asgary, S., M. J. Eghbal, M. Parirokh, F. Ghanavati, and H. Rahimi. 2008. "A Comparative Study of Histologic Response to Different Pulp Capping Materials and a Novel Endodontic Cement." *Oral Surgery, Oral Medicine, Oral Pathology, Oral Radiology, and Endodontics* 106 (4): 609–14. https://doi.org/10.1016/j.tripleo.2008.06.006.

Askar, H., J. Krois, G. Göstemeyer, P. Bottenberg, D. Zero, A. Banerjee, and F. Schwendicke. 2020. "Secondary Caries: What Is It, and How It Can Be Controlled, Detected, and Managed?" *Clinical Oral Investigations* 24 (5): 1869–76. https://doi.org/10.1007/s00784-020-03268-7.

Babensee, J. E., L. V. McIntire, and A. G. Mikos. 2000. "Growth Factor Delivery for Tissue Engineering." *Pharmaceutical Research* 17 (5): 497–504.

Baker, S. R., N. Bloom, S. J. Davis, K. J. Kost, M. C. Sammon, and T. Viratyosin. 2020. "The Unprecedented Stock Market Impact of COVID-19." *Working Paper 26945. Working Paper Series.* National Bureau of Economic Research. https://doi.org/10.3386/w26945.

Bakhtiar, H., M. H. Nekoofar, P. Aminishakib, F. Abedi, F. N. Moosavi, E. Esnaashari, A. Azizi, et al. 2017. "Human Pulp Responses to Partial Pulpotomy Treatment with TheraCal as Compared with Biodentine and ProRoot MTA: A Clinical Trial." *Journal of Endodontics* 43 (11): 1786–91. https://doi.org/10.1016/j.joen.2017.06.025.

Balhaddad, A. A., A. A. Kansara, D. Hidan, M. D. Weir, H. H. K. Xu, and M. A. S. Melo. 2019. "Toward Dental Caries: Exploring Nanoparticle-Based Platforms and Calcium Phosphate Compounds for Dental Restorative Materials." *Bioactive Materials* 4 (1): 43–55. https://doi.org/10.1016/j.bioactmat.2018.12.002.

Baras, B. H., M. A. S. Melo, J. Sun, T. W. Oates, M. D. Weir, X. Xie, Y. Bai, and H. H. K. Xu. 2019. "Novel Endodontic Sealer with Dual Strategies of Dimethylaminohexadecyl Methacrylate and Nanoparticles of Silver to Inhibit Root Canal Biofilms." *Dental Materials* 35 (8): 1117–29. https://doi.org/10.1016/j.dental.2019.05.014.

"Bioactive Materials Market Analysis | Global Industry Report, 2014–2025." n.d. Accessed May 5, 2020. https://www.grandviewresearch.com/industry -analysis/bioactive-materials-industry.

Buergers, R., M. Rosentritt, and G. Handel. 2007. "Bacterial Adhesion of Streptococcus Mutans to Provisional Fixed Prosthodontic Material." *The Journal of Prosthetic Dentistry* 98 (6): 461–69. https://doi.org/10.1016/S0022 -3913(07)60146-2.

Chatzistavrou, X., A. Lefkelidou, L. Papadopoulou, E. Pavlidou, K. M. Paraskevopoulos, J. C. Fenno, S. Flannagan, C. González-Cabezas, N. Kotsanos, and P. Papagerakis. 2018. "Bactericidal and Bioactive Dental Composites." *Frontiers in Physiology* 9: 103. https://doi.org/10.3389/fphys .2018.00103.

Chen, W., Y. Liu, H. S. Courtney, M. Bettenga, C. M. Agrawal, J. D. Bumgardner, and J. L. Ong. 2006. "In Vitro Anti-Bacterial and Biological Properties of Magnetron Co-Sputtered Silver-Containing Hydroxyapatite Coating." *Biomaterials* 27 (32): 5512–17. https://doi.org/10.1016/j.biomaterials.2006.07.003.

Chouirfa, H., H. Bouloussa, V. Migonney, and C. Falentin-Daudré. 2019. "Review of Titanium Surface Modification Techniques and Coatings for Antibacterial Applications." *Acta Biomaterialia* 83 (January): 37–54. https:// doi.org/10.1016/j.actbio.2018.10.036.

Colombo, S., and M. Beretta. 2018. "Dental Sealants Part 3: Which Material? Efficiency and Effectiveness." *European Journal of Paediatric Dentistry* 19 (3): 247–49. https://doi.org/10.23804/ejpd.2018.19.03.15.

Cramer, N. B., J. W. Stansbury, and C. N. Bowman. 2011. "Recent Advances and Developments in Composite Dental Restorative Materials." *Journal of Dental Research* 90 (4): 402–16. https://doi.org/10.1177/00220345103 81263.

Cury, J. A., and L. M. A. Tenuta. 2009. "Enamel Remineralization: Controlling the Caries Disease or Treating Early Caries Lesions?" *Brazilian Oral Research* 23 (June): 23–30. https://doi.org/10.1590/S1806-83242009000500005.

Del Curto, B., M. F. Brunella, C. Giordano, M. P. Pedeferri, V. Valtulina, L. Visai, and A. Cigada. 2005. "Decreased Bacterial Adhesion to Surface-Treated Titanium." *The International Journal of Artificial Organs* 28 (7): 718–30.

"Dental Fillings Market Size & Share | Industry Report, 2019–2026." n.d. Accessed May 5, 2020. https://www.grandviewresearch.com/industry-analysis/dental -fillings-market.

Dhir, G., D. W. Berzins, V. B. Dhuru, A. Raj Periathamby, and A. Dentino. 2007. "Physical Properties of Denture Base Resins Potentially Resistant to Candida Adhesion." *Journal of Prosthodontics* 16 (6): 465–72. https://doi.org /10.1111/j.1532-849X.2007.00219.x.

Dunn, C. A., Q. Jin, M. Taba, R. T. Franceschi, R. B. Rutherford, and W. V. Giannobile. 2005. "BMP Gene Delivery for Alveolar Bone Engineering at Dental Implant Defects." *Molecular Therapy: The Journal of the American Society of Gene Therapy* 11 (2): 294–99. https://doi.org/10.1016/j.ymthe.2004 .10.005.

Dziadek, M., J. Pawlik, E. Menaszek, E. Stodolak-Zych, and K. Cholewa-Kowalska. 2015. "Effect of the Preparation Methods on Architecture, Crystallinity, Hydrolytic Degradation, Bioactivity, and Biocompatibility of PCL/Bioglass Composite Scaffolds." *Journal of Biomedical Materials Research. Part B, Applied Biomaterials* 103 (8): 1580–93. https://doi.org/10.1002/jbm.b.33350.

Edelstein, B. L. 2006. "The Dental Caries Pandemic and Disparities Problem." *BMC Oral Health* 6 (Suppl 1, June): S2. https://doi.org/10.1186/1472-6831-6-S1-S2.

Engstrand, J., E. Unosson, and H. Engqvist. 2012. "Hydroxyapatite Formation on a Novel Dental Cement in Human Saliva." *ISRN Dentistry* 2012: 624056. https://doi.org/10.5402/2012/624056.

Gandolfi, M. G., F. Siboni, T. Botero, M. Bossù, F. Riccitiello, and C. Prati. 2015. "Calcium Silicate and Calcium Hydroxide Materials for Pulp Capping: Biointeractivity, Porosity, Solubility and Bioactivity of Current Formulations." *Journal of Applied Biomaterials & Functional Materials* 13 (1): 43–60. https://doi.org/10.5301/jabfm.5000201.

Garcia, I. M., S. B. Rodrigues, M. E. R. Gama, V. C. B. Leitune, M. A. Melo, and F. M. Collares. 2020. "Guanidine Derivative Inhibits C. Albicans Biofilm Growth on Denture Liner without Promote Loss of Materials' Resistance." *Bioactive Materials* 5 (2): 228–32. https://doi.org/10.1016/j.bioactmat.2020.02.007.

Giraud, T., P. Rufas, F. Chmilewsky, C. Rombouts, J. Dejou, C. Jeanneau, and I. About. 2017. "Complement Activation by Pulp Capping Materials Plays a Significant Role in Both Inflammatory and Pulp Stem Cells' Recruitment." *Journal of Endodontics* 43 (7): 1104–10. https://doi.org/10.1016/j.joen.2017.02.016.

Goldberg, M., and A. J. Smith. 2004. "Cells and Extracellular Matrices of Dentin and Pulp: A Biological Basis for Repair and Tissue Engineering." *Critical Reviews in Oral Biology and Medicine* 15 (1): 13–27.

Greenspan, D. C. 2016. "Glass and Medicine: The Larry Hench Story." *International Journal of Applied Glass Science* 7 (2): 134–38. https://doi.org/10.1111/ijag.12204.

Hamba, H., T. Nikaido, G. Inoue, A. Sadr, and J. Tagami. 2011. "Effects of CPP-ACP with Sodium Fluoride on Inhibition of Bovine Enamel Demineralization: A Quantitative Assessment Using Micro-Computed Tomography." *Journal of Dentistry* 39 (6): 405–13. https://doi.org/10.1016/j.jdent.2011.03.005.

Hench, L. L. 2006. "The Story of Bioglass." *Journal of Materials Science. Materials in Medicine* 17 (11): 967–78. https://doi.org/10.1007/s10856-006-0432-z.

Hench, L. L., R. J. Splinter, W. C. Allen, and T. K. Greenlee. 1971. "Bonding Mechanisms at the Interface of Ceramic Prosthetic Materials." *Journal of Biomedical Materials Research* 5 (6): 117–41. https://doi.org/10.1002/jbm.820050611.

Hill, E. E. 2007. "Dental Cements for Definitive Luting: A Review and Practical Clinical Considerations." *Dental Clinics of North America* 51 (3): 643–58, vi. https://doi.org/10.1016/j.cden.2007.04.002.

Ibrahim, M. S., A. A. Balhaddad, I. M. Garcia, F. M. Collares, M. D. Weir, H. H. K. Xu, and M. A. S. Melo. 2020. "PH-Responsive Calcium and Phosphate-Ion Releasing Antibacterial Sealants on Carious Enamel Lesions in Vitro." *Journal of Dentistry* (April): 103323. https://doi.org/10.1016/j.jdent.2020.103323.

Ibrahim, M. S., I. M. Garcia, T. Vila, A. A. Balhaddad, F. M. Collares, M. D. Weir, H. Xu, and M. A. Melo. 2020. "Multifunctional Antibacterial Dental Sealants Suppress Biofilms Derived from Children at High Risk of Caries." *Biomaterials Science* 8 (12): 3472–84. https://doi.org/10.1039/D0BM00370K.

Jatania, A., and B. M. Shivalinga. 2014. "An In Vitro Study to Evaluate the Effects of Addition of Zinc Oxide to an Orthodontic Bonding Agent." *European Journal of Dentistry* 8 (1): 112–17. https://doi.org/10.4103/1305-7456.126262.

Jefferies, S. R., A. E. Fuller, and D. W. Boston. 2015. "Preliminary Evidence That Bioactive Cements Occlude Artificial Marginal Gaps." *Journal of Esthetic and Restorative Dentistry* 27 (3): 155–66. https://doi.org/10.1111/jerd.12133.

Jin, Q. M., O. Anusaksathien, S. A. Webb, R. B. Rutherford, and W. V. Giannobile. 2003. "Gene Therapy of Bone Morphogenetic Protein for Periodontal Tissue Engineering." *Journal of Periodontology* 74 (2): 202–13. https://doi.org/10.1902/jop.2003.74.2.202.

Jin, Q., O. Anusaksathien, S. A. Webb, M. A. Printz, and W. V. Giannobile. 2004. "Engineering of Tooth-Supporting Structures by Delivery of PDGF Gene Therapy Vectors." *Molecular Therapy: The Journal of the American Society of Gene Therapy* 9 (4): 519–26. https://doi.org/10.1016/j.ymthe.2004.01.016.

Kim, S. G., M. Malek, A. Sigurdsson, L. M. Lin, and B. Kahler. 2018. "Regenerative Endodontics: A Comprehensive Review." *International Endodontic Journal* 51 (12): 1367–88. https://doi.org/10.1111/iej.12954.

Kitasako, Y., A. Sadr, H. Hamba, M. Ikeda, and J. Tagami. 2012. "Gum Containing Calcium Fluoride Reinforces Enamel Subsurface Lesions in situ." *Journal of Dental Research* 91 (4): 370–75. https://doi.org/10.1177/0022034512439716.

Kokubo, T., H. Kushitani, S. Sakka, T. Kitsugi, and T. Yamamuro. 1990. "Solutions Able to Reproduce In Vivo Surface-Structure Changes in Bioactive Glass-Ceramic A-W." *Journal of Biomedical Materials Research* 24 (6): 721–34. https://doi.org/10.1002/jbm.820240607.

Komabayashi, T., Q. Zhu, R. Eberhart, and Y. Imai. 2016. "Current Status of Direct Pulp-Capping Materials for Permanent Teeth." *Dental Materials Journal* 35 (1): 1–12. https://doi.org/10.4012/dmj.2015-013.

Kulkarni Aranya, A., S. Pushalkar, M. Zhao, R. Z. LeGeros, Y. Zhang, and D. Saxena. 2017. "Antibacterial and Bioactive Coatings on Titanium Implant Surfaces." *Journal of Biomedical Materials Research. Part A* 105 (8): 2218–27. https://doi.org/10.1002/jbm.a.36081.

Kunert, M., and M. Lukomska-Szymanska. 2020. "Bio-Inductive Materials in Direct and Indirect Pulp Capping—A Review Article." *Materials* 13 (5). https://doi.org/10.3390/ma13051204.

Laurent, P., J. Camps, and I. About. 2012. "Biodentine(T.M.) Induces TGF-B1 Release from Human Pulp Cells and Early Dental Pulp Mineralization."

International Endodontic Journal 45 (5): 439–48. https://doi.org/10.1111/j
.1365-2591.2011.01995.x.

Lawson, N. C., and A. Robles. 2017. "Tipping Point: An Update on Curing Lights,
Resin Composites, and Matrix Systems." *Compendium of Continuing
Education in Dentistry (Jamesburg, N.J.: 1995)* 38(2): 120–21.

Li, Z., L. Cao, M. Fan, and Q. Xu. 2015. "Direct Pulp Capping with Calcium
Hydroxide or Mineral Trioxide Aggregate: A Meta-Analysis." *Journal of
Endodontics* 41 (9): 1412–17. https://doi.org/10.1016/j.joen.2015.04.012.

Lim, B.-S., S.-J. Lee, J.-W. Lee, and S.-J. Ahn. 2008. "Quantitative Analysis of
Adhesion of Cariogenic Streptococci to Orthodontic Raw Materials."
American Journal of Orthodontics and Dentofacial Orthopedics 133 (6):
882–88. https://doi.org/10.1016/j.ajodo.2006.07.027.

Maktabi, H., A. A. Balhaddad, Q. Alkhubaizi, H. Strassler, and M. A. S. Melo.
2018. "Factors Influencing Success of Radiant Exposure in Light-Curing
Posterior Dental Composite in the Clinical Setting." *American Journal of
Dentistry* 31 (6): 320–28.

Malkondu, Ö., M. K. Kazandağ, and E. Kazazoğlu. 2014. "A Review on Biodentine,
a Contemporary Dentine Replacement and Repair Material." *BioMed
Research International* 2014: 160951. https://doi.org/10.1155/2014/160951.

Martins, M. T., F. Sardenberg, C. B. Bendo, M. H. Abreu, M. P. Vale, S. M. Paiva,
and I. A. Pordeus. 2017. "Dental Caries Remains as the Main Oral Condition
with the Greatest Impact on Children's Quality of Life." *PLoS One* 12 (10):
e0185365. https://doi.org/10.1371/journal.pone.0185365.

Melo, M. A. S., M. D. Weir, V. F. Passos, M. Powers, and H. H. K. Xu. 2017. "Ph-
Activated Nano-Amorphous Calcium Phosphate-Based Cement to Reduce
Dental Enamel Demineralization." *Artificial Cells, Nanomedicine, and
Biotechnology* 45 (8): 1778–85. https://doi.org/10.1080/21691401.2017.1290644.

Melo, M. A. S., S. F. F. Guedes, H. H. K. Xu, and L. K. A. Rodrigues. 2013.
"Nanotechnology-Based Restorative Materials for Dental Caries
Management." *Trends in Biotechnology* 31 (8): 459–67. https://doi.org/10
.1016/j.tibtech.2013.05.010.

Meng, H.-W., E. Y. Chien, and H.-H. Chien. 2016. "Dental Implant Bioactive
Surface Modifications and Their Effects on Osseointegration: A Review."
Biomarker Research 4 (1): 24. https://doi.org/10.1186/s40364-016-0078–z.

Mirizadeh, A., M. Atai, and S. Ebrahimi. 2018. "Fabrication of Denture Base
Materials with Antimicrobial Properties." *The Journal of Prosthetic Dentistry*
119 (2): 292–98. https://doi.org/10.1016/j.prosdent.2017.03.011.

Mohammadi, Z., and P. M. H. Dummer. 2011. "Properties and Applications
of Calcium Hydroxide in Endodontics and Dental Traumatology."
International Endodontic Journal 44 (8): 697–730. https://doi.org/10.1111/j
.1365-2591.2011.01886.x.

Monteiro, J. C., M. Stürmer, I. M. Garcia, M. A. Melo, S. Sauro, V. C. B. Leitune,
and F. M. Collares. 2020. "Dental Sealant Empowered by 1,3,5-Tri Acryloyl
Hexahydro-1,3,5-Triazine and α-Tricalcium Phosphate for Anti-Caries
Application." *Polymers* 12 (4). https://doi.org/10.3390/polym12040895.

Murray, P. E., F. Garcia-Godoy, and K. M. Hargreaves. 2007. "Regenerative Endodontics: A Review of Current Status and a Call for Action." *Journal of Endodontics* 33 (4): 377–90. https://doi.org/10.1016/j.joen.2006.09.013.

Nakashima, M., and A. Akamine. 2005. "The Application of Tissue Engineering to Regeneration of Pulp and Dentin in Endodontics." *Journal of Endodontics* 31 (10): 711–18.

Naumova, E. A., M. Staiger, O. Kouji, J. Modric, T. Pierchalla, M. Rybka, R. G. Hill, and W. H. Arnold. 2019. "Randomized Investigation of the Bioavailability of Fluoride in Saliva after Administration of Sodium Fluoride, Amine Fluoride and Fluoride Containing Bioactive Glass Dentifrices." *BMC Oral Health* 19 (1): 119. https://doi.org/10.1186/s12903-019-0805-6.

Nedeljkovic, I., J. De Munck, A.-A. Ungureanu, V. Slomka, C. Bartic, A. Vananroye, C. Clasen, W. Teughels, B. Van Meerbeek, and K. L. Van Landuyt. 2017. "Biofilm-Induced Changes to the Composite Surface." *Journal of Dentistry* 63 (August): 36–43. https://doi.org/10.1016/j.jdent.2017.05.015.

Nóbrega, D. F., C. E. Fernández, A. A. Del Bel Cury, L. M. A. Tenuta, and J. A. Cury. 2016. "Frequency of Fluoride Dentifrice Use and Caries Lesions Inhibition and Repair." *Caries Research* 50 (2): 133–40. https://doi.org/10.1159/000444223.

Norowski, P. A., and J. D. Bumgardner. 2009. "Biomaterial and Antibiotic Strategies for Peri-Implantitis: A Review." *Journal of Biomedical Materials Research. Part B, Applied Biomaterials* 88 (2): 530–43. https://doi.org/10.1002/jbm.b.31152.

Othman, H. F., C. D. Wu, C. A. Evans, J. L. Drummond, and C. G. Matasa. 2002. "Evaluation of Antimicrobial Properties of Orthodontic Composite Resins Combined with Benzalkonium Chloride." *American Journal of Orthodontics and Dentofacial Orthopedics* 122 (3): 288–94.

Park, S. E., A. R. Periathamby, and J. C. Loza. 2003. "Effect of Surface-Charged Poly (Methyl Methacrylate) on the Adhesion of Candida Albicans." *Journal of Prosthodontics* 12 (4): 249–54.

Petrini, P., C. R. Arciola, I. Pezzali, S. Bozzini, L. Montanaro, M. C. Tanzi, P. Speziale, and L. Visai. 2006. "Antibacterial Activity of Zinc Modified Titanium Oxide Surface." *The International Journal of Artificial Organs* 29 (4): 434–42.

Pitts, N. B., D. T. Zero, P. D. Marsh, K. Ekstrand, J. A. Weintraub, F. Ramos-Gomez, J. Tagami, S. Twetman, G. Tsakos, and A. Ismail. 2017. "Dental Caries." *Nature Reviews Disease Primers* 3 (May): 17030. https://doi.org/10.1038/nrdp.2017.30.

Polini, A., H. Bai, and A. P. Tomsia. 2013. "Dental Applications of Nanostructured Bioactive Glass and Its Composites." *Wiley Interdisciplinary Reviews. Nanomedicine and Nanobiotechnology* 5 (4): 399–410. https://doi.org/10.1002/wnan.1224.

Pratap, B., R. K. Gupta, B. Bhardwaj, and M. Nag. 2019. "Resin Based Restorative Dental Materials: Characteristics and Future Perspectives." *The Japanese Dental Science Review* 55 (1): 126–38. https://doi.org/10.1016/j.jdsr.2019.09.004.

Rabiee, S. M., N. Nazparvar, M. Azizian, D. Vashaee, and L. Tayebi. 2015. "Effect of Ion Substitution on Properties of Bioactive Glasses: A Review." *Ceramics International* 41 (6): 7241–51. https://doi.org/10.1016/j.ceramint.2015.02.140.

Ramseier, C. A., G. Rasperini, S. Batia, and W. V. Giannobile. 2012. "Advanced Reconstructive Technologies for Periodontal Tissue Repair." *Periodontology 2000* 59 (1): 185–202. https://doi.org/10.1111/j.1600-0757.2011.00432.x.

Reynolds, E. C., F. Cai, P. Shen, and G. D. Walker. 2003. "Retention in Plaque and Remineralization of Enamel Lesions by Various Forms of Calcium in a Mouthrinse or Sugar-Free Chewing Gum." *Journal of Dental Research* 82 (3): 206–11. https://doi.org/10.1177/154405910308200311.

Saleh, I. M., I. E. Ruyter, M. Haapasalo, and D. Ørstavik. 2004. "Survival of Enterococcus Faecalis in Infected Dentinal Tubules after Root Canal Filling with Different Root Canal Sealers In Vitro." *International Endodontic Journal* 37 (3): 193–98. https://doi.org/10.1111/j.0143-2885.2004.00785.x.

Schwendicke, F., F. Brouwer, A. Schwendicke, and S. Paris. 2016. "Different Materials for Direct Pulp Capping: Systematic Review and Meta-Analysis and Trial Sequential Analysis." *Clinical Oral Investigations* 20 (6): 1121–32. https://doi.org/10.1007/s00784-016-1802-7.

Sharon, E., R. Sharabi, A. Eden, A. Zabrovsky, G. Ben-Gal, E. Sharon, Y. Pietrokovski, Y. Houri-Haddad, and N. Beyth. 2018. "Antibacterial Activity of Orthodontic Cement Containing Quaternary Ammonium Polyethylenimine Nanoparticles Adjacent to Orthodontic Brackets." *International Journal of Environmental Research and Public Health* 15 (4). https://doi.org/10.3390/ijerph15040606.

Simonsen, R. J. 2002. "Pit and Fissure Sealant: Review of the Literature." *Pediatric Dentistry* 24 (5): 393–414.

Simonsen, R. J., and R. C. Neal. 2011. "A Review of the Clinical Application and Performance of Pit and Fissure Sealants." *Australian Dental Journal* 56 (Suppl 1, June): 45–58. https://doi.org/10.1111/j.1834-7819.2010.01295.x.

Sivakumar, I., K. S. Arunachalam, S. Sajjan, A. V. Ramaraju, B. Rao, and B. Kamaraj. 2014. "Incorporation of Antimicrobial Macromolecules in Acrylic Denture Base Resins: A Research Composition and Update." *Journal of Prosthodontics: Official Journal of the American College of Prosthodontists* 23 (4): 284–90. https://doi.org/10.1111/jopr.12105.

Skallevold, H. E., D. Rokaya, Z. Khurshid, and M. S. Zafar. 2019. "Bioactive Glass Applications in Dentistry." *International Journal of Molecular Sciences* 20 (23). https://doi.org/10.3390/ijms20235960.

Smeets, R., B. Stadlinger, F. Schwarz, B. Beck-Broichsitter, O. Jung, C. Precht, F. Kloss, A. Gröbe, M. Heiland, and T. Ebker. 2016. "Impact of Dental Implant Surface Modifications on Osseointegration." *BioMed Research International* 2016: 6285620. https://doi.org/10.1155/2016/6285620.

Sundqvist, G., D. Figdor, S. Persson, and U. Sjögren. 1998. "Microbiologic Analysis of Teeth with Failed Endodontic Treatment and the Outcome of Conservative Re-Treatment." *Oral Surgery, Oral Medicine, Oral Pathology, Oral Radiology, and Endodontology* 85 (1): 86–93. https://doi.org/10.1016/S1079-2104(98)90404-8.

Verran, J., and K. Whitehead. 2005. "Factors Affecting Microbial Adhesion to Stainless Steel and Other Materials Used in Medical Devices." *The International Journal of Artificial Organs* 28 (11): 1138–45.

Walsh, R. M., J. He, J. Schweitzer, L. A. Opperman, and K. F. Woodmansey. 2018. "Bioactive Endodontic Materials for Everyday Use: A Review." *General Dentistry* 66 (3): 48–51.

Wang, X., S. Song, L. Chen, C. M. Stafford, and J. Sun. 2018. "Short-Time Dental Resin Biostability and Kinetics of Enzymatic Degradation." *Acta Biomaterialia* 74 326–33. https://doi.org/10.1016/j.actbio.2018.05.009.

Wikesjö, U. M. E., A. V. Xiropaidis, R. C. Thomson, A. D. Cook, K. A. Selvig, and W. R. Hardwick. 2003. "Periodontal Repair in Dogs: RhBMP-2 Significantly Enhances Bone Formation under Provisions for Guided Tissue Regeneration." *Journal of Clinical Periodontology* 30 (8): 705–14.

Wikesjö, U. M. E., R. G. Sorensen, A. Kinoshita, X. J. Li, and J. M. Wozney. 2004. "Periodontal Repair in Dogs: Effect of Recombinant Human Bone Morphogenetic Protein-12 (RhBMP-12) on Regeneration of Alveolar Bone and Periodontal Attachment." *Journal of Clinical Periodontology* 31 (8): 662–70. https://doi.org/10.1111/j.1600-051X.2004.00541.x.

Xie, X., L. Wang, D. Xing, M. Qi, X. Li, J. Sun, M. A. S. Melo, et al. 2019. "Novel Rechargeable Calcium Phosphate Nanoparticle-Filled Dental Cement." *Dental Materials Journal* 38 (1): 1–10. https://doi.org/10.4012/dmj.2017–420.

Yitzhaki, S., L. Reshef, U. Gophna, M. Rosenberg, and N. Sterer. 2018. "Microbiome Associated with Denture Malodour." *Journal of Breath Research* 12 (2): 027103. https://doi.org/10.1088/1752-7163/aa95e0.

Zhang, N., M. A. S. Melo, M. D. Weir, M. A. Reynolds, Y. Bai, and H. H. K. Xu. 2016. "Do Dental Resin Composites Accumulate More Oral Biofilms and Plaque than Amalgam and Glass Ionomer Materials?" *Materials (Basel, Switzerland)* 9 (11). https://doi.org/10.3390/ma9110888.

Zhang, W., and P. C. Yelick. 2010. "Vital Pulp Therapy-Current Progress of Dental Pulp Regeneration and Revascularization." *International Journal of Dentistry* 2010: 856087. https://doi.org/10.1155/2010/856087.

Zhao, X., J. M. Courtney, and H. Qian. 2011. *Bioactive Materials in Medicine: Design and Applications.* Amsterdam: Elsevier.

Zhou, S., C. Sun, S. Huang, X. Wu, Y. Zhao, C. Pan, H. Wang, J. Liu, Q. Li, and Y. Kou. 2018. "Efficacy of Adjunctive Bioactive Materials in the Treatment of Periodontal Intrabony Defects: A Systematic Review and Meta-Analysis." *BioMed Research International* 2018: 8670832. https://doi.org/10.1155/2018/8670832.

Zhu, C., B. Ju, and R. Ni. 2015. "Clinical Outcome of Direct Pulp Capping with MTA or Calcium Hydroxide: A Systematic Review and Meta-Analysis." *International Journal of Clinical and Experimental Medicine* 8 (10): 17055–60.

2

Current Status and Role of Dental Polymeric Restorative Materials

Haohao Wang, Suping Wang, Xuedong Zhou,
Jiyao Li, Libang He, and Lei Cheng
Sichuan University

Contents

2.1 Introduction: Background and Overview

Dental caries is known as the destruction of dental hard tissues by acidic by-products from bacterial metabolism of dietary carbohydrates (Selwitz et al. 2007). Despite the great efforts in caries prevention, it is still one significant public health problem globally, and dental restorations are the most commonly used approach to restore decayed teeth (Selwitz et al. 2007). Apart from that, restorations also play an essential role in clinical treatment, including tooth wear, dental trauma, and esthetic purposes. Although all kinds of restorative materials emerge in an endless stream, there are generally two common categories of restorative dental materials: direct and indirect materials, both have their specific indications for clinical use (AFFAIRS ACOS 2003). The former category includes most commonly used filling materials like amalgam, resin composites, glass ionomer cement (GIC), etc., which are placed directly into a tooth cavity and shaped intraorally. The indirect restorations are fabricated outside of the mouth via dental impressions of a prepared tooth, such as crowns, inlays and onlays, bridgework, and veneers (Loomans and Özcan 2016).

Even though contemporary restorative materials provide fairly good functions and esthetic effects, none of them can fulfill all requirements for an ideal restorative material. Some drawbacks in their physical and chemical properties gradually come out in the course of clinical use, and the longevity of restorations is limited. According to information statistics, nearly 200 million dental restorations are placed annually in the U.S., and half of all dental restorations failed within ten years (Drummond 2008; Talib 1993). The subsequent replacements incur a heavy burden in medical expenditures (Deligeorgi et al. 2001). Faced up with the oncoming challenges, numerous attempts have been made to improve the performance of existing materials as well as the development of novel materials (Jokstad 2016). The ideal restorative material is expected to have characteristics of (1) physical and mechanical properties rivaling natural tooth structure in strength, adherence, and appearance; (2) biocompatibility with less adverse effects; (3) long-term effectiveness; (4) convenience in clinical operation; etc. (Dhar et al. 2015). While still under exploration, new strategies to solve current problems of dental materials are continuing to emerge and be bound to have a broad prospect.

This chapter outlines essential features and problems of current restorative dental biomaterials on purpose to serve as a background for understanding the facing challenges in the field.

2.2 Amalgam

Amalgam, a traditional material of dental restorations, has been successfully used for over 150 years and is still the choice in some places of the world because of its effectiveness and low cost (Spencer 2000). Amalgam mainly consists of liquid mercury with an alloy made of silver, tin, copper, and zinc solid particles (Anusavice et al. 2013). When mixing, the mercury and the alloy toundergo an amalgamation reaction and gradually condense and harden, forming a silver-grey mass (Anusavice et al. 2013). Because the material's color differs from a natural tooth's color, as illustrated in Figure 2.1, amalgam is mostly used for permanent posterior restorations. In long-term clinical application, amalgam showed higher longevity compared to composites (Moraschini et al. 2015). This may be because amalgam has a potential antimicrobial effect by releasing toxic mercury and results in low viability of oral biofilms on its surfaces (Busscher et al. 2010). However, the release of mercury is also the primary concern preventing the use of amalgam. An increasing attention has been

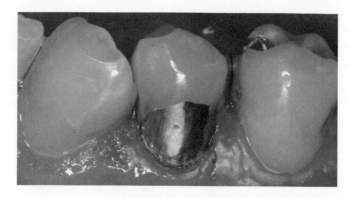

Figure 2.1 Clinical appearance of amalgam. The material's color differs from a natural tooth's color.

paid to the risk of mercury exposure from amalgam and the potential adverse effects (Reinhardt 1988).

Articles have reported a variety of directand indirect toxic effects from amalgam restorations on general body health, including neurotoxicity, kidney dysfunction, reduced immunocompetence, side effects on oral and intestinal bacterial flora, and so on (Edlich et al. 2007; Eley 1997; Eley and Cox 1993; Lygre et al. 2016). Conversely, other studies reported that the magnitude of mercury exposure for patients with several amalgam restorations is far below the toxicity threshold and can be considered as a "no effect" level (Anusavice et al. 2013). Although the merits of amalgam restorations are still prevailing, amalgam restorations have been gradually phased out, mainly because of their unsatisfied esthetic properties, mercury-releasing risks, and environmental pollution of their disposals.

2.3 Resin Composites

Composites have been introduced into the dental material field for nearly 50 years (Ilie and Hickel 2011). They are used for a variety of applications in restorative dentistry, including direct or indirect anterior and posterior cavity fillings, cosmetic restoration of anterior teeth, cavity liners, pit and fissure sealants, cores and buildups, inlays, onlays, crowns, and so on as illustrated in Figure 2.2 (Margeas 2013). Nowadays, composites are the dominant choice for dental restorations in most cases (Ferracane 2011). A literature survey performed 15 years ago ha already reported at the time that at least half of posterior direct restoration placements rely on

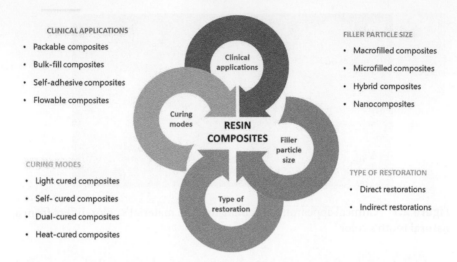

CLINICAL APPLICATIONS
- Packable composites
- Bulk-fill composites
- Self-adhesive composites
- Flowable composites

FILLER PARTICLE SIZE
- Macrofilled composites
- Microfilled composites
- Hybrid composites
- Nanocomposites

CURING MODES
- Light cured composites
- Self- cured composites
- Dual-cured composites
- Heat-cured composites

TYPE OF RESTORATION
- Direct restorations
- Indirect restorations

Figure 2.2   A variety of applications in restorative dentistry, including direct and indirect anterior and posterior cavity fillings, cosmetic restoration of anterior teeth, cavity liners, pit and fissure sealants, cores, and buildups, inlays, onlays, and crowns.

composite materials (Sadowsky 2006). Motivational reasons for the prevalent use of this relays on pleasant appearance, ability to be used as direct restorative material, satisfactory mechanical properties, and ability to preserve more natural tooth tissue during cavity preparation (Lu et al. 2006).

Resin composites consist of three major components: initiator system, resin matrix, and filler, each of which has its role in dictating material properties (Cramer et al. 2011). The initiator system can trigger a polymerization reaction, typically by light activating, and the resin matrix is thus converted from liquid monomers into a highly crosslinked polymer network, serving as the backbone of a composite. The filler plays essential roles in composite including modulus enhancement, radiopacity, optimizing wear, translucency, thermal expansion behavior improvement, and reduction of polymerization shrinkage (Cramer et al. 2011).

Each component represents an opportunity for tuning in the overall material properties of a composite. For example, by reducing the filler content of the mixture, composites could have a lower viscosity and become a prototype of a flowable composite. The modification of components in the composite has been the focus of intensive research in recent years, which yielded different classes of polymeric restorative materials with tuned formulations such as packable composites, flowable composites, polyacid modified resin composites (compomers), self-adhesive composites,

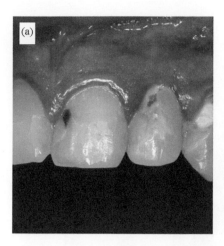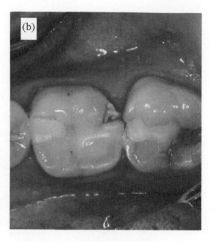

Figure 2.3   Clinical aspect of carious lesions around resin composites restorations located in anterior and posterior teeth.

infiltration resins, and bulk-fill resin composites (Baroudi and Rodrigues 2015; Talib 1993).

Although composites provide relatively good performance in clinical use, they still encounter significant challenges. One of the significant problems is secondary caries formation around the restorations, which usually lead to the failure of composites (Jokstad 2016). Figure 2.3 illustrates the appearance of carious lesions around resin composites restorations located in anterior and posterior teeth. Secondary caries incidence in composite restorations has been reported to be higher than other restorative materials (Nedeljkovic et al. 2015). The incidence of secondary caries has a multiplicity of influencing factors regarding the patient, the type of restorative material, operative technique, and others. One worth of discussion is the inherent fact that resin composites undergo shrinkage by volume when they are polymerized. This condition can be linked to the incidence of secondary caries, as illustrated in Figure 2.4.

Polymerization shrinkage is a volumetric shrink of composites due to the reduction of intermolecular distances during the chemical reaction between resin monomers. Polymerization shrinkage results in a poor sealing ability of composites and create microleakage between tooth-restoration interfaces (Jokstad 2016; Nedeljkovic et al. 2015). This could facilitate the invasion of bacteria at restoration margins and promote the development of secondary caries. Besides, a plethora of scientific articles have revealed that composites accumulate more plaque on their surface compared to other restorative materials (Skjörland 1973; Skjørland and Sønju 1982; Svanberg et al. 1990).

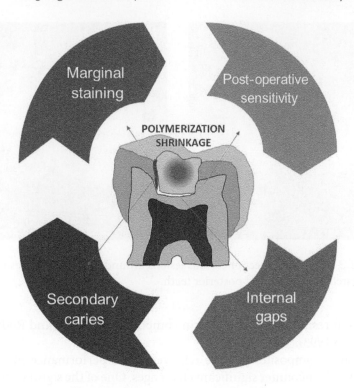

Figure 2.4 One of the inherent facts is that resin composites undergo shrinkage by volume when they are polymerized. This condition can be linked to the incidence of secondary caries.

2.4 Glass Ionomer Cements (GICs)

GICs are originally invented by Wilson and Kent in 1969 and have been widely used for dental restorations for over 40 years (Wilson and Kent 1973). GICs can adhere directly to the tooth structure and have an anti-caries property due to their fluoride release. Nevertheless, their long-term wear and strength are not as good as composites and amalgam. Therefore, GICs are more suitable for use in low stress-bearing areas. Also, GICs are not customarily used for aesthetic areas like anterior teeth due to their inadequate esthetic properties compared to composite. In summary, GICs are commonly used as liners and bases for approximal restorations, cervical restorations, occlusal, and small approximal restorations in deciduous teeth, microcavities, temporary restorations, and root perforation repairs (Sidhu 2011).

Simply speaking, glass ionomers are derived from a glass component and organic acids, which are referred to as acid-base reaction cements.

In particular, conventional GICs are composed of two formulations: a powder form of fluoroaluminosilicate glass mainly consisting of silica and alumina, and liquid solution of polyacrylic acid or polybasic acid coupled with acrylic acid, itaconic acid, and maleic acid (Smith 1998). There is also a small amount of tartaric acid in the liquid ingredients, mainly to improve its solidification (Smith 1998). In order to improve the physical characteristics, conventional GICs were modified and yielded two major categories: metal-modified glass-ionomer cements (MMGICs) and resin-modified glass-ionomer cement (RMGICs). MMGICs include the addition of fine metal particles and are often described as "packable" or "high powder:liquid ratio" GICs (Sidhu 2011).

Even though MMGICs are of improved physical properties and have been commercialized, their strength still does not match other posterior restorative materials (Naasan and Watson 1998; Yap et al. 2002). Their clinical performance in posterior teeth is not very well (Holst, 1996). RMGICs are developed by incorporating methacrylate components into the polyacrylic acid, supplementing the fundamental acid-base reaction by polymerization reaction as illustrated in Figure 2.5. Most of them were found to have the potential to release fluoride equivalent to that of conventional GICs (Wiegand et al. 2007). The introduction of polymerization reaction improved the mechanical strength of RMGICs to some extent, and they are mostly used as liners and bases and restorative materials in the clinic (Sidhu 2011).

Concerning the clinical performance, GICs show good features of adhesive properties, biocompatibility, and fluoride release. Unlike composites that require an adhesive system for bonding, GICs are capable of bonding

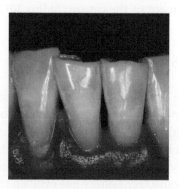

Figure 2.5 Clinical aspect of resin-modified glass ionomer cements (RMGICs). RMGICs are basically developed by incorporating methacrylate components into the polyacrylic acid, supplementing the fundamental acid-base reaction by polymerization.

themselves to teeth via mechanical interlocking and chemical bonding, typically ionic bonds between the carboxylate groups of the polyacid molecules and calcium ions on the tooth surface (Lin et al. 1992). Also, GICs show good biocompatibility because of their low setting exotherm, rapid neutralization, and release of generally benign ions (Nicholson and Czarnecka 2008). Reports in vivo have shown that GIC Fuji IX did not induce a harmful effect on pulp cells in rat's upper molars (Six et al. 2000). However, the biocompatibility of RMGICs is not as good as the conventional ones due to the addition of monomers, although the clinical results of RMGICs generally show no obvious adverse effects (Nicholson and Czarnecka 2008).

One of the most critical substantial advantages of GICs is their fluoride-releasing ability. It has been well documented that fluoride contributes to the reduction of demineralization, the enhancement of remineralization, and the inhibition of microbial growth and metabolism (Hamilton 1990; Rölla and Ekstrand 1996; Ten Cate and Featherstone 1996). Generally, fluoride release from GICs is considered to be clinically beneficial, and several in vitro studies found evidence for inhibition of demineralization by GICs (Glasspoole et al. 2001; Pereira et al. 1998; Tantbirojn et al. 1997; Wandera 1998; Yaman et al. 2004). However, clinical studies exhibited conflicting data on whether the fluoride concentration from restorations is sufficient to prevent secondary caries (Wiegand et al. 2007). Further clinical studies are critically needed to conclude. In terms of clinical drawbacks, GICs have a high sensitivity to moisture and inadequate wear and strength properties (Sidhu 2011; Sidhu et al. 2004). Although the modified RMGICs have improved performance, those drawbacks still exist, and there is still massive room for improvement in the future (Sidhu 2010; Sidhu et al. 2004).

2.5 Dental Bonding System

Bonding system is one of the branches of dental restorative dentistry, and its primary aim is to provide retention of restorations, typically composites, to the natural substance of teeth enamel and dentin. Historically, adhesive dentistry can be traced to 1955 when Dr. Michael Buonocore first demonstrated the bonding of acrylic resin to etched enamel (Buonocore 1955). Since then, adhesive technology has evolved rapidly in the following years. By now, the bonding system has evolved to the seventh generation, from no-etch (first-generation) to total-etch (fourth- and fifth-generation) to self-etch (sixth- and seventh-generation) systems (Freedman and Leinfelder 2002; Kugel and Ferrari 2000). These advances have led to a large number of commercial adhesives, providing great convenience and satisfactory performance in clinical applications Beyth et al. (2007), Breschi et al. (2010).

Adhesive systems usually contain resin monomers, an initiator system, solvents, and sometimes inorganic filler (Van Landuyt et al. 2007). Since both adhesive and composites are resin-based materials, they can bond to each other by copolymerization of residual double bonds. In the meanwhile, adhesive can bond to teeth by micromechanical interlocking into created porosities in prepared enamel and dentin, which is essentially an exchange process of replacing minerals in the dental tissue by resin monomers, forming the so-called resin tag structure (De Munck et al. 2005). Although a variety of adhesive products have appeared in the dental markets, they can generally be divided into two broad categories: etch-and-rinse adhesives and self-etch adhesives (Pashley et al. 2011; Van Meerbeek et al. 2011).

The etch-and-rinse adhesives have a separate etch-and-rinse step of removing the smear layer by applying an acid (mostly 30%–40% phosphoric acid) on the tooth and then rinsing. The self-etch adhesives eliminate the rinsing phase as they contain acidic monomers to treat the smear layer and maintain it as the substrate for the bonding. A comparison of these two categories shows that, in terms of durability, etch-and-rinse adhesives remain the "gold standard," and any kind of simplification in the clinical procedure may result in less bonding effectiveness (Breschi et al. 2008; De Munck et al. 2005). However, self-etch adhesives have unique features and are also widely used in clinical applications (Van Meerbeek et al. 2011).

Simplified procedures made them more user-friendly and time-saving. The elimination of the rinsing step also made them less technique-sensitive as they do not require wet-bonding techniques like etch-and-rinse adhesives (Perdigao 2010). Besides, lower incidence of postoperative sensitivity appears in self-etch adhesives as they are less aggressive in etching step (Perdigao et al. 2003; Unemori et al. 2004). Generally, in terms of enamel bonding, etch-and-rinse adhesives are still the choice of preference, while both etch-and-rinse adhesives and self-etch adhesives canbe a choice of dentin bonding according to the specific clinical situation (Van Meerbeek et al. 2011). With those approaches, the bonding effectiveness of modern adhesives are quite favorable, resulting in a reliable clinical performance (Akimoto et al. 2007; Peumans et al. 2010; van Dijken et al. 2007). However, there is still room for improvement Fan et al. (2011), Hansel et al. (1998), Imazato (2009), Jiao et al. (2017). Adhesives with better durability and anti-degradation properties are always desirable Wang et al. (2012,

2016), Weir et al. (2012),. Also, the development of composites with less shrink may improve the bonding effectiveness, as they could reduce the tension on the bonding layer caused by polymerization shrinkage stress (Kawai and Tsuchitani (2000), Liang et al. (2017), Neel et al. (2016), Riggs et al. (2000),).

2.6 Current Challenges

Restorative dentistry has been rapidly developed during the past few decades, accompanied by the vigorous new products in the dental market. With the evolution of caries management concepts from G.V. Black's "extension for prevention" to "minimally invasive," as well as increasing requirements for the aesthetics and health care, dental restorative materials are given more and more attention and expectations Chatzistavrou et al. (2014), Cocco et al. (2015),

None of the contemporary materials can fulfill the requirements of ideal restorative material. In the future, innovations in dental materials are faced with significant challenges and opportunities Xu et al. (2011), Zhang et al. (2014).

Through multidisciplinary partnerships and scientific advances, the restorative biomaterials are bound to have tremendous development prospects and great innovation space.

References

AFFAIRS ACOS. 2003. Direct and indirect restorative materials. *The Journal of the American Dental Association.* 134(4):463–472.

Akimoto N, Takamizu M, Momoi Y. 2007. 10-Year clinical evaluation of a self-etching adhesive system. *Operative Dentistry.* 32(1):3–10.

Anusavice KJ, Shen C, Rawls HR. 2013. *Phillips' science of dental materials.* Amsterdam: Elsevier Health Sciences. 365–378.

Baroudi K, Rodrigues JC. 2015. Flowable resin composites: A systematic review and clinical considerations. *Journal of Clinical and Diagnostic Research: JCDR.* 9(6):ZE18.

Beyth N, Domb AJ, Weiss EI. 2007. An in vitro quantitative antibacterial analysis of amalgam and composite resins. *Journal of Dentistry.* 35(3):201–206.

Breschi L, Mazzoni A, Nato F, Carrilho M, Visintini E, Tjäderhane L, Ruggeri A, Tay FR, Dorigo EDS, Pashley DH. 2010. Chlorhexidine stabilizes the adhesive interface: A 2-year in vitro study. *Dental Materials.* 26(4):320–325.

Breschi L, Mazzoni A, Ruggeri A, Cadenaro M, Di Lenarda R, De Stefano Dorigo E. 2008. Dental adhesion review: Aging and stability of the bonded interface. *Dental Materials*. 24(1):90–101.

Buonocore MG. 1955. A simple method of increasing the adhesion of acrylic filling materials to enamel surfaces. *Journal of Dental Research*. 34(6):849–853.

Busscher HJ, Rinastiti M, Siswomihardjo W, van der Mei HC. 2010. Biofilm formation on dental restorative and implant materials. *Journal of Dental Research*. 89(7):657–665.

Chatzistavrou X, Fenno JC, Faulk D, Badylak S, Kasuga T, Boccaccini AR, Papagerakis P. 2014. Fabrication and characterization of bioactive and antibacterial composites for dental applications. *Acta Biomaterialia*. 10(8):3723–3732.

Cocco AR, da Rosa WLdO, da Silva AF, Lund RG, Piva E. 2015. A systematic review about antibacterial monomers used in dental adhesive systems: Current status and further prospects. *Dental Materials*. 31(11):1345–1362.

Cramer N, Stansbury J, Bowman C. 2011. Recent advances and developments in composite dental restorative materials. *Journal of Dental Research*. 90(4):402–416.

De Munck JD, Van Landuyt K, Peumans M, Poitevin A, Lambrechts P, Braem M, Van Meerbeek B. 2005. A critical review of the durability of adhesion to tooth tissue: Methods and results. *Journal of Dental Research*. 84(2):118–132.

Deligeorgi V, Mjor I, Wilson N. 2001. An overview of reasons for the placement and replacement of restorations. *Primary Dental Care*. 8(1):5–11.

Dhar V, Hsu K, Coll J, Ginsberg E, Ball B, Chhibber S, Johnson M, Kim M, Modaresi N, Tinanoff N. 2015. Evidence-based update of pediatric dental restorative procedures: Dental materials. *Journal of Clinical Pediatric Dentistry*. 39(4):303–310.

Drummond JL. 2008. Degradation, fatigue, and failure of resin dental composite materials. *Journal of Dental Research*. 87(8):710–719.

Edlich R, Greene JA, Cochran AA, Kelley AR, Gubler KD, Olson BM, Hudson MA, Woode DR, Long III WB, McGregor W. 2007. Need for informed consent for dentists who use mercury amalgam restorative material as well as technical considerations in removal of dental amalgam restorations. *Journal of Environmental Pathology, Toxicology and Oncology*. 26(4):305–322.

Eley B, Cox S. 1993. The release, absorption and possible health effects of mercury from dental amalgam: A review of recent findings. *British Dental Journal*. 175(10):355–362.

Eley B. 1997. The future of dental amalgam: A review of the literature. Part 6: Possible harmful effects of mercury from dental amalgam. *British Dental Journal*. 182(12):455–459.

Fan Y, Nelson JR, Alvarez JR, Hagan J, Berrier A, Xu X. 2011. Amelogenin-assisted ex vivo remineralization of human enamel: Effects of supersaturation degree and fluoride concentration. *Acta Biomaterialia*. 7(5):2293–2302.

Ferracane JL. 2011. Resin composite—state of the art. *Dental Materials*. 27(1):29–38.

Freedman G, Leinfelder K. 2002. Seventh-generation adhesive systems. *Dentistry Today.* 21(11):106–111.

Glasspoole E, Erickson R, Davidson C. 2001. Demineralization of enamel in relation to the fluoride release of materials. *American Journal of Dentistry.* 14(1):8–12.

Hamilton I. 1990. Biochemical effects of fluoride on oral bacteria. *Journal of Dental Research.* 69(2_suppl):660–667.

Hansel C, Leyhausen G, Mai U, Geurtsen W. 1998. Effects of various resin composite (co) monomers and extracts on two caries-associated microorganisms in vitro. *Journal of Dental Research.* 77(1):60–67.

Holst A. 1996. A 3-year clinical evaluation of ketac-silver restorations in primary molars. *Swedish Dental Journal.* 20(6):209–214.

Ilie N, Hickel R. 2011. Resin composite restorative materials. *Australian Dental Journal.* 56(s1):59–66.

Imazato S. 2009. Bio-active restorative materials with antibacterial effects: New dimension of innovation in restorative dentistry. *Dental Materials Journal.* 28(1):11–19.

Jiao Y, Niu L-n, Ma S, Li J, Tay FR, Chen J-h. 2017. Quaternary ammonium-based biomedical materials: State-of-the-art, toxicological aspects and antimicrobial resistance. *Progress in Polymer Science.* 71:53–90.

Jokstad A. 2016. Secondary caries and microleakage. *Dental Materials.* 32(1):11–25.

Kawai K, Tsuchitani Y. 2000. Effects of resin composite components on glucosyltransferase of cariogenic bacterium. *Journal of Biomedical Materials Research Part A.* 51(1):123–127.

Kugel G, Ferrari M. 2000. The science of bonding: From first to sixth generation. *The Journal of the American Dental Association.* 131:20S–25S.

Liang K, Weir MD, Reynolds MA, Zhou X, Li J, Xu HH. 2017. Poly (amido amine) and nano-calcium phosphate bonding agent to remineralize tooth dentin in cyclic artificial saliva/lactic acid. *Materials Science and Engineering: C.* 72:7–17.

Lin A, McIntyre N, Davidson R. 1992. Studies on the adhesion of glass-ionomer cements to dentin. *Journal of Dental Research.* 71(11):1836–1841.

Loomans B, Özcan M. 2016. Intraoral repair of direct and indirect restorations: Procedures and guidelines. *Operative Dentistry.* 41(S7):S68–S78.

Lu H, Koh H, Alcaraz MGR, Schmidlin PR, Davis D. 2006. Direct composite resin fillings versus amalgam fillings for permanent or adult posterior teeth. Status and date: Edited (no change to conclusions), published in. (1).

Lygre GB, Haug K, Skjærven R, Björkman L. 2016. Prenatal exposure to dental amalgam and pregnancy outcome. *Community Dentistry and Oral Epidemiology.* 44(5):442–449.

Margeas R. 2013. Composite materials: Advances lead to ease of use, better performance. *Compendium of Continuing Education in Dentistry (Jamesburg, NJ: 1995).* 34(5):370–371.

Moraschini V, Fai CK, Alto RM, Dos Santos GO. 2015. Amalgam and resin composite longevity of posterior restorations: A systematic review and meta-analysis. *Journal of Dentistry.* 43(9):1043–1050.

Naasan M, Watson T. 1998. Conventional glass ionomers as posterior restorations. A status report for the American Journal of Dentistry. *American Journal of Dentistry*. 11(1):36–45.

Nedeljkovic I, Teughels W, De Munck J, Van Meerbeek B, Van Landuyt KL. 2015. Is secondary caries with composites a material-based problem? *Dental Materials*. 31(11):e247–e277.

Neel EAA, Aljabo A, Strange A, Ibrahim S, Coathup M, Young AM, Bozec L, Mudera V. 2016. Demineralization–remineralization dynamics in teeth and bone. *International Journal of Nanomedicine*. 11:4743.

Nicholson JW, Czarnecka B. 2008. The biocompatibility of resin-modified glass-ionomer cements for dentistry. *Dental Materials*. 24(12):1702–1708.

Pashley DH, Tay FR, Breschi L, Tjaderhane L, Carvalho RM, Carrilho M, Tezvergil-Mutluay A. 2011. State of the art etch-and-rinse adhesives. *Dental Materials*. 27(1):1–16.

Perdigao J, Geraldeli S, Hodges JS. 2003. Total-etch versus self-etch adhesive: Effect on postoperative sensitivity. *The Journal of the American Dental Association*. 134(12):1621–1629.

Perdigao J. 2010. Dentin bonding-variables related to the clinical situation and the substrate treatment. *Dental Materials*. 26(2):e24–e37.

Pereira P, Inokoshi S, Tagami J. 1998. In vitro secondary caries inhibition around fluoride releasing materials. *Journal of Dentistry*. 26(5–6):505–510.

Peumans M, De Munck J, Van Landuyt K, Poitevin A, Lambrechts P, Van Meerbeek B. 2010. Eight-year clinical evaluation of a 2-step self-etch adhesive with and without selective enamel etching. *Dental Materials*. 26(12):1176–1184.

Reinhardt JW. 1988. Risk assessment of mercury exposure from dental amalgams. *Journal of Public Health Dentistry*. 48(3):172–177.

Riggs P, Braden M, Patel M. 2000. Chlorhexidine release from room temperature polymerising methacrylate systems. *Biomaterials*. 21(4):345–351.

Rölla G, Ekstrand J. 1996. *Fluoride in oral fluids and dental plaque. Fluoride in dentistry*. 2nd ed. Copenhagen: Munksgaard. 215–229.

Sadowsky SJ. 2006. An overview of treatment considerations for esthetic restorations: A review of the literature. *The Journal of Prosthetic Dentistry*. 96(6):433–442.

Selwitz RH, Ismail AI, Pitts NB. 2007. Dental caries. *The Lancet*. 369(9555):51–59.

Sidhu SK, Pilecki P, Sherriff M, Watson TF. 2004. Crack closure on rehydration of glass-ionomer materials. *European Journal of Oral Sciences*. 112(5):465–469.

Sidhu SK. 2010. Clinical evaluations of resin-modified glass-ionomer restorations. *Dental Materials*. 26(1):7–12.

Sidhu SK. 2011. Glass-ionomer cement restorative materials: A sticky subject? *Australian Dental Journal*. 56(Suppl 1):23–30.

Six N, Lasfargues J-J, Goldberg M. 2000. In vivo study of the pulp reaction to Fuji IX, a glass ionomer cement. *Journal of Dentistry*. 28(6):413–422.

Skjørland KK, Sønju T. 1982. Effect of sucrose rinses on bacterial colonization on amalgam and composite. *Acta Odontologica Scandinavica*. 40(4):193–196.

Skjörland KK. 1973. Plaque accumulation on different dental filling materials. *European Journal of Oral Sciences*. 81(7):538–542.

Smith DC. 1998. Development of glass-ionomer cement systems. *Biomaterials.* 19(6):467–478.

Spencer A. 2000. Dental amalgam and mercury in dentistry. *Australian Dental Journal.* 45(4):224–234.

Svanberg M, Mjör I, Ørstavik D. 1990. Mutans streptococci in plaque from margins of amalgam, composite, and glass-ionomer restorations. *Journal of Dental Research.* 69(3):861–864.

Talib R. 1993. Dental composites: A review. *The Journal of Nihon University School of Dentistry.* 35(3):161–170.

Tantbirojn D, Douglas W, Versluis A. 1997. Inhibitive effect of a resin-modified glass ionomer cement on remote enamel artificial caries. *Caries Research.* 31(4):275–280.

Ten Cate J, Featherstone J. 1996. Physicochemical aspects of fluoride-enamel interactions. *Fluoride in Dentistry.* 2:252–272.

Unemori M, Matsuya Y, Akashi A, Goto Y, Akamine A. 2004. Self-etching adhesives and postoperative sensitivity. *American Journal of Dentistry.* 17(3):191–195.

van Dijken JW, Sunnegårdh-Grönberg K, Lindberg A. 2007. Clinical long-term retention of etch-and-rinse and self-etch adhesive systems in non-carious cervical lesions: A 13 years evaluation. *Dental Materials.* 23(9):1101–1107.

Van Landuyt KL, Snauwaert J, De Munck J, Peumans M, Yoshida Y, Poitevin A, Coutinho E, Suzuki K, Lambrechts P, Van Meerbeek B. 2007. Systematic review of the chemical composition of contemporary dental adhesives. *Biomaterials.* 28(26):3757–3785.

Van Meerbeek B, Yoshihara K, Yoshida Y, Mine A, De Munck J, Van Landuyt KL. 2011. State of the art of self-etch adhesives. *Dental Materials.* 27(1):17–28.

Wandera A. 1998. In vitro enamel effects of a resin-modified glass ionomer: Fluoride uptake and resistance to demineralization. *Pediatric Dentistry.* 20(7):411–417.

Wang S-P, Ge Y, Zhou X-D, Xu HH, Weir MD, Zhang K-K, Wang H-H, Hannig M, Rupf S, Li Q. 2016. Effect of anti-biofilm glass–ionomer cement on streptococcus mutans biofilms. *International Journal of Oral Science.* 8(2):76.

Wang Y, Samoei GK, Lallier TE, Xu X. 2012. Synthesis and characterization of new antibacterial fluoride-releasing monomer and dental composite. *ACS Macro Letters.* 2(1):59–62.

Weir M, Chow L, Xu H. 2012. Remineralization of demineralized enamel via calcium phosphate nanocomposite. *Journal of Dental Research.* 91(10):979–984.

Wiegand A, Buchalla W, Attin T. 2007. Review on fluoride-releasing restorative materials—fluoride release and uptake characteristics, antibacterial activity and influence on caries formation. *Dental Materials.* 23(3):343–362.

Wilson A, Kent B. 1973. Surgical cement. British patent. 1.

Xu HH, Moreau JL, Sun L, Chow LC. 2011. Nanocomposite containing amorphous calcium phosphate nanoparticles for caries inhibition. *Dental Materials.* 27(8):762–769.

Yaman SD, Er Ö, Yetmez M, Karabay GA. 2004. In vitro inhibition of caries-like lesions with fluoride-releasing materials. *Journal of Oral Science.* 46(1):45–50.

Yap A, Cheang P, Chay P. 2002. Mechanical properties of two restorative reinforced glass–ionomer cements. *Journal of Oral Rehabilitation.* 29(7):682–688.

Zhang J, Wu R, Fan Y, Liao S, Wang Y, Wen Z, Xu X. 2014. Antibacterial dental composites with chlorhexidine and mesoporous silica. *Journal of Dental Research.* 93(12):1283–1289.

3

Impact of Dental Caries on Survival of Polymeric Restorations

Maximiliano Sérgio Cenci, Tamires Timm Maske, and Françoise Hélène van de Sande

Federal University of Pelotas

Contents

3.1 Introduction

Dental caries is a well-recognized complex oral disease, with a behavioral-biofilm-sugar dependency (Marsh, 2003; Sheiham and James, 2015). In this chapter, the focus will be given to a small piece of the puzzle when addressing dental caries disease. As illustrated in Figure 3.1, the temporal disease progression of the non-idealized patient can be described in terms of trajectories of multiple influencing factors. Behavioral aspects and microbiological shifts can trigger a modification on biofilm toward to its pathogenicity. The triggered acidic, and acidogenic behaviors of the cariogenic biofilms can lead to caries progression. Thus, before discussing the role of dental materials, some remarks should be made.

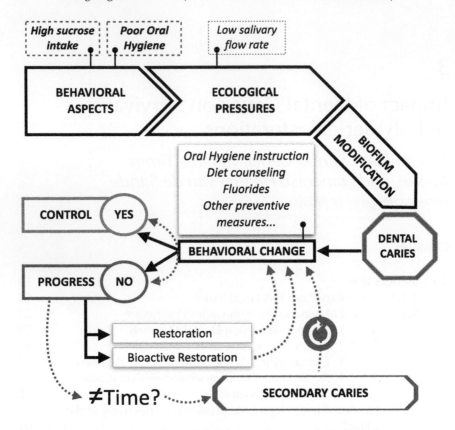

Figure 3.1 Schematic drawing illustrating the temporal disease progression of the non-idealized patient in terms of trajectories of multiple influencing factors. Behavioral aspects and microbiological shifts can trigger a modification on biofilm toward its pathogenicity. The trigged acidic and acidogenic behavior of the biofilm associated to the lack of caries management can lead to caries progression.

Although the broad usage of fluoride was responsible for a considerable reduction in caries prevalence across countries (Marthaler, 2004; Sheiham and James, 2014a), it is apparent that current approaches to control dental caries are failing to prevent high levels of caries in adults (Sheiham and James, 2014a,b). Findings from a systematic review have demonstrated the relationship between the level of sugar intake and caries increment, and as the effect of sugars on tooth structures is cumulative, dental caries progresses with age (Moynihan and Kelly, 2014). Results from a recently published cohort study have shown that although carious lesions increment was higher with higher levels of sugar-related feeding practices along

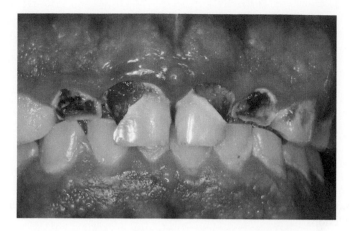

Figure 3.2 Clinical appearance of advanced carious lesions where the lack of restricted sugar intake and other preventive approaches were not implemented to prevent the disease's advance.

the life course, lower levels of sugar consumption were also related to an increment in caries experience, despite the use of fluoride (Peres et al., 2016). Therefore, restricting sugar intake seems mandatory to control dental caries (Sheiham and James, 2015) and to reduce the economic burden of sugar-related dental diseases (Meier et al., 2017).

By acknowledging that caries is a diet-related behavioral disease, it becomes understandable that localized approaches, targeting lesions, will fail to combat this dental disease. Figure 3.2 illustrates the clinical aspect of advanced carious lesions where the lack of restricted sugar intake and other preventive approaches were not implemented to prevent the disease's advance. Dentistry once accepted the concept of "extension for prevention" in which sound teeth structures should be removed and restored with dental materials to avoid the progression of carious lesions (Osborne and Summitt, 1998). Fortunately, with the advance in knowledge through research, utmost preservation of the tooth is advocated under the concepts of preventive, non-invasive, and minimally invasive dentistry (Ricketts et al., 2013; Schwendicke et al., 2016).

Sealing areas at risk of biofilm accumulation such as pits and fissures, and initial carious lesions, provide a physical barrier, the release of fluoride or other ions (bioactive materials) and enhance the cleaning ability at those sites (Ahovuo-Saloranta et al., 2013; Dorri et al., 2015; Meyer-Lueckel and Paris, 2016). Additionally, when needed, the removal of caries lesions is performed selectively, and the preservation of unsupported enamel is possible with direct adhesive materials. Figure 3.3 displays the use of

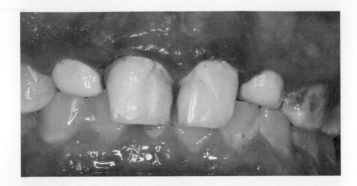

Figure 3.3   Photograph illustrating the use of fluoride-releasing material to fill cavitated lesions.

fluoride-releasing material to fill cavitated lesions (Schwendicke et al., 2016). In this sense, dental materials, including polymeric (methacrylate resin-based), may act as adjunct measures locally, helping to prevent, remineralize, arrest, and fill cavitated lesions.

3.1.1 Secondary Caries: A Local Issue?

There is still an ongoing debate whether carious lesions adjacent to restorations are, in fact, primary lesions or secondary lesions associated with interfacial gaps between the tooth and the restorative material (Brouwer et al., 2016; Jokstad, 2016). Here, the term secondary caries is used to designate the occurrence of carious lesions adjacent to restorations, as shown in Figure 3.4. Since resin composites have been associated with secondary caries more often than other materials (Rasines Alcaraz et al., 2014; Moraschini et al., 2015), and modifications are continually being proposed, the focus will be given to this material in particular.

When preventive measures or early diagnosis of the carious lesions has failed, and the diagnosis is made at later stages, a restoration is usually performed for lesion management. Dental biomaterials should be biologically safe and ideally should also be able to overcome the main reasons for direct restoration failure—secondary caries and fracture (Sarrett, 2005; Mjor, 2007; Opdam et al., 2014). Briefly, to overcome fracture, the mechanical properties of resin composites have been improved by modifying the inorganic phase, increasing filler content, altering particles shape, size and composition, as well as combining different monomers

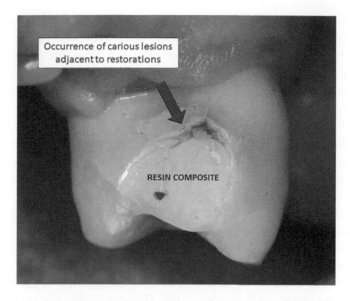

Figure 3.4 Photograph showing the clinical aspect of secondary caries:term used to designate the occurrence of carious lesions adjacent to restorations.

into the organic phase (Cramer et al., 2011; Ferracane, 2011). On the other hand, what would be the approach to overcome failure due to secondary caries?

In an attempt to reduce carious lesion formation next to resin composite restorations, some modifications were and are still being made into the organic phase of resin composites, to provide antimicrobial, remineralizing, stress-reducing, and degradation-resistant materials (Cheng et al., 2015, 2017; Fugolin and Pfeifer, 2017). Evaluations of most of these properties regarding secondary caries/mineral loss were mainly tested in in vitro/in situ studies.

Regrettably, no clinical trial was found investigating the effect of resin composite restorations with antibacterial properties for the prevention of secondary caries, maintaining the absence of evidence reported in the last updated publication on the subject in Cochrane database (Pereira-Cenci et al., 2013) and another review on the theme (do Amaral et al., 2015).

Regarding physical properties, the polymerization shrinkage/stress that may compromise the adhesive bonding between resin composite and tooth interfaces leading to gap formation, remains a concern (Nedeljkovic et al., 2015), and the presence of a gap has been related to secondary caries formation in vitro and in situ studies (Kuper et al., 2015a; Maske et al., 2017).

Low-shrinkage resin composites were introduced to minimize polymerization stress, which could reduce adhesive failures between tooth and restoration (Pitel, 2013). Nonetheless, overall failure rates, secondary caries, and marginal adaptation of low-shrinkage resin composites do not suggest that there is any improvement when compared to resin composites containing 2-hydroxyethyl methacrylate (HEMA), triethylene glycol dimethacrylate (TEGDMA), or other low-molecular-weight monomers (Magno et al., 2016; van Dijken and Pallesen, 2017). Besides, there is no clinical evidence showing that the presence of a gap would lead to secondary caries development (Mjor and Toffenetti, 2000; Heintze and Rousson, 2012; Ferracane and Hilton, 2016).

Systematic reviews, including solely controlled clinical trials, do not show high failure rates due to secondary caries (da Veiga et al., 2016), indicating that this failure type is related to factors (situations) not accessed in those studies. Operator variables including practice type (Laske et al., 2016) and diagnostic training to differentiate secondary caries from marginal discoloration (Mjor, 2005; Sarrett, 2005; Heintze, 2007), the caries risk of patients (van de Sande et al., 2016), and longer follow-up times (Opdam et al., 2014) may influence higher secondary caries outcomes in studies derived from practice-based research, which, in turn, reflect the daily clinical practice (Mjor, 2008). Nonetheless, the secondary caries problem is there in the clinical setting, as shown by a recent study that compared the clinical judgment carried out by general dentists to the experts' opinion based on the assessment of a sample of bitewing radiographs (Signori et al., 2018).

In general, resin composite restorations present annual failure rates (AFRs) between 1% and 5% (Demarco et al., 2017), and the replacement of restorations because of secondary caries ranges from 26% to 43% in posterior teeth (Gordan et al., 2015; Alvanforoush et al., 2017). It is worth noting that failure of resin composite restorations can vary significantly according to the caries risk of patients, showing AFRs of 4.6% for high-risk patients and 1.6% for low-risk patients in ten years of follow-up (Opdam et al., 2014). Additionally, failures due to secondary caries were shown to be much higher in high-risk caries patients compared to low-risk patients (van de Sande et al., 2013). In this perspective, future clinical studies addressing restorative material properties to inhibit secondary caries should be carried out with the inclusion of high caries risk patients. Moreover, the comprehension that patients hold responsibilities on treatment outcomes may assist the dentist in informing their patients about risks of failure, engaging patients on behavioral changes concerning diet and oral hygiene practices.

3.1.2 Dental Materials with Anti-Caries Proprieties

The replacement of dental structure lost due to caries disease or injuries represents a large part of general clinical practice worldwide. Dental materials can reconstruct the tooth structure lost and restore the function and aesthetic of the dental element. Moreover, it is assumed that dental materials can also play an additional function, i.e., helping in the control of (secondary) caries lesion incidence in tooth surface (Cenci et al., 2008, 2009; Weir et al., 2012, 2017; Melo et al., 2013). Figure 3.5 exemplifies the target location of investigated developing bioactive materials. Overall, the remineralizing and antibacterial polymeric materials are intended to act at the interface tooth/restoration.

Resin composite, amalgam, and glass ionomer cement (GIC) are materials widely used in dentistry to restore teeth. These dental restorations can fail for many reasons (Hickel et al., 2010), and secondary caries has been described as the principal reason for failures and replacement of these restorations (Mjor, 2005; Opdam et al., 2014). In an attempt to prevent secondary caries and improve the longevity of restorations, the development of new dental materials has been encouraged. Figure 3.6 highlights the main current strategies under development for improving the longevity of the polymeric restorations proposed as direct restorative materials. Manufactures and researches have been incorporating antimicrobials, using Ca-, P-, and F-releasing ions, and creating novel stress-reducing, degradation-resistant, and self-healing materials (by functional

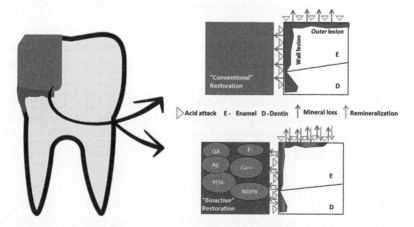

Figure 3.5 The target location of investigated developing bioactive materials. Overall, the remineralizing and antibacterial polymeric materials are intended to act at the interface tooth/restoration.

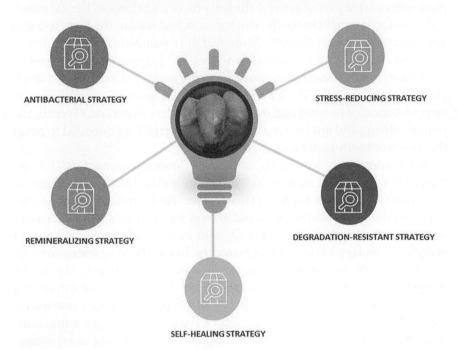

Cutting-Edge Developing Strategies to improve the longevity of restorations

ANTIBACTERIAL STRATEGY

STRESS-REDUCING STRATEGY

REMINERALIZING STRATEGY

DEGRADATION-RESISTANT STRATEGY

SELF-HEALING STRATEGY

Figure 3.6 Main current strategies under development for improving the longevity of the polymeric restorations proposed as direct restorative materials.

monomers incorporation) to overcome those limitations related to carious lesion development (Cramer et al., 2011; Fugolin and Pfeifer, 2017; Zhang et al., 2017).

In the following, a summary of the main pathways for polymeric restorative materials with anti-caries proprieties is provided. Possibilities and future perspectives of these dental materials for inhibiting secondary caries formation are shown.

3.1.2.1 Fluoride-Releasing Dental Materials
Fluoride is a well-known anti-caries agent interfering in the caries process, reducing the demineralization, and enhancing remineralization of enamel and dentin (Cury et al., 2016). Regardless of the ways that fluoride is used, its anti-caries effect is obtained by the same mode (acting on des-remineralization phenomena). By this assumption, several

fluoride-releasing dental materials have been claimed to help in the control of secondary caries lesion mainly in high caries risk patients (Benelli et al., 1993; Hara et al., 2006; Cenci et al., 2008).

GIC has been widely used in dentistry because of a variety of beneficial proprieties such as chemical adhesion to the dental substrate, biocompatibility, and fluoride release (Berg, 2002). GICs are composed of fluoride-containing silicate glass and polyalkenoic acid, which are set by an acid reaction between components. During the reaction, several ions (constituents of material) are released, including the fluoride ion (Wiegand et al., 2007). GICs are also capable of being recharged with fluoride ions by other sources; for example, fluoridated dentifrices (Vieira et al., 1999). By the F-release proprieties, GICs have been consistently showing inhibition to carious lesions around restoration margins (Benelli et al., 1993; Cenci et al., 2009; de Moraes et al., 2016). Other materials derived from GICs such as resin-modified glass-ionomer (RMGI) and polyacid-modified composites are also reported as fluoride-releasing and have been related to carious lesion control (de Moraes et al., 2016).

Resin composites have been developed as an attempt to promote F ion-release and therefore help in the carious lesion control. Different approaches to impart fluoride ion-releasing capability to composite materials have been reported. The initial reports address the incorporation of either water-soluble salts (NaF or SnF_2), matrix-bound fluoride, or fluoride-releasing filler systems (Arends et al., 1995). When soluble salts and matrix-bound fluoride are incorporated in the composite material, an easy washout of fluoride ions is related to the weakness of material proprieties. However, the incorporation of fluoride-releasing filler as strontium fluoride (SrF_2) or Ytterbium trifluoride (YbF_3) has shown good mechanical and physical proprieties (Wiegand et al., 2007).

The effect of fluoride-releasing composite resins on secondary caries lesions control has been evaluated on in vitro studies indicating that these composites tend to inhibit caries-like lesions compared to no-fluoride releasing composite, but it is not completely clear (Dijkman et al., 1994; Dionysopoulos et al., 1998; Yaman et al., 2004). Moreover, the fluoride levels leached from those composites are lower compared to levels released from conventional or RMGI or polyacid-modified composites (Preston et al., 1999; Asmussen and Peutzfeldt, 2002).

With the same intended capabilities of fluoride-releasing composites, adhesives with the potential to release fluoride ion have been developed and available in the dentistry market. Fluoride is incorporated in adhesive by the same methods used for resin composite, being the F-filler-incorporation approach with lower loss of material structural characteristics. These adhesives are expected to inhibit secondary caries lesions by promoting adhesion to tooth substrates and by releasing fluoride ions. In vitro studies have shown that fluoride-releasing adhesives were effective in inhibiting secondary lesions and enhancing the remineralization of decalcified dentin (Itota et al., 2002, 2003).

3.1.2.2 Ca- or P-Releasing Dental Materials

Another potential strategy to control secondary caries lesion is to drive the shift of demineralization to remineralization via calcium (Ca) or phosphate (P) ion release from particles of amorphous calcium phosphate (ACP). ACP is an intermediate in the hydroxyapatite formation and has been investigated as a bioactive additive for dental material (Combes and Rey, 2010; Zhao et al., 2011). The main advantages of ACP are its simplified formulation and biocompatibility with hard and soft tissues (Skrtic and Antonucci, 2011). Several studies have shown that ACP can release supersaturating levels of Ca^{2+} and PO_4^{-3}, which are ions favorable for hydroxyapatite formation (Cao et al., 2013; Zhou et al., 2014; Palaniswamy et al., 2016).

Considering the remineralization potential of ACP particles, experimental dental resin composites or adhesives containing these particles (micro or nano) have been shown to remineralize caries-like lesions (Skrtic et al., 1996; Langhorst et al., 2009; Melo et al., 2013; Zhang et al., 2015b; Weir et al., 2017) and have also been reported as a neutralizing agent to acids produced by cariogenic bacteria (Moreau et al., 2011).

Dental materials with ACP particles in their composition are considered useful in inhibiting secondary caries because they are able to release Ca^{+2} and PO_4^{-2} ions when the pH is decreased due to bacteria metabolism. By this mechanism, the carious lesion around composite ACP restoration is reduced in its progression (Melo et al., 2013). The release of those ions is diminished over time, lasting only a few months (Dickens et al., 2003; Langhorst et al., 2009). To achieve long-term and sustained Ca^{+2} and PO_4^{-2} ions release, new rechargeable materials have been researched (Zhang et al., 2015b, 2016). ACP rechargeable dental materials seem to be promising for caries-inhibiting restorations, but still, there is no clinical evidence for their use in clinical practice.

3.1.2.3 Dental Materials with Antimicrobial Proprieties

As described in the previous chapter, the two main components of polymeric restorative materials, here referred to as resin composites, are (1) filling material and (2) bonding systems applied to the tooth surface. The incorporation of antimicrobial agents in both components would have a role in the prevention of the effects caused by cariogenic bacteria located at the tooth-restoration interface (Pereira-Cenci et al., 2009).

The antimicrobial effects of resin composites would be relevant for inhibition of plaque accumulation on the surface of these materials and also at tooth around restorations. For bonding agents and systems, the role should be related to their antibacterial effects in terms of cavity disinfection or inactivation of bacteria that could invade the adhesive interface due to leakage (Imazato, 2003). Therefore, the presence of antimicrobial agents in the filling materials (composite or adhesive components) could be able to affect the secondary caries lesion initiation and progression.

Among the antimicrobial agents incorporated into dental restorative materials, 12-methacryloyloxydo-decylpyridium bromide (MDPB), quaternary of ammonium (QA), and metallic ions are frequently researched (Cocco et al., 2015; do Amaral et al., 2015).

MDPB was the first antimicrobial agent incorporated in the commercial adhesive (ClearFil Protect Bond™, Kuraray Co. Ltda., Japan). As a QA, MDPB exhibits biocide activity through a cationic agent that recharges the bacterial surface negatively and consequently damaging the cytoplasmic membrane of bacteria cells (Scheie, 1989). In situ studies using MDPB as commercial adhesives have demonstrated that the antibacterial materials can reduce the demineralization (secondary caries wall lesion) in dentin substrate (van de Sande et al., 2014; Kuper et al., 2015b; Montagner et al., 2015). This monomer was also able to slow down enamel demineralization around orthodontic brackets in vivo (Uysal et al., 2011). However, until the moment, there is no clinical evidence that this system incorporated into dental materials plays any role in the caries lesion development around restoration (Cocco et al., 2015).

Besides MPDB, other different kinds of quaternary of ammonium (QA) have also been investigated and have been proven to be effective in inhibiting the growth and metabolism of biofilms (Ge et al., 2015). The antibacterial mechanism of QA salts is due to their capability of causing bacteria lysis by binding to bacterial membranes (Namba et al., 2009; Xu et al., 2012). Moreover, the QA salts can copolymerize with other methacrylate monomers and could provide long-term antibacterial activity (Cheng et al., 2013). Experimental QA dental materials have shown antibacterial effects on complex biofilms formed in a laboratory (Zhang et al., 2013a, 2015a) and slowed down the progress of caries-like lesion (Han et al., 2017; Nascimento et al., 2017).

Another antimicrobial commonly used is silver particles that are incorporated into dental material as micro and nanoparticles (Cocco et al., 2015). The incorporation of this substance into adhesive systems (primer/bonding) has been shown to reduce the viability and metabolic activity of biofilm in vitro (Zhang et al., 2013b). Silver particles act on and inactivate bacterial enzymes, causing the loss of DNA's ability to replicate and leading to cell death (Morones et al., 2005). Microparticles of silver added to commercially available adhesive systems have shown reduced secondary caries formation in dentin margins of bonded resin composite restorations (Kramer et al., 2015). Although a reduction in secondary caries condition in vitro has mentioned, it is worth to be mentioned that the incorporation of these particles has been related to decrease mechanical and visual proprieties of material, leading to discoloration and reduced polymerization depth (Durner et al., 2011).

3.1.2.4 Stress-Reducing, Degradation-Resistant, and Self-Healing Materials

Shrinkage stress is often considered the most significant problem with current dental composites and a primary contributor to premature failure in these materials leading to gap formation (Ferracane, 2005). The presence of cariogenic biofilm associated to the gap at tooth-restoration interface has been related to secondary caries formation in vitro and in situ studies (Kuper et al., 2015a; Maske et al., 2017). A great effort has been made to develop novel dental materials with distinct polymerization methods that reduce shrinkage stress while maintaining all other desirable material properties (Cramer et al., 2011).

Stress-reducing materials have been proposed to reduce the gap formed between the tooth-restoration interface by modification on the polymer network that can simultaneously decrease stress and either maintain or enhance mechanical properties and monomer conversion (Fugolin and Pfeifer, 2017). Examples of these strategies are the incorporating of thio-urethanes (reducing 50% of polymerization stress), nano-sized prepoly-merized particles, and the use of functional monomers. Allyl disulfide as functional monomer has the capability to addition-fragmentation chain transfer (allyl bond can be broken and reformed as the radical propagates while keeping the net cross-linking density essentially unchanged) (Moraes et al., 2011; Park et al., 2012; Bacchi et al., 2016; Bacchi and Pfeifer, 2016). Capability to addition-fragmentation chain transfer is the strategy used by commercial bulk-fill material (Filtek Bulk Fill, 3M ESPE) (Fugolin and Pfeifer, 2017).

A recent randomized prospective study with five years of follow-up evaluating this material showed that the AFRs were 1.1% and 1.4% for classes I and II, respectively. The most common reasons for failure reported were fracture and secondary caries lesion. Even though the AFR was lower in bulk-fill restorations compared to conventional resin composite restoration, secondary caries was one of the main reasons for failures (van Dijken and Pallesen, 2016). These findings show and highlight that dental material per se may act as adjuvant in the prevention of secondary caries, but not in the control of dental caries disease.

Biodynamic in the oral cavity has been related to degradation of adhesive material into the tooth-restoration interface leading to marginal defects and subsequently to caries lesion formation around the restoration (Carvalho and Manso, 2016). New resistant-degradation materials have been researched to overcome this shortcoming. Materials using alternative paths for polymerization based on the vinyl bond of methacrylate monomers such as methacrylamides, vinyl ethers, azide-alkyne, thiol-vinyl sulfone, and improved thyolene chemistry have shown promising results (Fugolin and Pfeifer, 2017).

Another strategy used is the development of self-healing materials, which are capable of restoring mechanical integrity after small damage has occurred (Trask et al., 2007; Diesendruck et al., 2015). These materials usually are loaded with polymeric capsules with the healing agent. A polymerizable solution is encapsulated, and the reactants are released when the capsules are physically damaged (e.g., a crack within the matrix). An active catalyst kept out of contact with the monomer is also released by the rupturing of a capsule and is responsible for cross-linking the polymer (Diesendruck et al. 2015). New novel materials with incorporation of antimicrobial, remineralizing ions, and self-healing technology have been researched (Wu et al., 2015). However, there is until this moment shreds of evidence showing potential to secondary caries prevention, although the antimicrobial potential was showed.

3.1.3 Do Anti-Caries Dental Materials Work Effectively at the Clinic?

In the previous subsections, several dental materials with old and innovative proprieties to prevent (secondary) caries lesion development were described.

Anti-caries restorative materials are seen as attractive to the clinician because they could serve as a double purpose: repair the damage of caries lesion (cavity) and additionally help to prevent new caries lesion formation around restoration (Cury et al., 2016). Even considering the potential advantages of clinic situations, there are few clinical studies supporting their use based on the anti-caries effect. Most of the available evidence considering the caries lesion prevention comes from in vitro and in situ studies. Findings from these studies are considered essential for the feasibility of the proposed concepts and screening of potential formulations, but low in evidence level to support the best clinical decision-making. There is much need for randomized clinical trials to support the clinical translation of these materials.

Searching on the Cochrane database, only four systematic reviews discussing dental materials and their effect on caries lesion prevention were found. Two of these reviews considered the use of fluoride-releasing dental materials, and the others were focused on antimicrobial dental materials. Yengopal et al. (2009) evaluated different restorative materials used to treat caries in primary dentition, and secondary caries lesions were considered as one of the outcomes. In this systematic review, when a compomer (Dyract*; a resin composite modified by polyacid and fluoride-releasing material) was evaluated against amalgam restoration with 24 months of follow-up, it was noted that amalgam had three times more chance to develop secondary caries than compomer in class II cavities, thus favoring the anti-caries proprieties of that compomer. However, due to a low number of studies included in the review, the evidence is still insufficient to make any clinical recommendation. Besides, other independent systematic reviews showed that when resin-modified glass ionomer cement (RM-GIC) was evaluated against composite resin, there was no difference between both materials considering caries-preventive effect (Yengopal and Mickenautsch, 2011). According to these authors, the clinical meaning of the results remains uncertain due to bias risk and low quality of the studies included (Dorri et al., 2017).

In summary, clinical studies considering fluoride-releasing dental materials show contradictory results in secondary caries lesion prevention. It is worth to be pointed out that caries risk status of patients (low or high) included in those clinical trials was not described. Therefore, it may influence the outcome showing a high, small, or no anti-caries effect on preventing secondary caries. Clinical trials of dental materials with properties to inhibit secondary caries should be carried out with high caries risk patients where dental materials should present some positive effect.

Given the use of antimicrobial agents incorporated into composite restorations to prevent caries lesion development, two systematic reviews (previous and updated version) were found on the Cochrane database (Pereira-Cenci et al., 2009, 2013). In both versions, the authors were unable to identify any randomized controlled trials on the effects of antibacterial agents incorporated into composite restorations for the prevention of dental caries. The absence of high-level evidence for the effectiveness of this intervention emphasizes the need for well-designed, adequately powered, randomized controlled clinical trials.

No clinical trials or systematic reviews were found evaluating the other stress-reducing, degradation-resistant, and self-healing materials, and the available evidence to caries prevention is mainly based on laboratory studies.

To date, the lack of high-quality evidence to support the role of restorative materials on the management of primary and secondary caries led to uncertainty on the clinical performance of anti-caries restorative materials. Future clinical studies should address the role of anti-caries restorative materials at the tooth, individual, and community-based levels.

3.2 Final Conclusions

This chapter revealed extensive evidence showing that several dental materials with anti-caries properties have affected the secondary caries lesions development in vitro and situ studies. However, clinical evidence seems to be scarce and showing contradictory results. Are the "anti-caries dental materials" able to effectively control carious lesions around restorations? Future clinical studies should be carried out to address this question.

Carious lesions around restorations are considered as a consequence of a complex disease with behavioral-biofilm-sugar dependency and therefore considered as only a small piece of the puzzle that is dental caries disease. The lack of positive outcomes toward a reduced prevalence of secondary caries around the restorations when using "anti-caries dental materials" is explained by the rich complexity of the management of the caries disease.

Up-to-date, the effect of anti-caries dental materials alone may not be enough to avoid or combat dental caries disease. However, they could act as an adjuvant in the process helping locally on the caries lesion, especially in the cases where other preventive measures, such as the use of fluoride dentifrice, are not available. The management of caries disease is complicated and multi-strategic, and indeed involves strategies to change personal conduct and social behavior, especially regarding sugar consumption. If the dental caries control fails, dental restorative materials will inevitably fail as well.

References

Ahovuo-Saloranta A, Forss H, Walsh T, Hiiri A, Nordblad A, Makela M, Worthington HV: Sealants for preventing dental decay in the permanent teeth. *The Cochrane Database of Systematic Reviews* 2013;28(3);CD001830.

Alvanforoush N, Palamara J, Wong RH, Burrow MF: Comparison between published clinical success of direct resin composite restorations in vital posterior teeth in 1995–2005 and 2006–2016 periods. *Australian Dental Journal* 2017;62(2):132–145.

Arends J, Dijkman GEHM, Dijkman AG: Review of fluoride release and secondary caries reduction by fluoridating composites. *Advances in Dental Research* 1995;9:367–376.

Asmussen E, Peutzfeldt A: Long-term fluoride release from a glass ionomer cement, a compomer, and from experimental resin composites. *Acta Odontologica Scandinavica* 2002;60:93–97.

Bacchi A, Nelson M, Pfeifer CS: Characterization of methacrylate-based composites containing thio-urethane oligomers. *Dental Materials: Official Publication of the Academy of Dental Materials* 2016;32:233–239.

Bacchi A, Pfeifer CS: Rheological and mechanical properties and interfacial stress development of composite cements modified with thio-urethane oligomers. *Dental Materials: Official Publication of the Academy of Dental Materials* 2016;32:978–986.

Benelli EM, Serra MC, Rodrigues AL, Jr., Cury JA: In situ anticariogenic potential of glass ionomer cement. *Caries Research* 1993;27:280–284.

Berg JH: Glass ionomer cements. *Pediatric Dentistry* 2002;24:430–438.

Brouwer F, Askar H, Paris S, Schwendicke F: Detecting secondary caries lesions: A systematic review and meta-analysis. *Journal of Dental Research* 2016;95:143–151.

Cao Y, Mei ML, Xu J, Lo EC, Li Q, Chu CH: Biomimetic mineralisation of phosphorylated dentine by CPP-ACP. *Journal of Dentistry* 2013;41:818–825.

Carvalho RM, Manso AP: Biodegradation of resin-dentin bonds: A clinical problem? *Current Oral Health Reports* 2016;3:229–233.

Cenci MS, Pereira-Cenci T, Cury JA, Ten Cate JM: Relationship between gap size and dentine secondary caries formation assessed in a microcosm biofilm model. *Caries Research* 2009;43:97–102.

Cenci MS, Tenuta LM, Pereira-Cenci T, Del Bel Cury AA, ten Cate JM, Cury JA: Effect of microleakage and fluoride on enamel-dentine demineralization around restorations. *Caries Research* 2008;42:369–379.

Cheng L, Weir MD, Zhang K, Arola DD, Zhou X, Xu HH: Dental primer and adhesive containing a new antibacterial quaternary ammonium monomer dimethylaminododecyl methacrylate. *Journal of Dentistry* 2013;41:345–355.

Cheng L, Zhang K, Weir MD, Melo MA, Zhou X, Xu HH: Nanotechnology strategies for antibacterial and remineralizing composites and adhesives to tackle dental caries. *Nanomedicine (London, England)* 2015;10:627–641.

Cheng L, Zhang K, Zhang N, Melo MAS, Weir MD, Zhou XD, Bai YX, Reynolds MA, Xu HHK: Developing a new generation of antimicrobial and bioactive dental resins. *Journal of Dental Research* 2017;96:855–863.

Cocco AR, Rosa WL, Silva AF, Lund RG, Piva E: A systematic review about antibacterial monomers used in dental adhesive systems: Current status and further prospects. *Dental Materials: Official Publication of the Academy of Dental Materials* 2015;31:1345–1362.

Combes C, Rey C: Amorphous calcium phosphates: Synthesis, properties and uses in biomaterials. *Acta Biomaterialia* 2010;6:3362–3378.

Cramer NB, Stansbury JW, Bowman CN: Recent advances and developments in composite dental restorative materials. *Journal of Dental Research* 2011;90:402–416.

Cury JA, de Oliveira BH, dos Santos AP, Tenuta LM: Are fluoride releasing dental materials clinically effective on caries control? *Dental Materials: Official Publication of the Academy of Dental Materials* 2016;32:323–333.

da Veiga AM, Cunha AC, Ferreira DM, da Silva Fidalgo TK, Chianca TK, Reis KR, Maia LC: Longevity of direct and indirect resin composite restorations in permanent posterior teeth: A systematic review and meta-analysis. *Journal of Dentistry* 2016;54:1–12.

de Moraes MD, de Melo MA, Bezerra Dda S, Costa LS, Saboia Vde P, Rodrigues LK: Clinical study of the caries-preventive effect of resin-modified glass ionomer restorations: Aging versus the influence of fluoride dentifrice. *Journal of Investigative And Clinical Dentistry* 2016;7:180–186.

Demarco FF, Collares K, Correa MB, Cenci MS, Moraes RR, Opdam NJ: Should my composite restorations last forever? Why are they failing? *Brazilian Oral Research* 2017;31:e56.

Dickens SH, Flaim GM, Takagi S: Mechanical properties and biochemical activity of remineralizing resin-based ca-po4 cements. *Dental Materials: Official Publication of the Academy of Dental Materials* 2003;19:558–566.

Diesendruck CE, Sottos NR, Moore JS, White SR: Biomimetic self-healing. *Angewandte Chemie (International ed in English)* 2015;54:10428–10447.

Dijkman GE, de Vries J, Arends J: Secondary caries in dentine around composites: A wavelength-independent microradiographical study. *Caries Research* 1994;28:87–93.

Dionysopoulos P, Kotsanos N, Papadogiannis Y, Konstantinidis A: Artificial secondary caries around two new F-containing restoratives. *Operative Dentistry* 1998;23:81–86.

do Amaral GS, de Cassia NT, Maltz M, Arthur RA: Restorative materials containing antimicrobial agents: Is there evidence for their antimicrobial and anti-caries effects?—A systematic-review. *Australian Dental Journal* 2015;61(1):6–15.

Dorri M, Dunne SM, Walsh T, Schwendicke F: Micro-invasive interventions for managing proximal dental decay in primary and permanent teeth. *The Cochrane Database of Systematic Reviews* 2015:CD010431.

Dorri M, Martinez-Zapata MJ, Walsh T, Marinho VC, Sheiham Deceased A, Zaror C: Atraumatic restorative treatment versus conventional restorative treatment for managing dental caries. *The Cochrane Database of Systematic Reviews* 2017;12:CD008072.

Durner J, Stojanovic M, Urcan E, Hickel R, Reichl FX: Influence of silver nanoparticles on monomer elution from light-cured composites. *Dental Materials: Official Publication of the Academy of Dental Materials* 2011;27:631–636.

Ferracane JL, Hilton TJ: Polymerization stress—Is it clinically meaningful? *Dental Materials: Official Publication of the Academy of Dental Materials* 2016;32:1–10.

Ferracane JL: Developing a more complete understanding of stresses produced in dental composites during polymerization. *Dental Materials: Official Publication of the Academy of Dental Materials* 2005;21:36–42.

Ferracane JL: Resin composite—State of the art. *Dental Materials: Official Publication of the Academy of Dental Materials* 2011;27:29–38.

Fugolin APP, Pfeifer CS: New resins for dental composites. *Journal of Dental Research* 2017;96:1085–1091.

Ge Y, Wang S, Zhou X, Wang H, Xu HH, Cheng L: The use of quaternary ammonium to combat dental caries. *Materials (Basel, Switzerland)* 2015;8: 3532–3549.

Gordan VV, Riley JL, 3rd, Rindal DB, Qvist V, Fellows JL, Dilbone DA, Brotman SG, Gilbert GH: Repair or replacement of restorations: A prospective cohort study by dentists in the national dental practice-based research network. *Journal of the American Dental Association* 1939;2015(146):895–903.

Han Q, Li B, Zhou X, Ge Y, Wang S, Li M, Ren B, Wang H, Zhang K, Xu HHK, Peng X, Feng M, Weir MD, Chen Y, Cheng L: Anti-caries effects of dental adhesives containing quaternary ammonium methacrylates with different chain lengths. *Materials (Basel, Switzerland)* 2017;10(6):643

Hara AT, Turssi CP, Ando M, Gonzalez-Cabezas C, Zero DT, Rodrigues AL, Jr., Serra MC, Cury JA: Influence of fluoride-releasing restorative material on root dentine secondary caries in situ. *Caries Research* 2006;40:435–439.

Heintze SD, Rousson V: Clinical effectiveness of direct class ii restorations—A meta-analysis. *The Journal of Adhesive Dentistry* 2012;14:407–431.

Heintze SD: Systematic reviews: I. The correlation between laboratory tests on marginal quality and bond strength. II. The correlation between marginal quality and clinical outcome. *The Journal of Adhesive Dentistry* 2007;9(Suppl 1):77–106.

Hickel R, Peschke A, Tyas M, Mjor I, Bayne S, Peters M, Hiller KA, Randall R, Vanherle G, Heintze SD: FDI world dental federation: Clinical criteria for the evaluation of direct and indirect restorations-update and clinical examples. *Clinical Oral Investigations* 2010;14:349–366.

Imazato S: Antibacterial properties of resin composites and dentin bonding systems. *Dental Materials: Official Publication of the Academy of Dental Materials* 2003;19:449–457.

Itota T, Nakabo S, Iwai Y, Konishi N, Nagamine M, Torii Y: Inhibition of artificial secondary caries by fluoride-releasing adhesives on root dentin. *Journal of Oral Rehabilitation* 2002;29:523–527.

Itota T, Torii Y, Nakabo S, Tashiro Y, Konishi N, Nagamine M, Yoshiyama M: Effect of fluoride-releasing adhesive system on decalcified dentin. *Journal of Oral Rehabilitation* 2003;30:178–183.

Jokstad A: Secondary caries and microleakage. *Dental Materials: Official Publication of the Academy of Dental Materials* 2016;32:11–25.

Kramer N, Mohwald M, Lucker S, Domann E, Zorzin JI, Rosentritt M, Frankenberger R: Effect of microparticulate silver addition in dental adhesives on secondary caries in vitro. *Clinical Oral Investigations* 2015;19:1673–1681.

Kuper NK, Montagner AF, van de Sande FH, Bronkhorst EM, Opdam NJ, Huysmans MC: Secondary caries development in in situ gaps next to composite and amalgam. *Caries Research* 2015a;49:557–563.

Kuper NK, van de Sande FH, Opdam NJ, Bronkhorst EM, de Soet JJ, Cenci MS, Huysmans MC: Restoration materials and secondary caries using an in vitro biofilm model. *Journal of Dental Research* 2015b;94:62–68.

Langhorst SE, O'Donnell JN, Skrtic D: In vitro remineralization of enamel by polymeric amorphous calcium phosphate composite: Quantitative microradiographic study. *Dental Materials: Official Publication of the Academy of Dental Materials* 2009;25:884–891.

Laske M, Opdam NJ, Bronkhorst EM, Braspenning JC, Huysmans MC: Longevity of direct restorations in dutch dental practices. Descriptive study out of a practice based research network. *Journal of Dentistry* 2016;46:12–17.

Magno MB, Nascimento GC, Rocha YS, Ribeiro BD, Loretto SC, Maia LC: Silorane-based composite resin restorations are not better than conventional composites—A meta-analysis of clinical studies. *The Journal of Adhesive Dentistry* 2016;18:375–386.

Marsh PD: Are dental diseases examples of ecological catastrophes? *Microbiology (Reading, England)* 2003;149:279–294.

Marthaler TM: Changes in dental caries 1953–2003. *Caries Research* 2004;38:173–181.

Maske TT, Kuper NK, Cenci MS, Huysmans M: Minimal gap size and dentin wall lesion development next to resin composite in a microcosm biofilm model. *Caries Research* 2017;51:475–481.

Meier T, Deumelandt P, Christen O, Stangl GI, Riedel K, Langer M: Global burden of sugar-related dental diseases in 168 countries and corresponding health care costs. *Journal of Dental Research* 2017;96:845–854.

Melo MA, Weir MD, Rodrigues LK, Xu HH: Novel calcium phosphate nanocomposite with caries-inhibition in a human in situ model. *Dental Materials: Official Publication of the Academy of Dental Materials* 2013;29:231–240.

Meyer-Lueckel H, Paris S: When and how to intervene in the caries process. *Operative Dentistry* 2016;41:S35–S47.

Mjor IA, Toffenetti F: Secondary caries: A literature review with case reports. *Quintessence International (Berlin, Germany: 1985)* 2000;31:165–179.

Mjor IA: Clinical diagnosis of recurrent caries. *Journal of the American Dental Association (1939)* 2005;136:1426–1433.

Mjor IA: Controlled clinical trials and practice-based research in dentistry. *Journal of Dental Research* 2008;87:605.

Mjor IA: Minimum requirements for new dental materials. *Journal of Oral Rehabilitation* 2007;34:907–912.

Montagner AF, Kuper NK, Opdam NJ, Bronkhorst EM, Cenci MS, Huysmans MC: Wall-lesion development in gaps: The role of the adhesive bonding material. *Journal of Dentistry* 2015;43:1007–1012.

Moraes RR, Garcia JW, Barros MD, Lewis SH, Pfeifer CS, Liu J, Stansbury JW: Control of polymerization shrinkage and stress in nanogel-modified monomer and composite materials. *Dental Materials: Official Publication of the Academy of Dental Materials* 2011;27:509–519.

Moraschini V, Fai CK, Alto RM, Dos Santos GO: Amalgam and resin composite longevity of posterior restorations: A systematic review and meta-analysis. *Journal of Dentistry* 2015;43:1043–1050.

Moreau JL, Sun L, Chow LC, Xu HHK: Mechanical and acid neutralizing properties and bacteria inhibition of amorphous calcium phosphate dental nanocomposite. *Journal of Biomedical Materials Research Part B, Applied Biomaterials* 2011;98:80–88.

Morones JR, Elechiguerra JL, Camacho A, Holt K, Kouri JB, Ramirez JT, Yacaman MJ: The bactericidal effect of silver nanoparticles. *Nanotechnology* 2005;16:2346–2353.

Moynihan PJ, Kelly SA: Effect on caries of restricting sugars intake: Systematic review to inform who guidelines. *Journal of Dental Research* 2014;93:8–18.

Namba N, Yoshida Y, Nagaoka N, Takashima S, Matsuura-Yoshimoto K, Maeda H, Van Meerbeek B, Suzuki K, Takashiba S: Antibacterial effect of bactericide immobilized in resin matrix. *Dental Materials: Official Publication of the Academy of Dental Materials* 2009;25:424–430.

Nascimento P, Meereis CTW, Maske TT, Ogliari FA, Cenci MS, Pfeifer CS, Faria ESAL: Addition of ammonium-based methacrylates to an experimental dental adhesive for bonding metal brackets: Carious lesion development and bond strength after cariogenic challenge. *American Journal of Orthodontics and Dentofacial Orthopedics: Official Publication of the American Association of Orthodontists, its Constituent Societies, and the American Board of Orthodontics* 2017;151:949–956.

Nedeljkovic I, Teughels W, De Munck J, Van Meerbeek B, Van Landuyt KL: Is secondary caries with composites a material-based problem? *Dental Materials: Official Publication of the Academy of Dental Materials* 2015;31:e247–e277.

Opdam NJ, van de Sande FH, Bronkhorst E, Cenci MS, Bottenberg P, Pallesen U, Gaengler P, Lindberg A, Huysmans MC, van Dijken JW: Longevity of posterior composite restorations: A systematic review and meta-analysis. *Journal of Dental Research* 2014;93:943–949.

Osborne JW, Summitt JB: Extension for prevention: Is it relevant today? *American Journal of Dentistry* 1998;11:189–196.

Palaniswamy UK, Prashar N, Kaushik M, Lakkam SR, Arya S, Pebbeti S: A comparative evaluation of remineralizing ability of bioactive glass and amorphous calcium phosphate casein phosphopeptide on early enamel lesion. *Dental Research Journal* 2016;13:297–302.

Park HY, Kloxin CJ, Abuelyaman AS, Oxman JD, Bowman CN: Novel dental restorative materials having low polymerization shrinkage stress via stress relaxation by addition-fragmentation chain transfer. *Dental Materials: Official Publication of the Academy of Dental Materials* 2012;28:1113–1119.

Pereira-Cenci T, Cenci MS, Fedorowicz Z, Azevedo M: Antibacterial agents in composite restorations for the prevention of dental caries. *The Cochrane Database of Systematic Reviews* 2013:CD007819.

Pereira-Cenci T, Cenci MS, Fedorowicz Z, Marchesan MA: Antibacterial agents in composite restorations for the prevention of dental caries. *The Cochrane Database of Systematic Reviews* 2009:CD007819.

Peres MA, Sheiham A, Liu P, Demarco FF, Silva AE, Assuncao MC, Menezes AM, Barros FC, Peres KG: Sugar consumption and changes in dental caries from childhood to adolescence. *Journal of Dental Research* 2016;95:388–394.

Pitel ML: Low-shrink composite resins: A review of their history, strategies for managing shrinkage, and clinical significance. *Compendium of Continuing Education in Dentistry (Jamesburg, NJ: 1995)* 2013;34:578–590.

Preston AJ, Mair LH, Agalamanyi EA, Higham SM: Fluoride release from aesthetic dental materials. *Journal of Oral Rehabilitation* 1999;26:123–129.

Rasines Alcaraz MG, Veitz-Keenan A, Sahrmann P, Schmidlin PR, Davis D, Iheozor-Ejiofor Z: Direct composite resin fillings versus amalgam fillings for permanent or adult posterior teeth. *The Cochrane Database of Systematic Reviews* 2014:CD005620.

Ricketts D, Lamont T, Innes NP, Kidd E, Clarkson JE: Operative caries management in adults and children. *The Cochrane Database of Systematic Reviews* 2013:CD003808.

Sarrett DC: Clinical challenges and the relevance of materials testing for posterior composite restorations. *Dental Materials: Official Publication of the Academy of Dental Materials* 2005;21:9–20.

Scheie AA: Modes of action of currently known chemical anti-plaque agents other than chlorhexidine. *Journal of Dental Research* 1989;68:1609–1616.

Schwendicke F, Frencken JE, Bjorndal L, Maltz M, Manton DJ, Ricketts D, Van Landuyt K, Banerjee A, Campus G, Domejean S, Fontana M, Leal S, Lo E, Machiulskiene V, Schulte A, Splieth C, Zandona AF, Innes NP: Managing carious lesions: Consensus recommendations on carious tissue removal. *Advances in Dental Research* 2016;28:58–67.

Sheiham A, James WP: A new understanding of the relationship between sugars, dental caries and fluoride use: Implications for limits on sugars consumption. *Public Health Nutrition* 2014a;17:2176–2184.

Sheiham A, James WP: A reappraisal of the quantitative relationship between sugar intake and dental caries: The need for new criteria for developing goals for sugar intake. *BMC Public Health* 2014b;14:863.

Sheiham A, James WP: Diet and dental caries: The pivotal role of free sugars reemphasized. *Journal of Dental Research* 2015;94:1341–1347.

Signori C, Laske M, Mendes FM, Huysmans M, Cenci MS, Opdam NJM: Decision-making of general practitioners on interventions at restorations based on bitewing radiographs. *Journal of Dentistry* 2018;76:109–116.

Skrtic D, Antonucci JM: Bioactive polymeric composites for tooth mineral regeneration: Physicochemical and cellular aspects. *Journal of Functional Biomaterials* 2011;2:271–307.

Skrtic D, Hailer AW, Takagi S, Antonucci JM, Eanes ED: Quantitative assessment of the efficacy of amorphous calcium phosphate/methacrylate composites in remineralizing caries-like lesions artificially produced in bovine enamel. *Journal of Dental Research* 1996;75:1679–1686.

Trask RS, Williams HR, Bond IP: Self-healing polymer composites: Mimicking nature to enhance performance. *Bioinspiration & Biomimetics* 2007;2:P1–P9.

Uysal T, Amasyali M, Ozcan S, Koyuturk AE, Sagdic D: Effect of antibacterial monomer-containing adhesive on enamel demineralization around orthodontic brackets: An in-vivo study. *American Journal of Orthodontics and Dentofacial Orthopedics: Official Publication of the American Association of Orthodontists, Its Constituent Societies, and the American Board of Orthodontics* 2011;139:650–656.

van de Sande FH, Collares K, Correa MB, Cenci MS, Demarco FF, Opdam N: Restoration survival: Revisiting patients' risk factors through a systematic literature review. *Operative Dentistry* 2016;41:S7–S26.

van de Sande FH, Opdam NJ, Rodolpho PA, Correa MB, Demarco FF, Cenci MS: Patient risk factors' influence on survival of posterior composites. *Journal of Dental Research* 2013;92:78s–83s.

van de Sande FH, Opdam NJ, Truin GJ, Bronkhorst EM, de Soet JJ, Cenci MS, Huysmans MC: The influence of different restorative materials on secondary caries development in situ. *Journal of Dentistry* 2014;42:1171–1177.

van Dijken JW, Pallesen U: Posterior bulk-filled resin composite restorations: A 5-year randomized controlled clinical study. *Journal of Dentistry* 2016;51:29–35.

van Dijken JWV, Pallesen U: Durability of a low shrinkage TEGDMA/HEMA-free resin composite system in class II restorations. A 6-year follow up. *Dental Materials: Official Publication of the Academy of Dental Materials* 2017;33:944–953.

Vieira AR, de Souza IP, Modesto A: Fluoride uptake and release by composites and glass ionomers in a high caries challenge situation. *American Journal of Dentistry* 1999;12:14–18.

Weir MD, Chow LC, Xu HH: Remineralization of demineralized enamel via calcium phosphate nanocomposite. *Journal of Dental Research* 2012;91:979–984.

Weir MD, Ruan J, Zhang N, Chow LC, Zhang K, Chang X, Bai Y, Xu HHK: Effect of calcium phosphate nanocomposite on in vitro remineralization of human dentin lesions. *Dental Materials: Official Publication of the Academy of Dental Materials* 2017;33:1033–1044.

Wiegand A, Buchalla W, Attin T: Review on fluoride-releasing restorative materials—Fluoride release and uptake characteristics, antibacterial activity and influence on caries formation. *Dental Materials: Official Publication of the Academy of Dental Materials* 2007;23:343–362.

Wu J, Weir MD, Melo MA, Xu HH: Development of novel self-healing and antibacterial dental composite containing calcium phosphate nanoparticles. *Journal of Dentistry* 2015;43:317–326.

Xu X, Wang Y, Liao S, Wen ZT, Fan Y: Synthesis and characterization of antibacterial dental monomers and composites. *Journal of Biomedical Materials Research Part B: Applied Biomaterials* 2012;100:1151–1162.

Yaman SD, Er O, Yetmez M, Karabay GA: In vitro inhibition of caries-like lesions with fluoride-releasing materials. *Journal of Oral Science* 2004;46:45–50.

Yengopal V, Harneker SY, Patel N, Siegfried N: Dental fillings for the treatment of caries in the primary dentition. *The Cochrane Database of Systematic Reviews* 2009:CD004483.

Yengopal V, Mickenautsch S: Caries-preventive effect of resin-modified glass-ionomer cement (RM-GIC) versus composite resin: A quantitative systematic review. *European Archives of Paediatric Dentistry: Official Journal of the European Academy of Paediatric Dentistry* 2011;12:5–14.

Zhang K, Cheng L, Wu EJ, Weir MD, Bai Y, Xu HH: Effect of water-ageing on dentine bond strength and anti-biofilm activity of bonding agent containing new monomer dimethylaminododecyl methacrylate. *Journal of Dentistry* 2013a;41:504–513.

Zhang K, Li F, Imazato S, Cheng L, Liu H, Arola DD, Bai Y, Xu HH: Dual antibacterial agents of nano-silver and 12-methacryloyloxydodecylpyridinium bromide in dental adhesive to inhibit caries. *Journal of Biomedical Materials Research Part B, Applied Biomaterials* 2013b;101:929–938.

Zhang K, Wang S, Zhou X, Xu HH, Weir MD, Ge Y, Li M, Wang S, Li Y, Xu X, Zheng L, Cheng L: Effect of antibacterial dental adhesive on multispecies biofilms formation. *Journal of Dental Research* 2015a;94:622–629.

Zhang K, Zhang N, Weir MD, Reynolds MA, Bai Y, Xu HHK: Bioactive dental composites and bonding agents having remineralizing and antibacterial characteristics. *Dental Clinics of North America* 2017;61:669–687.

Zhang L, Weir MD, Chow LC, Antonucci JM, Chen J, Xu HH: Novel rechargeable calcium phosphate dental nanocomposite. *Dental Materials: Official Publication of the Academy of Dental Materials* 2016;32:285–293.

Zhang L, Weir MD, Hack G, Fouad AF, Xu HH: Rechargeable dental adhesive with calcium phosphate nanoparticles for long-term ion release. *Journal of Dentistry* 2015b;43:1587–1595.

Zhao J, Liu Y, Sun WB, Zhang H: Amorphous calcium phosphate and its application in dentistry. *Chemistry Central Journal* 2011;5:40.

Zhou C, Zhang D, Bai Y, Li S: Casein phosphopeptide-amorphous calcium phosphate remineralization of primary teeth early enamel lesions. *Journal of Dentistry* 2014;42(1):21–29.

4

Interactions between Oral Bacteria and Antibacterial Polymer-Based Restorative Materials

Fernando L. Esteban Florez and Sharukh S. Khajotia
The University of Oklahoma Health Sciences Center College of Dentistry

Contents

4.1 Introduction

The oral cavity is a habitat to a wide variety of microorganisms, including bacteria, yeasts, and viruses.[1] Bacteria are the most common type of microorganism present in the oral milieu. Over 700 bacterial species were detected in the oral microflora[2-6] using numerous cultural and molecular methods.[7,8] Studies have indicated that the variety of endogenously derived nutrients, the different types of niches available for bacterial attachment, and the establishment of the biofilm lifestyle are significant factors associated with the high variability of bacterial species found in the mouth.[1] Also, it is well known that commensal bacteria serve as an essential part of the host's immune system and, therefore, are considered as a barrier for the exogenous pathogenic colonization of oral surfaces.[9] These Gram-positive bacteria actively compete for the uptake of essential nutrients and adherence sites[10] and will produce inhibitory factors such as hydrogen peroxide[2] and bacteriocins,[11,12] thereby promoting adverse conditions for the survival and growth of antagonist bacterial species.[2,13]

Over the years, *Streptococcus mutans* has been considered the most cariogenic among all oral *streptococci* and has been implicated, by numerous authors, as the leading causative agent of both primary and secondary caries.[9,14] Figure 4.1 displays the image of *S. mutans'* biofilm and its main virulence factors linked to the caries disease. However, recent studies applying the pyrosequencing technique to polymerase chain reaction (PCR) products of the 16S rDNA gene have reported that bacterial communities extracted from distinct locations in the oral cavity (smooth, occlusal, or interproximal surfaces) and cavitation stages (shallow, medium, or deep) are comprised of a wide variety of bacterial species.[15,16] In addition, it was also shown that *S. mutans* only accounts for 1.6% of the total cariogenic biomass found in active carious lesions.[17] Therefore, its role as the primary causative of dental caries (tooth decay) has now been questioned.[18]

Other studies have demonstrated that the occurrence of these non-life-threatening oral infections is directly associated with the formation of multispecies biofilms[8,12,19] on the surfaces of teeth and with the accumulation

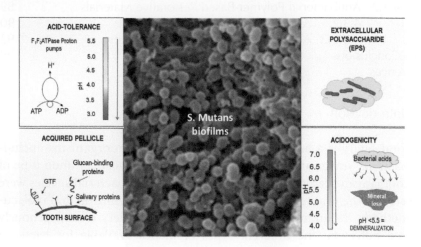

Figure 4.1   Image of *S. mutans'* biofilm and its main virulence factors linked to the caries disease.

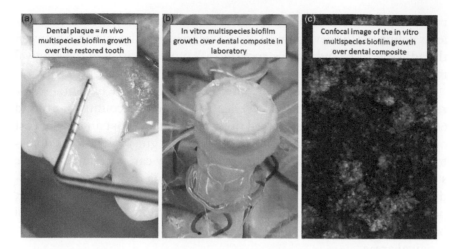

Figure 4.2 The clinical appearance of the multispecies biofilm, as known as dental plaque (a). The multispecies biofilms can be grown in laboratory studies (b) and assessed by laser confocal microscopy for the understanding of the material-biofilm interactions (c). Green color shows viable bacteria, whereas the red color shows bacteria that have been killed or are damaged.

of its acidic metabolites. Figure 4.2 spotlights the clinical appearance of the multispecies biofilm known as dental plaque (Figure 4.2a). The multispecies biofilms are grown in laboratory studies (Figure 4.2b) and assessed by laser confocal microscopy images for the understanding of the material-biofilm interactions (Figure 4.2c). Green color shows viable bacteria, whereas the red color shows bacteria that have been damaged or killed. These localized infections damage the hard tissues of teeth in a progressive and irreversible manner, and if not treated, will lead to the inflammation and death of pulpal tissues with consequent access of oral bacteria into the periapical areas of teeth and beyond.[1] Currently, the invasion of oral bacteria into the bloodstream poses as a severe health care concern, since positive and strong correlations have been found between oral bacteria and several systemic diseases such as bacterial endocardi-tis,[20,21] aspiration pneumonia,[22,23] osteomyelitis in children,[24] preterm low birth weight,[25,26] and cardiovascular diseases.[27-29]

Dental caries is one of the most common and costly bacterial infections affecting human beings.[3,4,30] It is estimated that the treatment of oral biofilm-related diseases cost approximately $81 billion in the U.S. alone.[31,32] A report from the National Center for Health Statistics (NCHS) published in May 2015 has indicated that 91% of U.S. adults (aged 20–64) had dental caries in permanent teeth in 2011 and 2012.[33] Secondary or recurrent caries is defined as the development of carious lesions at the interface between the adhesive resin and tooth structure,[34,35] more precisely, at the gingival margins of all types of Class II–V restorations.[36–38]

Secondary caries is the most common cause of failure of dental restorations.[39–44] The replacement of failed restorations accounts for around 60% of all restorations performed in the U.S. each year at an annual cost of over $5 billion.[30] Mjor et al.[34] indicated that gingival margins of restorations are more prone to failure by secondary caries because they are susceptible to contamination by oral fluids during the restorative procedures, lack of adaptation of the restorative material at the gingival floor, polymerization shrinkage, and the impossibility to effectively control biofilm formation and plaque accumulation at interproximal or subgingival areas.

The problem is exacerbated further on composite resin because these materials were demonstrated to have shorter service lives, accumulate more biofilms when compared to enamel[45] and other restorative materials,[46] and the biomass accumulated is more cariogenic in nature.[47–50] Hansel et al.,[51] while studying the effects of extractable components of composites over the growth of oral microorganisms, have demonstrated that some comonomers, such as Ethylene glycol dimethacrylate (ECDMA) and Triethylene glycol dimethacrylate (TEGDMA), upregulate the growth of acidogenic microorganisms. The pathogenic biofilm may play important roles in materials' biodegradation, hybrid layer deterioration, and pulpal irritation. Most importantly, the increased acidification of the microenvironment influences the selection of microorganisms with higher cariogenic potential, which predisposes to major shifts in the ecology of oral biofilms and triggers the development of oral diseases such as caries and periodontitis.

In this scenario, it becomes evident that the understanding of the interaction between oral biofilms and restorative polymer-based dental biomaterials is of paramount importance. The maintenance of oral health, decreasing the incidence of secondary caries, and improvement in the service lives of dental restorations can steer the research and development efforts in the direction of novel dental biomaterials having enhanced antibacterial and bioactive properties.

The present chapter is divided into three sections whereby relevant scientific evidence will be discussed with regard to the processes associated with early attachment of oral bacteria onto surfaces covered by saliva, the formation and growth of oral biofilms, and the interactions between antibacterial polymer-based restorative materials and oral biofilms.

4.2 Attachment of Oral Microorganisms

In general terms, bacteria can only exist as planktonic or biofilm populations.[52] Microbial adhesion is considered as the cornerstone step in the process of colonization of oral surfaces (biotic and abiotic),[53] which allows for the establishment and growth of oral biofilms. Figure 4.3 shows a schematic drawing of the diverse phases of oral biofilm formation. These firmly attached and highly organized (layered-stratified) communities of microorganisms are typically found embedded in a matrix of extracellular polymeric substances (EPS)[52,54,55] composed of exopolysaccharides of both bacterial and human origin. The deposition of EPS is currently regarded as a universal survival strategy among numerous bacteria[56]. EPS provides the necessary scaffolding for biofilm growth,[57] and also acts as a biologically active layer that offers protection against external aggressors such as antibiotics,[58] disinfectants,[59] and dynamic environments.[60] This matrix also serves as a reservoir for key molecules, enzymes, and nutrients that are necessary for the maintenance of cells' viability in conditions of nutrient deficiency.[61]

Garrett et al., while investigating bacterial adhesion and biofilms on oral surfaces, have suggested, based on previous scientific evidence,[56] that depending on the species considered, biofilms may be composed of 10%–25% cells and 75%–90% EPS.[52] According to Palmer and White,[62] biofilm growth is governed by several chemical and biological processes, including (1) formation of a conditioning layer, (2) reversible adhesion, (3) irreversible adhesion, (4) population growth, and (5) detachment of cells. Each of these processes will be discussed in more detail in the following subsections.

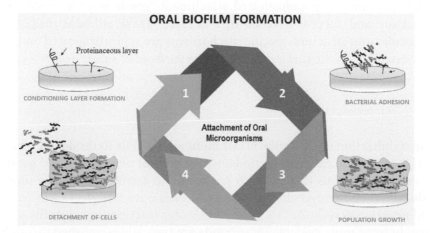

Figure 4.3 Schematic drawing of the diverse phases of oral biofilm formation.

4.2.1 Conditioning Layer Formation

The conditioning layer is a complex film that forms over the hard and non-shedding surfaces located in the oral cavity. This proteinaceous layer is composed of many polysaccharides, lipids, albumin, lysozymes, phosphoproteins, and glycoproteins from saliva and crevicular fluids,[63] and has been demonstrated to display a pivotal role in the process of bacterial adhesion and formation of biofilms. According to research findings accumulated over the years, the formation of such layer alters the physicochemical properties of surfaces while providing a source of nutrients and bond-promoting elements that upregulate early interactions between planktonic microorganisms and hard surfaces.[52,64,65] These nonspecific and reversible adhesive interactions were demonstrated to be governed by well-established processes within fluid dynamics such as mass transport (by Brownian motion), molecular diffusion and gravitational effects, physicochemical interactions (long-range van der Waals), and electrical double-layer forces.[66] The hydrophilicity of a substrate has also been shown to influence early interactions between bacteria and materials wherein hydrophobic surfaces (nonpolar) are associated with faster and higher accumulation of bacteria, and hydrophilic surfaces (polar) are demonstrated to accumulate fewer bacteria at a slower rate.[67]

According to Dunne,[66] bacteria and inert surfaces are typically negatively charged. Therefore, the final determination on the chances for initial adhesion will depend on the net sum of attractive and repulsive forces generated between the two surfaces. If the resultant net charges are repulsive, then the initial adhesion is energetically unfavorable. Microorganisms have developed very sophisticated attachment "machinery" to overcome this issue and survive attached to a surface. These adhesins-mediated molecular and structure-specific mechanisms are typically located on pili that extend from the surface of cells to the surfaces of substrates.[68]

4.2.2 Bacterial Adhesion

The stabilization of the initial attachment allows cells to reside at a given surface for more extended periods, where critical phenotypic and genotypic modifications take place to promote the establishment of a more substantial and irreversible anchoring of cells onto the surfaces of teeth and dental materials. At this point, molecular reactions between the surfaces become more evident. These bonds are typically established through molecular, structural (capsules, fimbriae, or fibrillae), or receptor-specific mechanisms (e.g., component of the surfaces of materials or tissues) mediated by the production of exopolysaccharides and adhesins (F71, F8, F13, K88).

Previous studies have demonstrated the importance of specific adhesion mechanisms on the virulence of oral microorganisms.[69-72] According to these studies, all bacteria seem to be competent to fabricate multiple types of adhesins, thereby increasing their chances of attachement onto a wide variety of substrata.[68] Planktonic microorganisms will then be able to attach to early colonizers to form aggregates on the surface of the substratum. The replication of firmly attached cells and the recruitment of additional bacteria result in higher levels of EPS deposition and microcolony formation, which, in turn, further facilitates the attachment of different species of planktonic cells. As this process evolves, a layered structure (early biofilm) is then formed wherein bacterial cells become physically separated from the remaining cells due to their EPS embedment. Such a sessile lifestyle then triggers the expression of a number of genes that alter cells' morphologies and surface properties. These important changes enable EPS-immobilized cells to establish synergic cooperation, by diffusion and quorum sensing, with surround bacteria to facilitate the exchange of nutrients and metabolites, which in turn results in spatial heterogeneities in term of structure and function throughout the biofilm.[65]

4.2.3 Population Growth

The availability and permeability of nutrients within biofilms have been demonstrated to directly impact the growth and maturation potential of most of bacterial biofilm.[66] The formation of channels is believed to be an important bacterial strategy for the maintenance and growth of sessile cells because it allows for the swift movement of molecules in and out of biofilms.[52] In addition, bacterial metabolism along with the formation of mushroom-like structures ensures the establishment of an optimum hydrodynamic flow across the biofilm that results in a current regulation of internal pH and improved perfusion profiles for nutrients and oxygen, which, in turn, favors biofilm growth rather than erosion of biofilms' outermost layers.[57,73,74] According to Vroom et al.[75] and Marsh et al.,[57] the heterogeneity of dental biofilms in conjunction with the development of gradients of key biochemical parameters explains why microorganisms of apparently incompatible metabolism and growth requirements (e.g., aerobic and anaerobic) may coexist and thrive at the same site.

After the initial growth period (lag phase), biofilms tend to grow very fast by the multiplication of sessile cells alongside the recruitment of additional planktonic bacteria. At the exponential growth stage, physical and chemical contributions to promote initial attachment end, and biological processes tend to dominate. At this point, microorganisms start to produce and excrete polysaccharide polymers and divalent cations to promote the establishment of stronger and long-lasting cell-to-cell bonds.[66] The final stages of biofilm development are then characterized by high cell concentrations where equilibrium is established between the rates of division and death of cells.[76]

Quorum sensing is a very sophisticated cell-to-cell communication system in which Gram-positive and Gram-negative bacteria within biofilms secrete small peptides[77] and acyl-homoserine lactones (AHLs)[78] to regulate changes in cells' genotypic expression, which, in turn, promote several phenotypic alterations, including physiological, metabolic, molecular, and surface changes. These are typically observed as a significant reduction in cell susceptibility to biocides (antibiotics) and antimicrobial agents.[57] Depending on the density of cells within a biofilm, the bacteria may produce enzymes, such as N-acetyl-heparosanlyase and hyaluronidase,[79] to break down polysaccharides (both soluble and insoluble; located at the outermost regions of biofilms) and release surface bacteria for the colonization of fresh and non-colonized substrates. Released cells are then upregulated to function again as planktonic microorganisms. Several operons coding for flagella proteins become highly expressed, which allows them to develop the machinery required for motility and attachment. At the same time, genes expressing a number of porins become down-regulated, thus completing biofilm's genetic cycle for adhesion and cohesion.[52]

4.2.4 Detachment of Cells

The final stage in the development of biofilms is typically associated with the release of cells from the biofilm community into the environment. Such an essential stage in the lifecycle of biofilms (1) accounts for the increased biological heterogeneity observed in the oral cavity, (2) is known to contribute to the survival of bacteria actively, and ultimately, (3) leads to the transmission of bacterial-originated oral diseases.[80] As for the example of the phases previously described, bacterial detachment is typically regulated by many complex mechanisms involving numerous environmental signals, transduction pathways, and effectors.[81] Passive mechanisms may include quorum-sensing, matrix-degrading enzymes (*dpsB*, *hyaluronidase*), and external agents, such as fluid shear forces, abrasion by the collision of solid particulates, predator grazing, and human intervention. [82-84] Active mechanisms, on the other hand, are controlled by the bacteria and include the excretion of inter-species antimicrobial compounds, competition, mutualism, and parasitism.

Other factors, such as nutrient levels, oxygen concentration, pH, and temperature, have also been correlated with the dispersion of biofilms in a great variety of bacterial species.[81] According to Lee et al.[85] the cariogenic *S. mutans* bacterium also produces an enzyme to mediate microorganisms released from dental plaque. This surface-protein-releasing (SPR) enzyme is capable of mediating the release of cells by degrading P1 salivary receptors (*Pac*), which then promotes the attachment of *S. mutans* to the surface of teeth.[86] Therefore, detachment of biofilms plays a critical role in the exacerbation and spread of bacterial infections within a single host, and it has been currently recognized to be responsible for indirect and direct host-to-host contaminations.

4.3 Interactions between Oral Bacteria and Antibacterial Polymer-Based Restorative Materials

Tooth-colored, polymer-based direct restorative materials, such as resin composites and dental bondings, polyacid-modified composite resins (PMCR), and resin-modified glass ionomer (RMGI) were demonstrated to have superior esthetic properties when compared to metallic restorations. Despite their clinical success and global acceptance among dentists and patients, these materials were shown to display important and significant limitations in the oral cavity's harsh conditions, thereby critically reducing the longevity of these types of restorations.[87] Such limitations are mainly related to processes of biodegradation, polymerization shrinkage, solvation, and hydrolysis.

Biodegradation, as defined by Oilo,[88], is *a gradual breakdown of a material mediated by specific biological activity*. Fúcio et al.,[89] while investigating the interaction between *S. mutans* and esthetic restorative materials, such as resin composites, have stated that biodegradation is a complex problem based on chemical and physical degradation (thermolysis, oxidation, solvolysis, photolysis, and radiolysis) of materials' properties caused by disintegration in saliva, wear and erosion by food, chewing, and bacterial activity. In this direction, the surface-topography changes promoted by *S. mutans* biofilms of distinct maturation levels (one-day, one-week, and one-month) were investigated by Beyth et al.[90], who demonstrated, using atomic force microscopy (AFM),

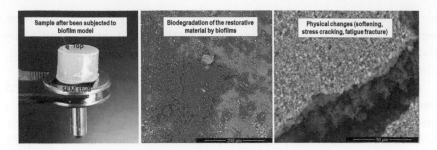

Figure 4.4   Illustrative images of the biodegradation caused by biofilm formation by scanning electronic microscopy images.

that acidic metabolites produced by cariogenic biofilms can cause damage to the surface of most restorative materials.[91] Figure 4.4 illustrates the biodegradation caused by biofilm formation with the help of scanning electronic microscopy images.

According to Bourbia et al.,[92] physical processes associated with biodegradation of restorative materials can be further classified under material loss and uptake (sorption, extraction, dissolution, and mineralization) and physical changes (softening, stress cracking, fatigue fracture, etc.). Hydrolysis is defined as the chemical process by which water molecules break down siloxane and ester bonds present in the organic matrix and coupling agents of dental polymers. These chemical processes were shown to be catalyzed in the presence of salivary enzymes, such as cholesterol esterases, pseudocholinesterase, and oral bacteria,[92-94] and are accounted as one of the significant factors associated with the overall decrease in optical, mechanical, and physical properties of direct esthetic restorative materials during their service lives.

Figure 4.5 displays clinical images of failed resin composites in the smile zone. The presence of marginal staining and secondary caries lesions are clinical signs of failure of the dental restorations.

Several clinical studies have demonstrated that polymer-based bonded restorations are more prone to failure by secondary caries when compared to amalgam restorations.[43,87,95] A study comparing the bacterial microflora growing on different restorative materials found that polymeric composite restorations support eight times more bacteria than amalgams. Besides, the authors stated that the quantity and variety of microorganisms found on composite were comparable to those found in infected root canals, while those found on amalgam restorations were similar to those found in carious dentin and dental plaque.[96] Other studies that focused

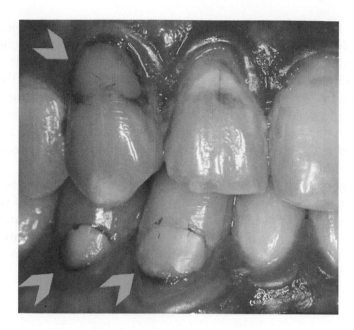

Figure 4.5 Clinical images of failed resin composites in the smile zone. The presence of marginal staining is a clinical sign of failure of the dental restorations.

on the effects of restorative materials on dental biofilms reported that biofilms grown over amalgams are typically thicker but less viable than biofilms grown against composite.[97]

These findings have demonstrated that long-term interactions between restorative materials and dental biofilms influence both the restorative materials (biodegradation) and bacteria (upregulation). From there, several studies[98] were conducted to determine the effect of polymer degradation by-products on the growth rates of biofilm-forming cariogenic oral bacteria. Gregson et al.,[99] while investigating the impact of three oral bacteria strains (*S. mutans*, *S. gordonii*, and *S. sanguis*) on the surface and mechanical properties of a composite containing Bis-GMA, TEGDMA, and dimethylamino ethyl methacrylate, reported that *S. mutans* and *S. gordonii* promoted the degradation of ester bonds significantly, as measured by Fourier-transformed infrared spectroscopy (FTIR). Still, according to the authors, such chemical degradation results in increased surface roughening, the release of polymer by-products, such as TEG and methacrylates resulting in the upregulation of both *S. mutans* and *S. gordonii*.

These findings suggest that (1) polymer materials may be subjected to surface deterioration by bacterial accumulation and (2) surface chemical composition plays a major role in the attachment, growth, and selection of pathogenic biofilms.[97] Also, in vivo studies have demonstrated that biofilms attached to composite restorations typically produce higher levels of lactic acid as compared to biofilms grown either on amalgam or glass ionomer restorations.[51] These findings combined could be used as a supporting hypothesis as to why composites tend to fail more by secondary caries than any other type of dental restoration.

The significant limitations of current polymer compositions, associated with shorter service lives ($\approx$ 6 years)[87] and higher incidences of secondary caries,[100] have precipitated the need for a new generation of polymer-based materials for direct restorative applications. Great attention has been given to the development of multi-functional "smart" materials with enhanced antibacterial, self-healing, tissue mineralization, and biocompatibility properties.

4.3.1 Low-Shrinkage Composite Resins

Since Bowen's report in 1962,[101] resin composites have been subjected to an extensive and continuous development process. Under the oral cavity's harsh conditions, current methacrylate-based restorative biomaterials display interesting physical resistance, adequate stability, and superior esthetic properties when compared to metallic restorative materials. However, despite all the remarkable improvements implemented over the years, these materials display some significant shortcomings that limit their clinical applications.[102,103] In this direction, polymerization shrinkage and subsequent contraction stresses continue to challenge the scientific community and manufacturers around the world. These important material-related limitations have been clinically correlated to restorations with imperfect margins, microleakage,[104] marginal staining, postoperative sensitivity, secondary caries, debonding,[103] cuspal displacement, and even with crack initiation and growth in healthy tooth structure.[105] Therefore, eliminating or significantly reducing the amount of polymerization contraction is one of the most important issues in the development of novel resin composites and dental bondings.[106]

From the organic matrix standpoint, polymerization contraction occurs due to a molecular densification process whereby van der Waals' distances between monomer molecules are replaced by covalent bonds during the formation of polymer chains, thereby resulting in significantly smaller intermolecular distances.[107] As the polymerization process progresses, cured areas of the polymer network tend to restrict the Brownian motion of monomers by competing with the kinetics of polymerization, which results in pendant methacrylate groups, unreacted monomers, and low degrees of conversion.[108] Weinmann et al.[105] stated that the density of reactive sites could be reduced by increasing both the molecular weight per reactive group and the filler load fraction. Although useful, these strategies are limited by the poor rheological properties (i.e., increased viscosity and stickiness) associated with high-molecular-weight monomers and the consequently reduced amounts of the organic matrix that cannot provide chemical-physical incorporation of very high concentrations of filler particles (>82 wt%).

Recent efforts have been directed towards the development of low-shrinkage resin composites based on the use of siloranes,[105] spirorthocarbonates (SOC),[106] high-molecular-weight dimer acid-based dimethacrylates,[109] tricyclodecane-urethane (TCD), ormorcers,[110–112] oxiranes,[113,114] silsesquioxanes (SSQ),[115] dimethyl-diethoxysilane (DMDES),[116] tetraethoxysilane (TEOS),[116] 4-epoxycyclohexylmetyl-(3,4-epoxy) cyclohexane carboxylate (ERL4221),[117] and epoxy-polyols.[118] Other approaches, such as the development of stress-decreasing resins (SDR)[119] and nanofilled composites[120], have also been reported in the literature with varying degrees of success.

Lien et al.[108] investigated the physical properties of a new silorane-based restorative system (Filtek LS, 3M ESPE, St. Paul, U.S.A.) in comparison to traditional methacrylate-based restorative materials such as Beautifil-II (Giomer; Shofu, San Marcos, U.S.A.), Dyract eXtra (Compomer; Dentsply, York, U.S.A.), Esthet-X (Microhybrid, Dentsply, York, U.S.A.), Filtek Supreme (Nanocomposite; 3M ESPE, St. Paul, U.S.A.), and Filtek Z250 (Hybrid; 3M ESPE, St. Paul, U.S.A.). The results reported have demonstrated that Filtek LS displayed better flexural strength and fracture toughness properties in association with lower compressive strength and microhardness values. Filtek LS was also shown to have the lowest polymerization shrinkage among all materials tested.

Fu et al.[106] studied the degree of conversion, volumetric shrinkage, contraction stress, and compressive strength properties of an experimental low-shrinkage resin composites containing bismethylene spiroorthocarbonate expanding monomer. The results reported have indicated that the addition of unsaturated bismethylene spiroorthocarbonate and bisS-GMA resulted in experimental materials with improved mechanical and wettability properties with reduced polymerization shrinkage and low concentration of stress.

High-molecular-weight dimer acid dimethacrylates (h-DA) derived from the cyclodimerization and hydrogenation of linoleic acid have been developed to address the issues of methacrylate-based materials. h-Da is in a linear and acyclic aliphatic structure that provides for the attainment of monomers with amorphous aliphatic cores and reduced double-bond concentrations per unit volume. Such molecular structure was shown to result in polymer materials with reduced polymerization shrinkage, high degrees of conversion, low glass-transition temperatures, and good flexibility. Also, the aliphatic core's hydrophobic nature is expected to maximize the long-term chemical and mechanical stability of materials by reducing the hydrolysis of siloxane and ether bonds present in the polymer's organic matrix.[109]

Ormocers (organically modified ceramics) were developed to overcome some drawbacks of conventional dimethacrylate-based resin composites (e.g., elution, polymerization shrinkage, and polymerization-induced stress). These materials were obtained from the mixture of inorganic polymers (glass-like) and organic networks that are copolymerized with polysiloxanes. These low-shrinkage copolymer materials are produced based on sol-gel manufacturing processes that allow to control many variables such as the density of inorganic/organic networks, position of cross-linking sites, and dimension of interparticle spacing.

Montanaro et al.,[121] while assessing the in vitro *S. mutans* adhesion to different restorative materials [Filtek Flow, Tetric Flow, Arabesk Flow, Clearfil APX, Solitaire 2, Z250, Fuji IX, Fuji IX Fast, F2000 (compomer) and Admira (ormocer)], had demonstrated that Admira and Fuji IX Fast supported the highest levels of bacterial adherence among all materials investigated. Rosin et al. performed a one-[122] and two-year[123] multi-practice clinical study to assess the clinical performance of an ormocer restorative material (Definite; Degussa, Germany). Toward that objective, 356 restorations (48 class-I, 150 class-II, 63 class-III, 32 class-IV, and 63 class-V) were placed. Their findings demonstrated high rates of marginal deterioration, staining, and class V restorations loss (6 out 63), thereby suggesting that further research should be performed to improve the clinical performance of these hybrid materials. Hiyasat et al.[124] investigated the biocompatibility (in terms of cytotoxicity levels) of resin composites and their flowable derivatives (Admira, Z250, Tetric Ceram, Admira Flow, Tetric Flow, and Celtic Flow) using an ISO-approved fibroblast cell line (3T3, Clone A31; European Collection of Cell Culture, U.K.) and the MTT assay. Their results demonstrated that materials of distinct compositions leached different chemicals in concentrations considered potentially dangerous for the pulp cells. Besides, their results indicated that ormocer materials (Admira and Admira Flow) were significantly more cytotoxic when compared to traditional methacrylate-based materials.

Oxiranes (either aliphatic or aromatic) are epoxy-based materials that polymerize through ring-opening reactions and display low levels of polymerization shrinkage (>1% vol.). Such dimensional stability has been demonstrated to result from the association between the low-speed polymerization reactions and the material's ability to relax curing stresses. [125] These hydrophobic and oxygen-inhibition-resistant materials typically display high degrees of conversion and low water uptake levels. These properties combined have resulted in materials with promising properties against hydrolysis and biodegradation.[126]

Only one resin composite using a silorane variation of the oxirane technology was commercialized (Filtek LS, 3M ESPE). Despite these advantages, the requirement for a proprietary dental bonding agents associated with impractical curing times and inferior handling properties (challenging to insert, condense, and shape) significantly limited the widespread use of oxiranes by clinicians around the world, which has recently resulted in the removal of this material from the market.[125]

4.3.2 Antibacterial Polymer-Based Restorative Materials

The use of polymer-based materials for direct restorative applications in dentistry was first reported in 1962.[101] Since then, these materials have gone through a constant evolutionary process that resulted in modern resin composites with improved optical, mechanical, physical, and chemical properties. Currently available resin composites can be used either as preventive (e.g., pit and fissure sealants) or restorative materials in virtually all regions of the oral cavity and types of cavity preparation. These materials were previously demonstrated to have comparable annual failure rates when compared to dental amalgams (1% and 3%, Classes I and II)[95,127–129] and indirect restorations,[128] and have also been currently used in minimally invasive cosmetic techniques to improve the esthetic properties of discolored and malpositioned teeth.

However, contrasting reports have shown that when compared to dental amalgams, resin composites restorations have shorter service lives and higher failure rates due to secondary caries. In fact, Seemann et al.[130] have used the Delphi method to forecast the trends in restorative dentistry over the next 20 years and to identify treatment goals and related properties of restorative materials. This study demonstrated that bioactivity toward the pulp-dentin complex and prevention of secondary caries, along with a significant reduction in technical sensitivity, were rated as key properties for the development of future restorative materials. Such need has precipitated the development of several polymer-based restorative materials displaying antibacterial and bioactive functionalities. Two main strategies for the development of antibacterial restorative dental materials (leaching and non-leaching) have been proposed in the literature and, therefore, will be discussed in the following subsections.

4.3.2.1 Antibacterial Leaching Strategy

Initial attempts to decrease the incidence of secondary caries adjacent to resin composites restorations were based on the development of antibacterial-releasing materials that were obtained by the simple incorporation of agents such as fluoride, chlorhexidine, hydrocortisone, triclosan, and octenidine into resin composites and dental bonding agents. These materials were demonstrated to display interesting short-term antibacterial activity against a number of oral pathogenic bacteria including *S. mutans* and *Lactobacillus acidophilus*. The incorporation of fluoride into polymer-based dental materials can be considered as the initial development in the era of restorative dental materials with antibacterial functionalities. Fluoride's anticaries properties are based on a two-fold mechanism, namely: (1) the inhibition of bacterial biosynthetic metabolism and (2) interaction and accumulation of fluoride in the hard tissues of teeth.

In the former mechanism, bacterial cells uptake hydrogen fluoride (H.F.) freely available in the EPS. Inside of cells, H.F. dissociates into H^+ and F^- ions where fluoride ions adversely impact the function of proton-extruding enzymes to result in the progressive acidification of the cytoplasm. This irreversible process tends to inhibit the function of several other important enzymes involved with the maintenance of life and the metabolism of fermentable carbohydrates into acids (mainly lactic).

Numerous studies have shown the ability of fluoride to downregulate some essential virulence factors of *S. mutans*, such as the ability to produce acids and glucans (both soluble and insoluble).[131–133] The latter anti-cariogenic mechanism of fluoride is associated with the formation of fluorapatite [$Ca_5(PO_4)_3F$] and calcium fluoride (CaF_2), which are species with reduced solubility levels in lactic acid and were demonstrated to favor the remineralization of the tooth structure.[134–136] Principal examples of antibacterial materials containing fluoride include polyacid-modified composite resins, glass-ionomer cements (conventional and resin-modified), giomers, and glass carbomers.

Polyacid-modified composite resins, also known as compomers, were produced in an attempt to develop a material displaying the fluoride-releasing capabilities of traditional GICs[137] associated with the esthetics and mechanical properties of resin composites.[138] These materials are composed of acid-functional monomers (di-ester of 2-hydroxyethyl methacrylate with butane tetracarboxylic acid),[139] inorganic filler particles, large monomer molecules (BisGMA and UDMA), traditional diluents (TEGDMA), and photoinitiators (camphoroquinone). These materials are typically polymerized through standard free-radical addition polymerization upon visible-light irradiation of appropriate wavelength and photon energy ($\approx$450 nm, 2.76 eV).[140] Their fluoride-releasing properties are attained from the reaction between water (from saliva) and alumina-silicate particles that, through an acid-base reaction,[141,142] makes fluoride ions available for transport from the surface of the reactive inorganic filler particles to areas adjacent to the restoration,[143] thereby displaying a buffering effect when exposed to acidic conditions. Such property is considered clinically relevant because it could reduce the incidence of secondary caries by decreasing the acidity of *S. mutans* metabolic by-products.

Giomers can be classified as a flowable resin composites containing polyacrylic acid pre-reacted fluoro-alumino-silicate glass particles to render a stable glass-ionomer phase that is then incorporated into the resin composites organic matrix.[138] Due to the reduced amount of pre-reacted filler particles incorporated, these materials tend to display only moderate fluoride-releasing properties. Glass carbomers, or complex glass-ionomer cements, are dialkyl siloxane-modified materials that were engineered to promote the remineralization of the tooth structure in preventive and restorative applications. Such interesting property was achieved due to the presence of mineralizing ions such as calcium fluorapatite nanocrystals and hydroxyapatite. The main disadvantage of glass carbomers is related to their long setting times. To overcome this limitation, manufacturers recommend irradiating the newly placed material with high-intensity, light-curing units to increase the internal temperature of the material to promote its complete setting.

Resin-modified glass-ionomer cements contain the traditional ion-leachable glass powder associated with water-soluble monomers (2-hydroxyethyl methacrylate, HEMA) and a polymeric acid, that combined with a light-sensitive activator-initiator system, results in traditional free-radical addition polymerization reactions. Even though these materials were initially designed to be used as liners and bases, other applications in restorative dentistry (such as core build-ups) have also been reported. Even though several reports have demonstrated the antibacterial and bacteriostatic effects of fluoride, it has been recently stated that fluoride-releasing restorative materials cannot sustain the minimum fluoride concentration (>10 ppm) to reduce the viability of cells within biofilms.[144]

Bell et al. investigated the fluoride-releasing properties of GIC specimens (thickness=1.5 mm, diameter r=6.0 mm) immersed in saliva for 20 days using an ion analyzer (Orion EA940, Orion Research, Inc.). The results reported demonstrating that specimens released approximately 1 ppm within the first 10 min after immersion, and a total of nearly 15 ppm accumulated over 24 h.[145] Other studies have demonstrated that after the initial burst, the fluoride release rapidly decreased after 24–72 h,[146] reaching almost constant levels after 10–20 days.[147]

Chlorhexidine (CHX) has been demonstrated to have a broad-spectrum efficacy against oral bacteria (Gram-positive and Gram-negative), and therefore, has been considered the "gold standard" biocide during the assessment of novel antimicrobial agents.[148] This biguanide organic molecule[149] also displays high substantivity and low cytotoxicity to mammalian cells, which are properties of clinical relevance during the control of biofilm-related oral infections (such as caries and periodontal diseases). In general terms, CHX antibacterial behavior is based on the suppression of several transmembrane factors that result in increased drug uptake, membrane lysis, and cell death. In an attempt to overcome the limitations of fluoride-releasing materials, several forms of chlorhexidine (acetate, diacetate, gluconate, and hydrochloride) were incorporated into restorative dental materials.[150]

Even though these materials displayed varying degrees of antibacterial activity against cariogenic bacteria, the effectiveness of chlorhexidine-releasing polymers was not directly correlated with the amount of drug-loaded into the material, but rather with monomer compositions, degree of cross-linking, particle sizes, dispersion pattern, and loading methods.[151,152] One of the major drawbacks associated with these materials results from the fact that CHX is immiscible with monomers currently used in dentistry. The simple incorporation of CHX into dental polymers leads to the formation of large aggregates within the composite's organic matrix and has been correlated with the attainment of porous structures,[151,153] rough surfaces, and low mechanical and physical properties.[154] Finally, CHX-containing materials are not capable of meeting the minimum requirements for long-term dental applications and have been associated with increased staining and bacterial accumulation.[155]

4.3.2.2 Antibacterial Non-Leaching Strategy

Modern multi-functional polymer-based restorative materials have been developed to overcome the significant and critical limitations associated with materials containing leachable antibacterial agents (fluoride, chlorhexidine, antibiotics, etc.). These novel dental biomaterials were engineered based on the immobilization of antibacterial agents (monomers, salts, or nanoparticles) to result in materials with long-lasting functionalities and superior chemical, physical, mechanical, and optical properties. The first description of the use of an immobilized and non-leachable antibacterial monomer was made by Imazato et al.[156] who developed a quaternary ammonium dimethacrylate (12-methacryloyloxydodecyl-pydidinium bromide, MDPB) that was functionalized within the polymer matrix by covalent copolymerization. Since then, other quaternary ammonium monomers (QAMs) such as 2-dimethyl-2-dodecyl-1-methacryloxyethyl ammonium iodine (DDMAI), 2-methacryloyloxyethyl dimethylammonium (IDMA1), and 2,2-bis(methacryloxyloxyethyl dimethylammonium, IDMA2) were developed and tested for their utility as antibacterial agents.

The biocide mechanism of action associated with cationic polymers containing QAMs is based on the interaction between positively charged moieties and negatively charged components from bacterial cell membranes. Such interaction adversely impacts the transmembrane electrical potential, which in turn leads bacterial cells to lyse under their own osmotic pressure.[157,158] This structure-specific activity was demonstrated to be dependent on QAMs' concentration and chain length, polymer hydrophobicity, and electrical charge (positive).[159]

A recent study investigated the development of QAMs-induced resistance in cariogenic (*S. mutans*, *S. sanguis*, and *S. gordonii*), endodontic (*E. faecalis*), and periodontal (*A. actinomycetemcomitans*, *F. nucleatum*, *P. gingivalis*, and *P. intermedia*) bacterial species.[160] The results reported have demonstrated that antibacterial monomers used did not result in resistant bacteria, whereas species of bacteria (*S. gordonii*, *E. faecalis*, *F. nucleatum*, and *P. gingivalis*) became resistant after being treated with CHX. The addition of cetylpyridinium chloride (CPC), a well-known and effective antibacterial agent (FDA-approved in oral hygiene aids), to resin composites and dental bondings has also been reported. According to previous studies, the addition of small concentrations of CPC (1%–3%) resulted in the complete inhibition of *S. mutans* in a 12 h period, thereby demonstrating that immobilized bactericides are still capable of displaying significant antibacterial functionalities.[157]

Novel antimicrobial carboxyl-modified BisGMA analogs (BisGMA-COOH1, BisGMA-COOH2, and BisGMA-COOH3) were synthesized, characterized (SEM, FTIR, mechanical properties, and water sorption and solubility), and tested for antibacterial activity against *S. mutans* (CECT 479) and *Candida albicans* (ATCC 10231) in a recent study.[161] According to the results reported, experimental compositions containing acidic carboxyl-modified monomers and silver nanoparticles displayed interesting degrees of conversion (up to 83.7%) and antibacterial functionalities when compared to commercially available dental bonding agents. Despite these promising results, the addition of acidic groups (pH: 3.23–2.24) to traditional monomers (such as BisGMA and TEGDMA) resulted in very hydrophilic materials with lower flexural strength values. It can be suggested that carboxyl-modified materials may be more susceptible to degradation by water, enzymes, and bacteria because these materials were demonstrated to be very hydrophilic.

Rupf et al.,[162] while investigating the impact of bispyridines-containing resin composites (octenidine dihydrochloride, ODH) over the adhesion and growth of oral biofilms (in situ), by SEM and fluorescence microscopy, have shown that experimental materials (containing either 3% or 6%, wt/wt) significantly reduced total biofilm formation. The fluorescence microscopy findings have also demonstrated that biofilms grown against experimental materials were less viable when compared to biofilms grown on commercially available resin composites, thereby corroborating the short-term antibacterial effects of ODH-containing materials in preventive, restorative, and prosthetic dentistry applications.

Antimicrobial peptides (AMPs) derived from histatin 5, lactoferrin, and parotid secretory proteins (P113, hLf-11, and GL13K, respectively)[163–167] have also been recently incorporated and immobilized into experimental polymer-based materials. As previously reviewed, the objective of using these orally expressed peptides (from both organic and synthetic origins) is to develop dental biomaterials with strong antimicrobial functionalities, minimum cytotoxicity to mammalian cells, and low ability to induce resistant bacterial strains.[168] In general terms, these positively charged molecules express their antibacterial behavior through a structure-specific mechanism that preferentially targets the outer membrane and cell wall (both negatively charged) in Gram-positive and Gram-negative bacteria, and results in membrane perforation with consequent disruption of cellular integrity and cell death.[169] Balhara et al.,[166] while investigating the membrane selectivity to GL13K AMP, have demonstrated that these molecules are capable of disrupting the lipid bilayers through a partial micellization and transient pore mechanism. Their results have indicated that GL13K is effective against biofilm-forming bacteria (both Gram-positive and Gram-negative).

Silver nanoparticles have been demonstrated to display outstanding properties against a broad spectrum of bacteria, viruses, and fungi[170–172] when incorporated into dental polymers (prosthodontics and restorative) and implants.[173-176] The antibacterial mechanism associated with silver nanoparticles remains to be fully elucidated. The generation of reactive species of oxygen (ROS) and leaching of silver ions (Ag+) have been previously recognized to promote damage to multiple bacterial molecules such as DNA (binary fission),[177] ribosomes (the 70S), proteins, and lipids that may lead to cell inactivation, membrane disruption, and subsequent cell death.

The release of Ag+, by a surface-dissolution process, has been recently accepted as the principal-agent implicated with the antibacterial utility of silver nanoparticles.[178] Peretyazhko et al.,[179] while investigating the dissolution of silver nanoparticles of different sizes (6, 9, 13, and 70 nm) coated with functionalized ligands (methoxyl polyethylene glycol, PEGSH) at neutral and acidic pH conditions, have demonstrated the establishment of a size-dependent mechanism, whereby nanoparticles of smaller sizes dissolved at faster rates (increased surface-to-volume ratio) when compared to nanoparticles of larger sizes. Noronha et al.[178] stated, based on previous scientific evidence, that nanoparticles' dissolution also depends on the ionic strength of the medium, pH, concentration of dissolved oxygen, temperature, presence of complexing ligands, surface coatings, and nanoparticles' shapes and sizes.[180,181]

The addition of silver nanoparticles to polymer-based restorative materials has been correlated with significant reductions in caries-producing bacteria. The majority of reports indicate minor impact on their mechanical properties[182-185] and dentin shear strength values.[174]

Durner et al., while investigating the influence of silver nanoparticles on monomer elution from light-cured composites through gas chromatography and mass spectroscopy, have demonstrated that the incorporation of silver nanoparticles (0.0125%–0.3%) into a commercial composite resulted in adverse impacts over the material's degree of polymerization, where experimental materials released higher quantities of elutable species when compared to commercial materials.[186]

The release of uncured monomers (BisGMA, HEMA, and TEGDMA) and additives (camphoroquinone) from experimental materials is of serious concern because elutable substances are known to cause DNA strand breakage (induced by ROS generation)[187] and potent allergic reactions, thereby adversely impacting the material's biocompatibility and cytotoxicity behavior.[188-191]

A recent study published by Natale et al.[192] has successfully demonstrated the in situ formation of silver and calcium phosphate mixed particles (1.2% and 24.8% wt/wt, respectively), through a photoreduction process mediated by visible light irradiation (peak emission: 470 nm), to result in experimental dimethacrylate-based restorative materials with combined antibacterial and remineralizing properties. According to the results reported, experimental materials displayed a promising degree of conversion (83%–86%), significant reductions in *S. mutans* viable colony counts (3-log or 99.9% reductions), decreased flexural strength, and higher color differences when compared to unfilled materials.

Metal oxides based on nickel, zinc, copper, tungsten, and titanium have also been tested for their efficacy as antibacterial agents in polymer-based restorative dental biomaterials. These metallic nanoparticles have been documented to display interesting antibacterial behavior against several opportunistic oral pathogens such as *Aggregatibacter actinomycetem-comitans, Fusobacterium nucleatum, Porphyromonas gingivalis, Prevotella intermedia, Streptococcus mitis, S. mutans, Streptococcus sanguis, Rothia dentocariosa*, and *Rothia mucilaginosa*.[193]

However, due to lower production costs and better biocompatibility properties, the large body of research available has focused on oxides of zinc and titanium as potential alternatives for the development of novel antibacterial dental biomaterials. Metal oxide nanoparticles (size average $\cong$25–35 nm) are typically present in cosmetic ingredients, food packaging, paints, and medical devices. In dentistry, they are present in the formulation of endodontic materials, and their accepted mechanism of action is based on the production of reactive oxygen species (ROS). Liu et al.[194] investigated the utility of ZnO nano-solutions (3, 6, and 12 mmol/l, 70 nm; Alfa Aesar, Ward Hill, USA) against *Escherichia coli* (O157:H7). Their findings (SEM, TEM, and Raman spectroscopy) have clearly demonstrated the establishment of a concentration-dependent mechanism where higher concentrations of nanoparticles resulted in more substantial antimicrobial properties. In regard to their mechanism of action, their findings have demonstrated that cells were grown in the presence of ZnO nanoparticles (12 mmol/l) displayed deformed cell walls, altered membrane components (lipids and proteins), disorganized intracellular structures, and leakage of intracellular components.

Titanium dioxide nanoparticles ($nTiO_2$) have also been shown to have significant antimicrobial activity against several Gram-positive and Gram-negative microorganisms that are relevant for both oral and public health. Due to their abundance, low production costs, biocompatibility, high refractive index, resistance to discoloration, and widespread use, $nTiO_2$ have been incorporated into several products including personal care (cosmetics, sunscreen, pressed powders), food (chewing gums, candies), and health (sunscreen, toothpaste, shampoos, deodorants) products. Weir et al.,[195] while investigating the use of $nTiO_2$ in food and personal care products using Monte Carlo computer modeling, have demonstrated that U.S. adults are typically exposed to 1 mg/kg$_{(body weight)}$ of nTiO$_2$ from food products. Their results have also indicated that children have the highest exposure chances because of the higher nTiO$_2$ content present in sweets and chewing gums.

According to Cai et al.,[196] lipid peroxidation of bacterial cell walls (mediated by ROS) upon light irradiation (typically U.V. wavelengths) is the primary process by which nTiO$_2$ express their antibacterial mode of action. Other studies have demonstrated that nTiO$_2$ are capable of spontaneously producing ROS in nonirradiated conditions because of their (1) unique surface properties, (2) interaction with cellular components, or (3) capability of activating the NADPH-oxidase enzyme.[197,198]

A recent publication[199] has demonstrated that experimental dental bonding agents containing varying concentrations of nTiO$_2$ displayed interesting antibacterial functionalities against S. mutans biofilms when irradiated with U.V. (either 8.4 or 43.0 J/cm^2). According to the authors, such antibacterial behavior could be primarily attributed to the generation of hydrogen peroxide molecules.[200] Welch et al.[201] investigated the tensile bond strength of experimental dental bonding agents with on-demand antibacterial and bioactive functionalities containing varying concentrations of nTiO$_2$ (5, 10, 20, and 30 wt%). Their results have clearly demonstrated that experimental dental bonding agents displayed tensile strength values that were similar to those observed for commercially available materials, thereby demonstrating that the incorporation of nTiO$_2$ in the concentrations investigated did not result in materials with lower mechanical properties.

Cai et al.[202] investigated the influence of U V-driven photocatalysis on the surface roughness, hydrophobicity, morphology, cytotoxicity, bacteria and fibroblast cell adhesion, and bioactivity (ability to form hydroxyapatite) properties of an experimental dental adhesive resin containing Bis-GMA and HEMA (55/45 wt/wt ratio) and nTiO$_2$ (20 wt%, P25, Evonik Industries, AG Germany). In their study, specimens fabricated with experimental materials were light-irradiated (1, 3, and 12 h) either in water or in air. The results reported have demonstrated that experimental materials were significantly impacted (both positively and negatively) by U.V. photocatalysis. Concerning their surface properties (wettability and morphology), it becomes clear that the use of U.V. wavelengths resulted in surfaces that were significantly more hydrophilic and rougher when compared to control group samples (nTiO$_2$-free). It can be hypothesized from the results reported that UV-driven surface degradation might result in restorative materials that are more susceptible to bacterial accumulation and biodegradation. With regard to cell adhesion (both bacteria and dermal fibroblasts), antibacterial activity, and bioactivity, the results have shown that experimental materials were less cytotoxic, more antibacterial, and capable of promoting the formation of significant amounts of hydroxyapatite on the surface of experimental $nTiO_2$-containing materials.

4.4 Conclusions

Despite the remarkable advances made in the past few decades, problems such as polymerization shrinkage, higher accumulation of oral biofilms, upregulation of pathogenic bacteria, and secondary caries continue to plague these essential restorative materials.

Multidisciplinary science teams composed of dentists, materials scientists, polymer chemists, and engineers are now trying to solve these limitations by developing multi-functional and stimuli-responsive "smart" materials with long-lasting antibacterial and bioactive properties to decrease the incidence of secondary caries and costs associated with oral health care. The nano-revolution seen in the field of materials science may help to solve these current and significant problems in dentistry.

References

1. R. P. Allaker *The Use of Antimicrobial Nanoparticles to Control Oral Infections*, Nano-Antimicrobials. 2011 Aug 26: 395–425 Vol. (Ed. M. R. Nicola Cioffi), Springer-Verlag Berlin Heidelberg, Berlin, (2012).
2. K. Hojo, S. Nagaoka, T. Ohshima, N. Maeda *Journal of Dental Research*. 88, 982–990 (2009).
3. J. A. Aas, B. J. Paster, L. N. Stokes, I. Olsen, F. E. Dewhirst *Journal of Clinical Microbiology*. 43, 5721–5732 (2005).
4. S. D. Forssten, M. Björklund, A. C. Ouwehand *Nutrients*. 2, 290–298 (2010).
5. M. Faveri, M. P. Mayer, M. Feres, L. C. de Figueiredo, F. E. Dewhirst, B. J. Paster *Oral Microbiology and Immunology*. 23, 112–118 (2008).
6. B. J. Paster, I. Olsen, J. A. Aas, F. E. Dewhirst *Periodontology 2000*. 42, 80–87 (2006).
7. P. M. Wilson, P. M. Wilson *Journal of Periodontal Research*. 33, 438–438 (1998).
8. S. S. Socransky, C. Smith, A. D. Haffajee *Journal of Clinical Periodontology*. 29, 260–268 (2002).
9. J. A. Banas *Frontiers in Bioscience: A Journal and Virtual Library*. 9, 1267–1277 (2004).
10. A. H. Nobbs, Y. Zhang, A. Khammanivong, M. C. Herzberg *Journal of Bacteriology*. 189, 3106–3114 (2007).
11. J. Kreth, J. Merritt, W. Shi, F. Qi *Molecular Microbiology*. 57, 392–404 (2005).

12. A. Pepperney, M. Chikindas *Probiotics and Antimicrobial Proteins*. 3, 68–96 (2011).
13. P. D. Marsh *Caries Research*. 38, 204–211 (2004).
14. D. Ajdic, W. M. McShan, R. E. McLaughlin, G. Savic, J. Chang, M. B. Carson, C. Primeaux, R. Tian, S. Kenton, H. Jia, S. Lin, Y. Qian, S. Li, H. Zhu, F. Najar, H. Lai, J. White, B. A. Roe, J. J. Ferretti *Proceedings of the National Academy of Sciences of the United States of America*. 99, 14434–14439 (2002).
15. A. Simon-Soro, M. Guillen-Navarro, A. Mira *Journal of Oral Microbiology*. 6, 25443 (2014).
16. E. L. Gross, C. J. Beall, S. R. Kutsch, N. D. Firestone, E. J. Leys, A. L. Griffen *PLoS One*. 7, e47722 (2012).
17. Á. Simón-Soro, P. Belda-Ferre, R. Cabrera-Rubio, L. D. Alcaraz, A. Mira *Caries Research*. 47, 591–600 (2013).
18. M. A. Munson, A. Banerjee, T. F. Watson, W. G. Wade *Journal of Clinical Microbiology*. 42, 3023–3029 (2004).
19. M. R. Becker, B. J. Paster, E. J. Leys, M. L. Moeschberger, S. G. Kenyon, J. L. Galvin, S. K. Boches, F. E. Dewhirst, A. L. Griffen *Journal of Clinical Microbiology*. 40, 1001–1009 (2002).
20. E. F. Berbari, F. R. Cockerill III, J. M. Steckelberg *Mayo Clinic Proceedings*. 72, 532–542 (1997).
21. A. Zbinden, N. J. Mueller, P. E. Tarr, G. Eich, B. Schulthess, A. S. Bahlmann, P. M. Keller, G. V. Bloemberg *Journal of Clinical Microbiology*. 50, 2969–2973 (2012).
22. F. A. Scannapieco *Journal of Periodontology*. 70, 793–802 (1999).
23. J. F. Morris, D. L. Sewell *Clinical Infectious Diseases: An Official Publication of the Infectious Diseases Society of America*. 18, 450–452 (1994).
24. T. Dodman, J. Robson, D. Pincus *Journal of Paediatrics and Child Health*. 36, 87–90 (2000).
25. N. Buduneli, H. Baylas, E. Buduneli, O. Turkoglu, T. Kose, G. Dahlen *Journal of Clinical Periodontology*. 32, 174–181 (2005).
26. Y. W. Han, Y. Fardini, C. Chen, K. G. Iacampo, V. A. Peraino, J. M. Shamonki, R. W. Redline *Obstetrics and Gynecology*. 115, 442–445 (2010).
27. J. Beck, R. Garcia, G. Heiss, P. S. Vokonas, S. Offenbacher *Journal of Periodontology*. 67, 1123–1137 (1996).
28. M. C. Herzberg, M. W. Meyer *Journal of Periodontology*. 67, 1138–1142 (1996).
29. T. Dietrich, P. Sharma, C. Walter, P. Weston, J. Beck *Journal of Periodontology*. 84, S70–S84 (2013).
30. M. A. S. Melo, S. F. F. Guedes, H. H. K. Xu, L. K. A. Rodrigues *Trends in Biotechnology*. 31, 10.1016/j.tibtech.2013.05.010 (2013).
31. B. Horev, M. I. Klein, G. Hwang, Y. Li, D. Kim, H. Koo, D. S. Benoit *ACS Nano*. 9, 2390–2404 (2015).
32. T. F. Flemmig, T. Beikler *Periodontology 2000*. 55, 9–15 (2011).

33. B. A. Dye, G. Thornton-Evans, L. Xianfen, T. J. Lafolla *Dental Caries and Tooth Loss in Adults in the United States, 2011-2012*, Vol. 197 Centers for Disease Control and Prevention, National Center for Health Statistics, Bethesda, MD, 2015.
34. I. A. Mjor *Journal of the American Dental Association (1939)*. 136, 1426-1433 (2005).
35. I. A. Mjor, F. Toffenetti *Quintessence International (Berlin, Germany: 1985)*. 31, 165-179 (2000).
36. I. A. Mjor *Operative Dentistry*. 10, 88-92 (1985).
37. I. A. Mjor, V. Qvist *Journal of Dentistry*. 25, 25-30 (1997).
38. I. A. Mjor *Quintessence International (Berlin, Germany: 1985)*. 29, 313-317 (1998).
39. R. L. Sakaguchi *Dental Materials: Official Publication of the Academy of Dental Materials*. 21, 3-6 (2005).
40. H. J. Healey, R. W. Phillips *Journal of Dental Research*. 28, 439-446 (1949).
41. T. Fusayama, H. Hosoda, T. Iwamoto *The Journal of Prosthetic Dentistry*. 14, 537-553 (1964).
42. I. A. Mjor, J. E. Moorhead, J. E. Dahl *International Dental Journal*. 50, 361-366 (2000).
43. M. Bernardo, H. Luis, M. D. Martin, B. G. Leroux, T. Rue, J. Leitao, T. A. DeRouen *Journal of the American Dental Association (1939)*. 138, 775-783 (2007).
44. J. L. Drummond *Journal of Dental Research*. 87, 710-719 (2008).
45. N. Konishi, Y. Torii, A. Kurosaki, T. Takatsuka, T. Itota, M. Yoshiyama *Journal of Oral Rehabilitation*. 30, 790-795 (2003).
46. R. Hahn, R. Weiger, L. Netuschil, M. Bruch *Dental Materials: Official Publication of the Academy of Dental Materials*. 9, 312-316 (1993).
47. T. Sönju, P. O. Glantz *Archives of Oral Biology*. 20, 687-691 (1975).
48. D. Orstavik, J. Orstavik *Journal of Oral Rehabilitation*. 3, 139-144 (1976).
49. K. K. Skjorland *Acta Odontologica Scandinavica*. 40, 129-134 (1982).
50. M. Svanberg, I. A. Mjor, D. Orstavik *Journal of Dental Research*. 69, 861-864 (1990).
51. C. Hansel, G. Leyhausen, U. E. Mai, W. Geurtsen *Journal of Dental Research*. 77, 60-67 (1998).
52. T. R. Garrett, M. Bhakoo, Z. Zhang *Progress in Natural Science*. 18, 1049-1056 (2008).
53. K. Hori, S. Matsumoto *Biochemical Engineering Journal*. 48, 424-434 (2010).
54. A. Heydorn, B. K. Ersboll, M. Hentzer, M. R. Parsek, M. Givskov, S. Molin *Microbiology (Reading, England)*. 146 (Pt 10), 2409-2415 (2000).
55. J. W. Costerton *International Journal of Antimicrobial Agents*. 11, 217-221; discussion 237-219 (1999).
56. J. W. Costerton, K. J. Cheng, G. G. Geesey, T. I. Ladd, J. C. Nickel, M. Dasgupta, T. J. Marrie *Annual Review of Microbiology*. 41, 435-464 (1987).
57. P. D. Marsh *Journal of Clinical Periodontology*. 32 (Suppl 6), 7-15 (2005).

58. J. Goldberg Biofilms and antibiotic resistance: a genetic linkage *Trends in Microbiology*. 10, 264 (2002).
59. J.-S. Peng, W.-C. Tsai, C.-C. Chou *International Journal of Food Microbiology*. 77, 11–18 (2002).
60. M. J. Chen, Z. Zhang, T. R. Bott *Biotechnology Techniques*. 12, 875–880 (1998).
61. B. Koch, J. Worm, L. E. Jensen, O. Hojberg, O. Nybroe *Applied and Environmental Microbiology*. 67, 3363–3370 (2001).
62. R. J. Palmer Jr., D. C. White *Trends in Microbiology*. 5, 435–440 (1997).
63. P. D. Marsh, D. J. Bradshaw *Journal of Industrial Microbiology*. 15, 169–175 (1995).
64. S. L. Percival, S. Malic, H. Cruz, D. W. Williams *Introduction to Biofilms*, Vol. (Eds. S. Percival, D. Knottenbelt, C. Cochrane), Springer Berlin Heidelberg, Berlin, Heidelberg, 2011, 41–68.
65. N. J. Lin *Dental Materials*. 33, 667–680 (2017).
66. W. M. Dunne *Clinical Microbiology Reviews*. 15, 155–166 (2002).
67. H. J. Busscher, M. Rinastiti, W. Siswomihardjo, H. C. van der Mei *Journal of Dental Research*. 89, 657–665 (2010).
68. Y. H. An, R. B. Dickinson, R. J. Doyle *Mechanisms of Bacterial Adhesion and Pathogenesis of Implant and Tissue Infections*, Vol. (Eds. Y. H. An, R. J. Friedman), Humana Press, Totowa, NJ, 2000, 1–27.
69. C. J. Whittaker, C. M. Klier, P. E. Kolenbrander *Annual Review of Microbiology*. 50, 513–552 (1996).
70. H. F. Jenkinson *Journal of Industrial Microbiology*. 15, 186–192 (1995).
71. H. F. Jenkinson, R. J. Lamont *Critical Reviews in Oral Biology and Medicine: An Official Publication of the American Association of Oral Biologists*. 8, 175–200 (1997).
72. A. H. Nobbs, R. J. Lamont, H. F. Jenkinson *Microbiology and Molecular Biology Reviews: MMBR*. 73, 407–450 (2009).
73. B. Carpentier, O. Cerf *Journal of Applied Bacteriology*. 75, 499–511 (1993).
74. L. Marcotte, H. Therien-Aubin, C. Sandt, J. Barbeau, M. Lafleur *Biofouling*. 20, 189–201 (2004).
75. J. M. Vroom, K. J. De Grauw, H. C. Gerritsen, D. J. Bradshaw, P. D. Marsh, G. K. Watson, J. J. Birmingham, C. Allison *Applied and Environmental Microbiology*. 65, 3502–3511 (1999).
76. B. L. Bassler *Current Opinion in Microbiology*. 2, 582–587 (1999).
77. M. H. Sturme, M. Kleerebezem, J. Nakayama, A. D. Akkermans, E. E. Vaugha, W. M. de Vos *Antonie van Leeuwenhoek*. 81, 233–243 (2002).
78. N. A. Whitehead, A. M. Barnard, H. Slater, N. J. Simpson, G. P. Salmond *FEMS Microbiology Reviews*. 25, 365–404 (2001).
79. I. W. Sutherland *Carbohydrate Polymers*. 38, 319–328 (1999).
80. J. B. Kaplan *Journal of Dental Research*. 89, 205–218 (2010).
81. E. Karatan, P. Watnick *Microbiology and Molecular Biology Reviews: MMBR*. 73, 310–347 (2009).

82. J. R. Lawrence, B. Scharf, G. Packroff, T. R. Neu *Microbial Ecology*. 44, 199–207 (2002).
83. Y. C. Choi, E. Morgenroth *Water Science and Technology: A Journal of the International Association on Water Pollution Research*. 47, 69–76 (2003).
84. P. Ymele-Leki, J. M. Ross *Applied and Environmental Microbiology*. 73, 1834–1841 (2007).
85. S. F. Lee, Y. H. Li, G. H. Bowden *Infection and Immunity*. 64, 1035–1038 (1996).
86. N. Vats, S. F. Lee *Archives of Oral Biology*. 45, 305–314 (2000).
87. J. A. Soncini, N. N. Maserejian, F. Trachtenberg, M. Tavares, C. Hayes *Journal of the American Dental Association (1939)*. 138, 763–772 (2007).
88. G. Oilo *Advances in Dental Research*. 6, 50–54 (1992).
89. S. B. P. Fúcio, A. B. de Paula, J. C. O. Sardi, C. Duque, L. Correr-Sobrinho, R. M. Puppin-Rontani *Brazilian Dental Journal*. 27, 681–687 (2016).
90. N. Beyth, R. Bahir, S. Matalon, A. J. Domb, E. I. Weiss *Dental Materials: Official Publication of the Academy of Dental Materials*. 24, 732–736 (2008).
91. S. B. Fucio, F. G. Carvalho, L. C. Sobrinho, M. A. Sinhoreti, R. M. Puppin-Rontani *Journal of Dentistry*. 36, 833–839 (2008).
92. M. Bourbia, D. Ma, D. G. Cvitkovitch, J. P. Santerre, Y. Finer *Journal of Dental Research*. 92, 989–994 (2013).
93. Y. Finer, F. Jaffer, J. P. Santerre *Biomaterials*. 25, 1787–1793 (2004).
94. Y. Finer, J. P. Santerre *Journal of Dental Research*. 83, 22–26 (2004).
95. N. J. Opdam, E. M. Bronkhorst, B. A. Loomans, M. C. Huysmans *Journal of Dental Research*. 89, 1063–1067 (2010).
96. C. Splieth, O. Bernhardt, A. Heinrich, H. Bernhardt, G. Meyer *Quintessence International (Berlin, Germany: 1985)*. 34, 497–503 (2003).
97. T. M. Auschill, N. B. Arweiler, M. Brecx, E. Reich, A. Sculean, L. Netuschil *European Journal of Oral Sciences*. 110, 48–53 (2002).
98. D. Senadheera, D. G. Cvitkovitch *Advances in Experimental Medicine and Biology*. 631, 178–188 (2008).
99. K. S. Gregson, H. Shih, R. L. Gregory *Clinical Oral Investigations*. 16, 1095–1103 (2012).
100. T. Thomé, M. C. G. Erhardt, A. A. Leme, I. Al Bakri, A. K. Bedran-Russo, L. E. Bertassoni *Emerging Polymers in Dentistry*, Vol. (Ed. F. Puoci), Springer International Publishing, Cham, 2015, 265–296.
101. R. L. Bowen *Dental Filling Material Comprising Vinyl Silane Treated Fused Silica and a Binder Consisting of the Reaction Product of Bis Phenol and Glycidyl Acrylate*, Vol. Google Patents, 1962.
102. N. Moszner, U. Salz *Progress in Polymer Science*. 26, 535–576 (2001).
103. J. L. Ferracane *Operative Dentistry*. 33, 247–257 (2008).
104. J. L. Ferracane, J. C. Mitchem *American Journal of Dentistry*. 16, 239–243 (2003).
105. W. Weinmann, C. Thalacker, R. Guggenberger *Dental Materials: Official Publication of the Academy of Dental Materials*. 21, 68–74 (2005).

106. J. Fu, W. Liu, Z. Hao, X. Wu, J. Yin, A. Panjiyar, X. Liu, J. Shen, H. Wang *International Journal of Molecular Sciences.* 15, 2400–2412 (2014).

107. J. P. Santerre, L. Shajii, B. W. Leung *Critical Reviews in Oral Biology & Medicine.* 12, 136–151 (2001).

108. W. Lien, K. S. Vandewalle *Dental Materials.* 26, 337–344 (2010).

109. M. Trujillo-Lemon, J. Ge, H. Lu, J. Tanaka, J. W. Stansbury *Journal of Polymer Science Part A: Polymer Chemistry.* 44, 3921–3929 (2006).

110. S. Kalra, A. Singh, M. Gupta, V. Chadha *Contemporary Clinical Dentistry.* 3, 48–53 (2012).

111. N. Moszner, A. Gianasmidis, S. Klapdohr, U. K. Fischer, V. Rheinberger *Dental Materials.* 24, 851–856 (2008).

112. H. Wolter, W. Storch, H. Ott, *New Inorganic/Organic Copolymers (ORMOCER{reg_sign}s) for Dental Applications.* Materials Research Society, Pittsburgh, PA, 1994.

113. A. R. Aleixo, R. D. Guiraldo, A. P. Fugolin, S. B. Berger, R. L. Consani, A. B. Correr, A. Gonini-Junior, M. B. Lopes *Photomedicine and Laser Surgery.* 32, 267–273 (2014).

114. N. Beyth, I. Yudovin-Farber, R. Bahir, A. J. Domb, E. I. Weiss *Biomaterials.* 27, 3995–4002 (2006).

115. M. S. Soh, A. U. Yap, A. Sellinger *European Journal of Oral Sciences.* 115, 230–238 (2007).

116. K. H. Lee, S. H. Rhee *Biomaterials.* 30, 3444–3449 (2009).

117. M. H. Chen, C. R. Chen, S. H. Hsu, S. P. Sun, W. F. Su *Dental Materials: Official Publication of the Academy of Dental Materials.* 22, 138–145 (2006).

118. D. A. Tilbrook, R. L. Clarke, N. E. Howle, M. Braden *Biomaterials.* 21, 1743–1753 (2000).

119. N. Ilie, R. Hickel *Australian Dental Journal.* 56 (Suppl 1), 59–66 (2011).

120. V. Uskokovic, L. E. Bertassoni *Materials (Basel, Switzerland).* 3, 1674–1691 (2010).

121. L. Montanaro, D. Campoccia, S. Rizzi, M. E. Donati, L. Breschi, C. Prati, C. R. Arciola *Biomaterials.* 25, 4457–4463 (2004).

122. M. Rosin, H. Steffen, C. Konschake, U. Greese, D. Teichmann, A. Hartmann, G. Meyer *Clinical Oral Investigations.* 7, 20–26 (2003).

123. M. Rosin, C. Schwahn, B. Kordass, C. Konschake, U. Greese, D. Teichmann, A. Hartmann, G. Meyer *Quintessence International (Berlin, Germany: 1985).* 38, e306–e315 (2007).

124. A. S. Al-Hiyasat, H. Darmani, M. M. Milhem *Clinical Oral Investigations.* 9, 21–25 (2005).

125. B. L. Hoedebecke *The University of Texas Health Science Center at San Antonio,* 2016.

126. H. R. Rawls, A. D. Johnston, B. K. Norling, K. Whang *Restorative Resin Compositions and Methods of Use,* Vol. Google Patents, 2015.

127. J. Manhart, H. Chen, G. Hamm, R. Hickel *Operative Dentistry.* 29, 481–508 (2004).

128. F. F. Demarco, M. B. Correa, M. S. Cenci, R. R. Moraes, N. J. Opdam *Dental Materials: Official Publication of the Academy of Dental Materials.* 28, 87–101 (2012).
129. N. J. Opdam, E. M. Bronkhorst, J. M. Roeters, B. A. Loomans *Dental Materials: Official Publication of the Academy of Dental Materials.* 23, 2–8 (2007).
130. R. Seemann, S. Flury, F. Pfefferkorn, A. Lussi, M. J. Noack *Dental Materials: Official Publication of the Academy of Dental Materials.* 30, 442–448 (2014).
131. G. H. Bowden *Journal of Dental Research.* 69, 653–659; discussion 682–653 (1990).
132. I. R. Hamilton *Journal of Dental Research.* 69, 660–667; discussion 682–663 (1990).
133. A. Tatevossian *Journal of Dental Research.* 69, 645–652; discussion 682–643 (1990).
134. W. Nicholson John Fluoride-Releasing Dental Restorative Materials: An Update, *Balkon Journal of Dental Medicine* 18, 60 (2014). Health and Applied Science, Twickenham, United Kingdom.
135. J. M. ten Cate *British Dental Journal.* 214, 161–167 (2013).
136. J. Berg, A. L. Seminario *Journal of Dental Education.* 73, 527 (2009).
137. L. M. Tenuta, J. A. Cury *Brazilian Oral Research.* 24 (Suppl 1), 9–17 (2010).
138. A. Wiegand, W. Buchalla, T. Attin *Dental Materials.* 23, 343–362 (2007).
139. G. Eliades, A. Kakaboura, G. Palaghias *Dental Materials.* 14, 57–63 (1998).
140. J. M. Meyer, M. A. Cattani-Lorente, V. Dupuis *Biomaterials.* 19, 529–539 (1998).
141. N. D. Ruse *Journal (Canadian Dental Association).* 65, 500–504 (1999).
142. J. W. Nicholson, M. A. McKenzie *Journal of Oral Rehabilitation.* 26, 767–774 (1999).
143. B. J. Millar, F. Abiden, J. W. Nicholson *Journal of Dentistry.* 26, 133–136 (1998).
144. J. A. Cury, B. H. de Oliveira, A. P. dos Santos, L. M. Tenuta *Dental Materials: Official Publication of the Academy of Dental Materials.* 32, 323–333 (2016).
145. A. Bell, S. L. Creanor, R. H. Foye, W. P. Saunders *Journal of Oral Rehabilitation.* 26, 407–412 (1999).
146. P. Karantakis, M. Helvatjoglou-Antoniades, S. Theodoridou-Pahini, Y. Papadogiannis *Operative Dentistry.* 25, 20–25 (2000).
147. H. Yli-Urpo, P. K. Vallittu, T. O. Narhi, A. P. Forsback, M. Vakiparta *Journal of Biomaterials Applications.* 19, 5–20 (2004).
148. J. F. Zhang, R. Wu, Y. Fan, S. Liao, Y. Wang, Z. T. Wen, X. Xu *Journal of Dental Research.* 93, 1283–1289 (2014).
149. G. McDonnell, A. D. Russell *Clinical Microbiology Reviews.* 12, 147–179 (1999).
150. C. Farrugia, J. Camilleri *Dental Materials: Official Publication of the Academy of Dental Materials.* 31, e89–e99 (2015).
151. X. Xu, S. Costin Antimicrobial Polymeric Dental Materials, Vol. The Royal Society of Chemistry, Washington, DC, 2014, 279–309. Polymeric Materials with Antimicrobial Activity: From Synthesis to Applications.
152. D. Leung, D. A. Spratt, J. Pratten, K. Gulabivala, N. J. Mordan, A. M. Young *Biomaterials.* 26, 7145–7153 (2005).

153. K. J. Anusavice, N. Z. Zhang, C. Shen *Journal of Dental Research*. 85, 950–954 (2006).

154. D. E. Slot, N. C. Vaandrager, C. Van Loveren, W. H. Van Palenstein Helderman, G. A. Van der Weijden *Caries Research*. 45, 162–173 (2011).

155. V. Deligeorgi, I. A. Mjor, N. H. Wilson *Primary Dental Care: Journal of the Faculty of General Dental Practitioners (U.K.)*. 8, 5–11 (2001).

156. S. Imazato, R. R. Russell, J. F. McCabe *Journal of Dentistry*. 23, 177–181 (1995).

157. N. Namba, Y. Yoshida, N. Nagaoka, S. Takashima, K. Matsuura-Yoshimoto, H. Maeda, B. Van Meerbeek, K. Suzuki, S. Takashiba *Dental Materials: Official Publication of the Academy of Dental Materials*. 25, 424–430 (2009).

158. N. Beyth, S. Farah, A. J. Domb, E. I. Weiss *Reactive and Functional Polymers*. 75, 81–88 (2014).

159. F. Li, M. D. Weir, J. Chen, H. H. Xu *Dental Materials: Official Publication of the Academy of Dental Materials*. 29, 450–461 (2013).

160. S. Wang, H. Wang, B. Ren, H. Li, M. D. Weir, X. Zhou, T. W. Oates, L. Cheng, H. H. K. Xu *Dental Materials*. 33, 1127–1138 (2017).

161. V. Melinte, T. Buruiana, A. Chibac, M. Mares, H. Aldea, E. C. Buruiana *Dental Materials: Official Publication of the Academy of Dental Materials*. 32, e314–e326 (2016).

162. S. Rupf, M. Balkenhol, T. O. Sahrhage, A. Baum, J. N. Chromik, K. Ruppert, D. K. Wissenbach, H. H. Maurer, M. Hannig *Dental Materials*. 28, 974–984 (2012).

163. D. M. Rothstein, P. Spacciapoli, L. T. Tran, T. Xu, F. D. Roberts, M. Dalla Serra, D. K. Buxton, F. G. Oppenheim, P. Friden *Antimicrobial Agents and Chemotherapy*. 45, 1367–1373 (2001).

164. M. Godoy-Gallardo, C. Mas-Moruno, M. C. Fernández-Calderón, C. Pérez-Giraldo, J. M. Manero, F. Albericio, F. J. Gil, D. Rodríguez *Acta Biomaterialia*. 10, 3522–3534 (2014).

165. M. Abdolhosseini, S. R. Nandula, J. Song, H. Hirt, S. U. Gorr *Peptides*. 35, 231–238 (2012).

166. V. Balhara, R. Schmidt, S. U. Gorr, C. Dewolf *Biochimica et Biophysica Acta*. 1828, 2193–2203 (2013).

167. H. Hirt, S.-U. Gorr *Antimicrobial Agents and Chemotherapy*. 57, 4903–4910 (2013).

168. B. Bechinger, S. U. Gorr *Journal of Dental Research*. 96, 254–260 (2017).

169. T. Anunthawan, C. de la Fuente-Núñez, R. E. W. Hancock, S. Klaynongsruang *Biochimica et Biophysica Acta (BBA)—Biomembranes*. 1848, 1352–1358 (2015).

170. M. Rai, A. P. Ingle, A. K. Gade, M. C. Duarte, N. Duran *IET Nanobiotechnology*. 9, 280–287 (2015).

171. M. Rai, K. Kon, A. Ingle, N. Duran, S. Galdiero, M. Galdiero *Applied Microbiology and Biotechnology*. 98, 1951–1961 (2014).

172. G. C. Padovani, V. P. Feitosa, S. Sauro, F. R. Tay, G. Duran, A. J. Paula, N. Duran *Trends in Biotechnology*. 33, 621–636 (2015).

173. K. Zhang, M. A. Melo, L. Cheng, M. D. Weir, Y. Bai, H. H. Xu *Dental Materials: Official Publication of the Academy of Dental Materials*. 28, 842–852 (2012).

174. M. A. Melo, L. Cheng, K. Zhang, M. D. Weir, L. K. Rodrigues, H. H. Xu *Dental Materials: Official Publication of the Academy of Dental Materials*. 29, 199–210 (2013).

175. Y. Liu, Z. Zheng, J. N. Zara, C. Hsu, D. E. Soofer, K. S. Lee, R. K. Siu, L. S. Miller, X. Zhang, D. Carpenter, C. Wang, K. Ting, C. Soo *Biomaterials*. 33, 8745–8756 (2012).

176. V. E. Santos Jr., A. Vasconcelos Filho, A. G. Targino, M. A. Flores, A. Galembeck, A. F. Caldas Jr., A. Rosenblatt *Journal of Dentistry*. 42, 945–951 (2014).

177. K. Chaloupka, Y. Malam, A. M. Seifalian *Trends in Biotechnology*. 28, 580–588 (2010).

178. V. T. Noronha, A. J. Paula, G. Duran, A. Galembeck, K. Cogo-Muller, M. Franz-Montan, N. Duran *Dental Materials: Official Publication of the Academy of Dental Materials*. 33, 1110–1126 (2017).

179. T. S. Peretyazhko, Q. Zhang, V. L. Colvin *Environmental Science & Technology*. 48, 11954–11961 (2014).

180. C. Levard, E. M. Hotze, G. V. Lowry, G. E. Brown *Environmental Science & Technology*. 46, 6900–6914 (2012).

181. S. K. Misra, A. Dybowska, D. Berhanu, S. N. Luoma, E. Valsami-Jones *The Science of the Total Environment*. 438, 225–232 (2012).

182. L. Cheng, M. D. Weir, H. H. Xu, J. M. Antonucci, A. M. Kraigsley, N. J. Lin, S. Lin-Gibson, X. Zhou *Dental Materials: Official Publication of the Academy of Dental Materials*. 28, 561–572 (2012).

183. A. L. S. Borges, T. P. Sato, C. Conjo, R. D. Rossoni, J. C. Junqueira, P. D. Marcato, N. E. D. Caballero, S. M. Rode, R. M. Melo *Dental Materials*. 30, e42.

184. P. B. das Neves, J. A. Agnelli, C. Kurachi, C. W. de Souza *Brazilian Dental Journal*. 25, 141–145 (2014).

185. A. Akhavan, A. Sodagar, F. Mojtahedzadeh, K. Sodagar *Acta Odontologica Scandinavica*. 71, 1038–1042 (2013).

186. J. Durner, M. Stojanovic, E. Urcan, R. Hickel, F.-X. Reichl *Dental Materials*. 27, 631–636 (2011).

187. J. Volk, C. Ziemann, G. Leyhausen, W. Geurtsen *Dental Materials: Official Publication of the Academy of Dental Materials*. 25, 1556–1563 (2009).

188. A. T. Goon, M. Isaksson, E. Zimerson, C. L. Goh, M. Bruze *Contact Dermatitis*. 55, 219–226 (2006).

189. J. Durner, H. Kreppel, J. Zaspel, H. Schweikl, R. Hickel, F. X. Reichl *Biomaterials*. 30, 2066–2071 (2009).

190. E. Urcan, H. Scherthan, M. Styllou, U. Haertel, R. Hickel, F. X. Reichl *Biomaterials*. 31, 2010–2014 (2010).

191. J. Durner, M. Debiak, A. Burkle, R. Hickel, F. X. Reichl *Archives of Toxicology*. 85, 143–148 (2011).

192. L. C. Natale, Y. Alania, M. C. Rodrigues, A. Simões, D. N. de Souza, E. de Lima, V. E. Arana-Chavez, T. L. R. Hewer, R. Hiers, F. L. Esteban-Florez, G. E. S. Brito, S. Khajotia, R. R. Braga *Materials Science and Engineering: C*. 76, 464–471 (2017).

193. S. T. Khan, A. A. Al-Khedhairy, J. Musarrat *Journal of Nanoparticle Research*. 17, 276 (2015).

194. Y. Liu, L. He, A. Mustapha, H. Li, Z. Q. Hu, M. Lin *Journal of Applied Microbiology*. 107, 1193–1201 (2009).

195. A. Weir, P. Westerhoff, L. Fabricius, K. Hristovski, N. von Goetz *Environmental Science & Technology*. 46, 2242–2250 (2012).

196. Y. Cai, Doctoral thesis, comprehensive summary, Acta Universitatis Upsaliensis, 2013.

197. P. Gajjar, B. Pettee, D. W. Britt, W. Huang, W. P. Johnson, A. J. Anderson *Journal of Biological Engineering*. 3, 9 (2009).

198. T. Xia, M. Kovochich, M. Liong, L. Mädler, B. Gilbert, H. Shi, J. I. Yeh, J. I. Zink, A. E. Nel *ACS Nano*. 2, 2121–2134 (2008).

199. Y. Cai, M. Stromme, A. Melhus, H. Engqvist, K. Welch *Journal of Biomedical Materials Research. Part B, Applied Biomaterials*. 102, 62–67 (2014).

200. Y. Cai, M. Strømme, K. Welch *Journal of Biomaterials and Nanobiotechnology*. 5, 200–209 (2014).

201. K. Welch, Y. Cai, H. Engqvist, M. Strømme *Dental Materials*. 26, 491–499 (2010).

202. Y. Cai, M. Stromme, P. Zhang, H. Engqvist, K. Welch *RSC Advances*. 4, 57715–57723 (2014).

5

Biomaterial, Host, and Microbial Interactions
Factors to Consider When Developing Resin-Based Restorative Materials

Kimberly Ngai and Yoav Finer
University of Toronto

Contents

5.1 Resin Composite Restorations

Resin composites are the most commonly used restorative materials in dentistry today due to growing demands for tooth-colored restorations, increasing concern regarding exposure to mercury in dental amalgams (Khalichi et al. 2009; Mackert and Berglund 1997), and its varied applications in day-to-day practice (Ferracane 2011). Despite its growing popularity, resin-based composites lack the durability of amalgam fillings and tend to have higher failure rates, primarily due to the development of microleakage along the margins of restorations and subsequent recurrent decay (Bernardo et al. 2007; Murray et al. 2002; Soncini et al. 2007).

The integrity of the resin-dentin bond is compromised over time due to thermal changes, mastication stresses, and chemical degradation by acids and enzymes (Shokati et al. 2010). These factors contribute to shorter longevity and higher frequency of replacement in composite restorations, as compared to amalgam (Bernardo et al. 2007; Derouen et al. 2016; Khalichi et al. 2009; Soncini et al. 2007). The shorter lifespan has also been attributed to monomer composition, polymerization shrinkage, marginal discoloration, and degradation, compromised adhesion and bonding, cyclic fatigue through mastication and fracture (Bouillaguet 2004; Li et al. 2014; Santerre et al. 2001; Shokati et al. 2010).

5.2 Resin Composite Formulation

A composite material, by definition, is a product that is formed by the interatomic interactions between two or more components, resulting in superior properties to those of the individual components alone (Dogon 1990). The four major components of dental resin composites are (1) a polymeric matrix, (2) inorganic filler particles, (3) coupling agents such as silanes, for binding the filler to the matrix, and (4) an initiator/inhibitor polymerization system (Santerre et al. 2001).

5.2.1 Polymeric Matrix

The predominant base monomer used for the polymeric matrix is 2,2-bis[4(2-hydroxy-3-methacryloxypropoxy)-phenyl] propane, also known as bisphenol A glycidyl methacrylate (BisGMA) (Bowen 1956). BisGMA is a high-molecular-weight monomer that has low chain mobility due to the hydrophobic aromatic rings in its backbone (Delaviz et al. 2014). The high viscosity of BisGMA, due to the pi-pi interactions between the aromatic rings and the hydrogen bonding within the molecule, prevents a high amount of filler from being added and reduces the degree of conversion in the polymer. To overcome this, diluent monomers, such as triethylene glycol dimethacrylate (TEGDMA), urethane dimethacrylate (UDMA), and ethoxylated bisphenol A based dimethacrylate (Bis-EMA) (Figure 5.1), are mixed with BisGMA to increase the efficiency of polymerization, decrease the overall viscosity, and enhance resin mobility, thereby improving the handling and manipulation of the material (Delaviz et al. 2014; Ferracane 2011; Santerre et al. 2001; Smith 1985).

TEGDMA, a low-molecular-weight di-vinyl monomer, is the most commonly used diluent monomer in current resin restorations (Delaviz et al. 2014). However, since the addition of this monomer or other lower molecular and/or hydrophilic diluent monomers in resin composites greatly increases water sorption and polymerization shrinkage, there is a limit to the amount of diluent that can be incorporated (Deb 1998).

5.2.2 Inorganic Fillers

Filler particles, commonly glass, quartz, or ceramic oxide, are the significant constituents by weight and volume of resin composites and can be classified according to their chemical composition, average particle size, and manufacturing method (Dogon 1990; Santerre et al. 2001; Ferracane 2011). Filler particles are essential in providing the composite with improved mechanical properties. The improvements on the mechanical performance includes an increase in compressive strength and modulus of elasticity, along with a reduction in polymerization shrinkage after curing, water sorption, and the coefficient of thermal expansion (Santerre et al. 2001; Dogon 1990).

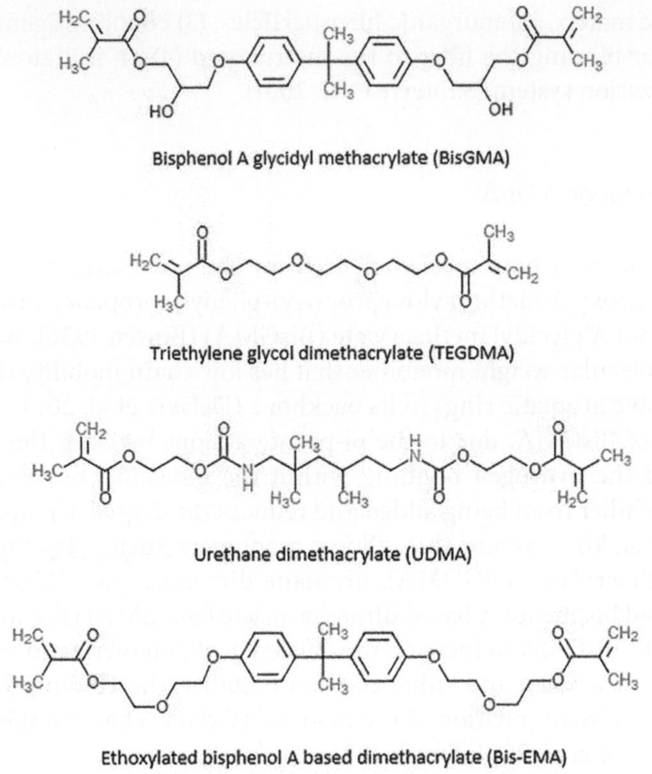

Bisphenol A glycidyl methacrylate (BisGMA)

Triethylene glycol dimethacrylate (TEGDMA)

Urethane dimethacrylate (UDMA)

Ethoxylated bisphenol A based dimethacrylate (Bis-EMA)

Figure 5.1   Common methacrylate-based monomers used in resin composite materials.

5.3   Resin Adhesive Systems

The purpose of resin adhesive systems is to bond the resin composite material to the tooth structure for retention of the restoration while providing an impermeable seal at the resin-tooth interface (Delaviz et al. 2014). There are currently two main adhesive systems used: (1) total-etch (etch-and-rinse) and (2) self-etch (Bourbia et al. 2013; Delaviz et al. 2014). The composition and steps for each technique are demonstrated in Figure 5.2.

5.3.1   Total-Etch Adhesive Systems/Etch and Rinse Technique

The total-etch adhesive system involves separate acid-etching and priming/bonding steps (Liu et al. 2011) and can be applied in either a

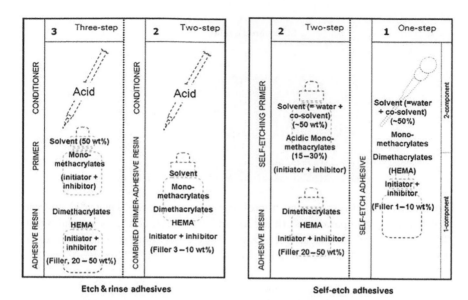

Figure 5.2 Chemical composition and application procedures for etch and rinse (a) vs. self-etch (b) adhesives systems. (Used with permission from Van Landuyt et al. (2007).)

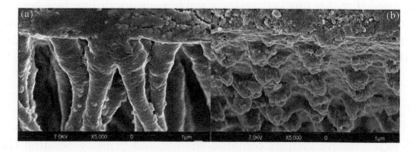

Figure 5.3 Scanning electron microscopy images of a total-etch (a) and self-etch (b) adhesive system. (Used with permission from Breschi et al. (2008).)

two- or three-step technique, depending on whether the primer and adhesive resin are combined or not (Figures 5.2a and 5.3a) (Delaviz et al. 2014). Acid conditioning is the first step of the etch and rinse technique. In many systems, 37% phosphoric acid is applied to the tooth for 15–30 s in order to demineralize and remove the smear layer. The smear layer is a thin film left on the superficial dentin surface following dental instrumentation that

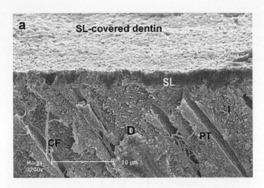

Figure 5.4 Scanning electron microscopy image of smear layer (SL)-covered dentin after wet preparation with a diamond bur. SL thickness is around 3 μm. (SL, smear layer; CF, collagen fiber; D, dentin; PT, peritubular dentin; I, intertubular dentin). (Used with permission from Bortolotto et al. (2009).)

consists of microcrystalline and organic particles and debris (Figure 5.4) (Bortolotto et al. 2009; Delaviz et al. 2014). This is followed by rinsing the acid with water, priming with hydrophilic methacrylate monomers that can prevent collagen collapse by rewetting the dentin, and application of a more hydrophobic methacrylate bonding agent (Delaviz et al. 2014). It was suggested that this process creates a stable resin-tooth interface because the more hydrophobic adhesive resin is able to penetrate and mechanically interlock with the created micropores on the enamel and dentin surface (Nakabayashi et al. 1991).

5.3.2 Self-Etch Adhesive Systems/Self-Etch Technique

Self-etch adhesive systems combine etching and priming/bonding (Liu et al. 2011), eliminating the rinsing step (Figures 5.2b and 5.3b). Either etching and priming or etching, priming, and bonding are combined to create a two- or one-step technique, respectively (Delaviz et al. 2014). Self-etch adhesive systems contain resin monomers that are both hydrophilic and acidic (Bourbia et al. 2013).

Therefore, they can etch and prime simultaneously and either modify or remove the smear layer completely to enhance bonding (Bortolotto et al. 2009). However, this hydrophilicity could make self-etch techniques more vulnerable to water sorption, and potentially more susceptible to degradation, compared to conventional total-etch adhesive systems (Hashimoto et al. 2008).

5.4 Resin-Dentin Interface

The resin-dentin interface consists of the composite resin restoration, resin adhesive system, and tooth substrate. This interface is created from the two-way bonding of the adhesive to enamel/dentin by micromechanical interlocking between resin and tooth substrate (Hashimoto et al. 2000; Wang and Spencer 2003) and to the lining composite by copolymerization of the methacrylate monomers in composite and adhesive resins (Delaviz et al. 2014; Huang, Cvitkovitch et al. 2018).

5.5 Biodegradation of the Resin-Dentin Interface

The biological interface between composite and dentin is called the hybrid layer, which is a resin-reinforced layer formed from the infiltration of adhesive resin into a demineralized dentin surface and entanglement with exposed collagen fibrils (Figure 5.5) (Hashimoto et al. 2000; Nakabayashi et al. 1991; Spencer et al. 2010; Wang and Spencer 2003). Several factors inhibit the formation of a robust adhesive-dentin bond, and an inadequate seal at the resin-dentin interface is susceptible to break down and considered as the weak link in the composite restoration (Spencer et al. 2010).

One of the main reasons for resin degradation at this interface is water sorption and the chemical hydrolysis of the ester bonds within the polymer (Tay and Pashley 2003). Other factors include incomplete monomer/polymer conversion of the adhesive, inadequate resin infiltration, and insufficient solvent evaporation (Breschi et al. 2008; Ferracane 2006; Wang et al. 2007). Resin composites and adhesives can also undergo a significant

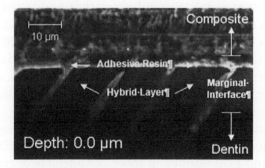

Figure 5.5 Confocal laser scanning microscopy image of the interfacial margin of a resin-dentin specimen demonstrating the hybrid layer. (Used with permission from Kermanshahi et al. (2010).)

amount of biological breakdown, catalyzed by acids, bases, or enzymes present in the oral cavity (Delaviz et al. 2014). This is often referred to as biodegradation and is due to the hydrolysis of condensation type bonds within the resin (Delaviz et al. 2014; Finer et al. 2004; Santerre et al. 2001; Serkies et al. 2016; Shokati et al. 2010).

Biodegradation is a significant contributor to the loss of integrity at restoration margins, resulting in bacterial microleakage along the interface and limiting the overall longevity of resin-based restorations (Kermanshahi et al. 2010; Spencer et al. 2010). Other sequelae of bacterial microleakage include postoperative sensitivity, secondary caries, pulp inflammation, and pulpal necrosis (Bouillaguet 2004).

5.5.1 Biodegradation by Salivary Esterases

Since the early 1990s, the focus of research on resin composite degradation shifted from wear and mechanical function toward the chemical breakdown of restorative materials by enzymes in the oral cavity (Delaviz et al. 2014). Several studies have investigated the role of salivary-like enzymes that cleave susceptible condensation linkages in resin composites and adhesives (Finer et al. 2004; Finer and Santerre 2004; Kermanshahi et al. 2010).

There are several enzymes present in human saliva that may participate in this degradative process (Shokati et al. 2010; Spencer et al. 2010). Human salivary-derived esterases are the most commonly associated enzymes involved (Finer et al. 2004; Shokati et al. 2010). Previous studies have shown that human saliva samples contain cholesterol esterase-like (CE) and pseudocholinesterase (PCE) activities in sufficient quantity to have strong degradative effects on the methacrylate-based organic matrix of resin composite materials, particularly on the unprotected ester linkages in major matrix monomeric segments such as BisGMA and TEGDMA, as shown in Figure 5.6 (Finer et al. 2004; Finer and Santerre 2004; Jaffer et al. 2002; Serkies et al. 2016; Shokati et al. 2010). This degradation has been suggested to decrease the interfacial fracture toughness, and therefore compromise the mechanical integrity of the resin-dentin interface (Serkies et al. 2016; Shokati et al. 2010).

Also, Kermanshahi et al. (2010) showed that increased incubation time and exposure to simulated salivary esterase activities (SHSE) composed mainly of CE and PCE resulted in more considerable degradation of the resin-dentin interface that leads to cariogenic bacterial biofilm formation along with the compromised resin-dentin interface (Kermanshahi et al. 2010).

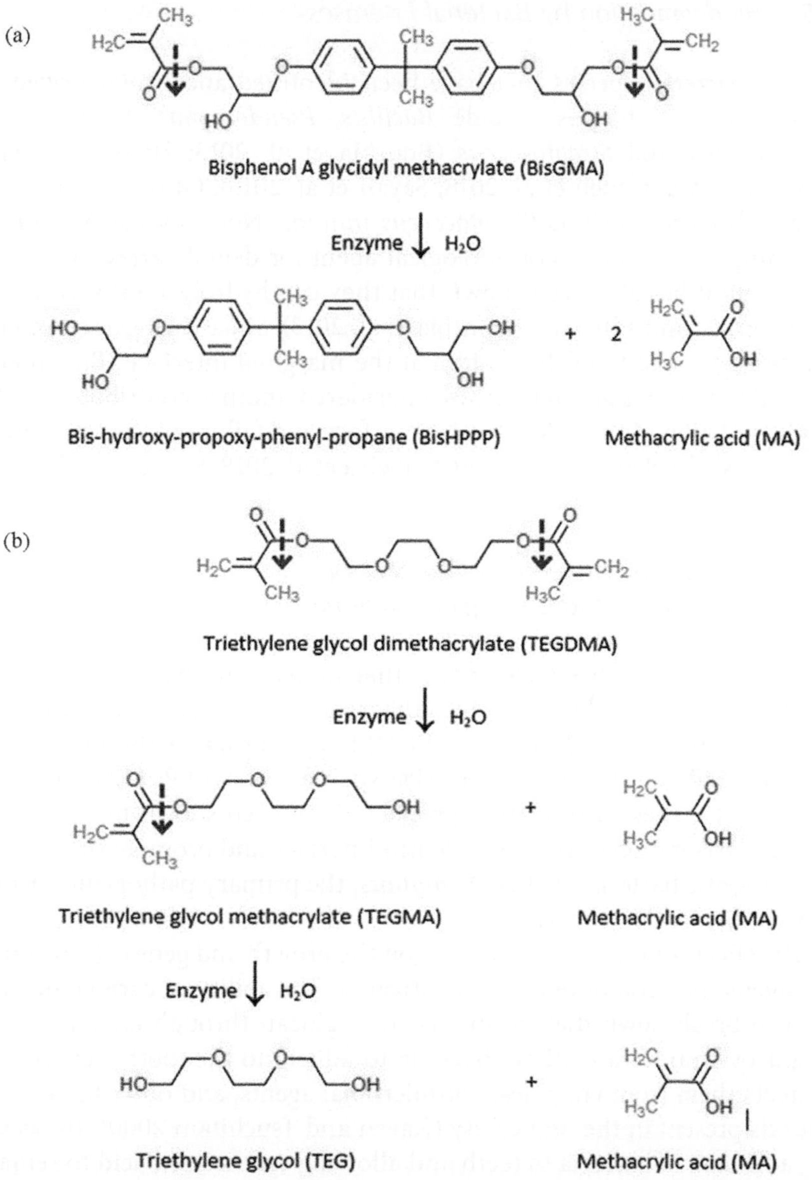

Figure 5.6 Enzymatic degradation of BisGMA (a) and TEGDMA (b) by esterases.

5.5.2 Biodegradation by Bacterial Esterases

Several bacterial species that have been identified and characterized to have esterase activities include *Bacillus, Pseudomonas, Streptomyces, Enterococcus*, and *Streptococcus* (Bourbia et al. 2013; Huang, Siqueira et al. 2018; Marashdeh et al. 2018; Sayali et al. 2013). Of interest are cariogenic bacteria, such as *Streptococcus mutans*. Not only has *S. mutans* been implicated as a major etiological agent for dental caries (Aas et al. 2008), but it has also been shown that they can hydrolyze resin composite materials and adhesives (Bourbia et al. 2013). Since cariogenic bacteria comprise a majority of the biofilm at the marginal interface (Buchmann et al. 1990), bacterial esterases are considered another contributor to the biodegradation of the resin-dentin interface and failure of the restoration (Kermanshahi et al. 2010; Huang, Siqueira et al. 2018; Spencer et al. 2010).

5.5.3 Interaction between Biodegradation
By-Products and Cariogenic Bacteria

Biodegradation studies have shown that human and bacterial esterases catalyze the hydrolysis of the methacrylate resin-based monomers of composite resin, BisGMA, and TEGDMA, resulting in the production of biodegradation by-products (BBPs) such as Bis-HPPP, TEG, and MA (Figure 5.6). These degradation products have been shown to contribute to the deterioration of the resin-dentin interface and promote the growth of cariogenic bacteria, such as *S. mutans*, the primary pathogenic species responsible for dental caries.

The effects of Bis-HPPP and TEG on the growth and gene expression of cariogenic bacteria have been investigated. The ability of cariogenic bacteria to break down dietary sucrose into glucan through enzymes such as glucosyltransferase allows bacteria to adhere to the tooth surface and protects them from enzymes, antimicrobial agents, and other toxic compounds present in the oral cavity (Kawai and Tsuchitani 2000). By securing adhesion of bacteria to teeth and allowing synthesized acid to remain in contact with the enamel, glucosyltransferase activity, therefore, has a crucial role in the onset of biofilm and caries formation (Singh et al. 2009; Tsumori and Kuramitsu 1997).

Glucosyltransferase (gtf) genes have been found to encode glucosyltransferase enzymes in *S. mutans*, which are responsible for the synthesis of glucans and function in bacterial attachment and biofilm formation on the surface of teeth (Khalichi et al. 2009). Singh et al. (2009) showed that both Bis-HPPP and MA upregulated *glucosyltransferase B* (*gtfB*) gene expression in *S. mutans NG8 cells*. It is believed that the elevated levels of these BBPs create environmental stress that stimulates a bacterial response that promotes the transcription of genes needed for glucan production (Jefferson 2004). In addition to an increased ability for bacterial adhesion and biofilm formation, another bacterial response to BBPs is enhanced SMU_118c gene expression. SMU_118c is a dominant esterase from *S. mutans* capable of hydrolyzing the constitutive monomers of composite resin, and therefore increased SMU_118c esterase production may accelerate the biodegradation of the resin-dentin interface, ultimately contributing to the failure of resin composite restorations (Huang, Sadeghinejad et al. 2018).

Khalichi et al. (2004) conducted a study investigating the effects of TEG and MA on the growth of *S. mutans NG8*, *S. mutans JH1005*, and *S. salivarius AT2*. Their findings showed that the growth of all three strains of oral bacteria was modified in a pH- and concentration-dependent manner by both TEGDMA degradation by-products. Furthermore, TEG has been shown to upregulate *gtfB* expression in both planktonic and biofilm cultures, at relevant in vivo concentrations (Khalichi et al. 2009). The potential mechanism by which TEG may contribute to the cariogenicity of *S. mutans* was explored by Sadeghinejad et al. (2016), and their findings suggest that TEG can upregulate various virulence genes, such as *gtfB*, *gtfC*, and *gbpB*, and corresponding proteins, as well as activate specific adaptation mechanisms including biofilm formation, acid tolerance, and stress response pathways. Therefore, upregulation of *gtfB* and *gtfC* and their related proteins by TEG could have a large impact on the cariogenic potential of *S. mutans* by producing a stickier and thicker biofilm at the resin-dentin interface, which is another factor that may lead to premature restoration failures (Sadeghinejad et al. 2016).

5.5.4 Biodegradation by Collagenolytic Enzymes

The resin-dentin interface is susceptible to degradation by matrix metalloproteinases (MMPs), a group of proteolytic enzymes that are calcium- and zinc-dependent (Verma and Hansch 2007). MMPs are present in human saliva and are secreted by various connective tissues and pro-inflammatory cells, including fibroblasts, endothelial cells, and odontoblasts (Delaviz et al. 2014; Verma and Hansch 2007). MMPs can also be found bound to mineralized collagen fibrils in dentin, including stromelysin-1 (MMP-3) (Boukpessi et al. 2008), true collagenase (MMP-8) (Sulkala et al. 2007), and gelatinases A and B (MMP-2 and MMP-9, respectively) (Huang, Cvitkovitch et al. 2018; Martin-De Las Heras et al. 2000; Mazzoni et al. 2007). MMPs play a role in many physiological and pathological processes (Chaussain-Miller et al. 2006; Verma and Hansch 2007).

MMPs have been suggested to take part in the formation of the dentin organic matrix, as well as its destruction following demineralization by bacterial acids (Chaussain-Miller et al. 2006). MMPs, therefore, could be involved in the progression of carious lesions (Chaussain-Miller et al. 2006). Besides, activation of dentinal MMPs in the presence of water can lead to hydrolyzation of exposed collagen fibrils within the hybrid layer, compromising its stability and reducing the fracture toughness of the interface (Chaussain-Miller et al. 2006; Huang, Cvitkovitch et al. 2018; Serkies et al. 2016).

Activation of MMPs from saliva and the dentinal matrix can occur under acidic conditions, such as during acid etching of a bonding procedure, or upon acid production by oral microorganisms (Chaussain-Miller et al. 2006; Delaviz et al. 2014; Liu et al. 2011).

Cysteine cathepsins are enzymes identified in dentin that may work alongside MMPs to degrade collagen and play a role in caries pathogenesis (Nascimento et al. 2011; Tersariol et al. 2010). Like MMPs, cysteine cathepsins may become activated under the abovementioned acidic conditions (Delaviz et al. 2014). It is suggested that the proteolytic activity of MMPs and cysteine cathepsins may have synergistic and adjunctive effects on the caries process and in the degradation of the resin-dentin interface (Nascimento et al. 2011).

5.6 Strategies to Improve the Longevity of Resin Composite Restorations

5.6.1 Enhancing Biostability of Resin Composites

5.6.1.1 Reducing Polymerization Shrinkage
Achieving an adequate seal at the resin-tooth marginal surface will reduce the number of salivary enzymes and bacteria able to penetrate the resin-dentin interface, as well as activation of MMPs and cysteine cathepsins, thus improving the longevity of the restoration. One way to achieve this is by reducing the volumetric shrinkage of the composite upon curing by methods such as the use of bulkier monomers, hyperbranched structures, and ring-opening polymerization (Delaviz et al. 2014). However, even after incorporating these formulations, the problem of marginal breakdown

and recurrent caries may still be significant, and therefore the lifespan of the restoration may still be limited.

A randomized clinical trial (Popoff et al. 2012) compared the clinical performance between silorane-based resin and resins with conventional monomers. The results showed that the reduction in initial volumetric shrinkage did not have any significant effect in clinical performance after one year, suggesting that polymerization shrinkage may not be the sole factor in marginal degradation and secondary caries (Delaviz et al. 2014; Popoff et al. 2012).

5.6.1.2 Shielding Unprotected Bonds

The addition of monomers that are capable of shielding susceptible bonds in resin composite and adhesives may be beneficial in inhibiting the hydrolysis of the resinous matrix. Fluorinated monomers and fluorinated BisGMA derivatives have been investigated for this purpose (Figure 5.7) (Delaviz et al. 2014). Fluorinated monomers have water repellent properties, are chemically stable, and are resistant to stain and discoloration (Kadoma 2010). However, they require longer curing times at room temperature that may limit its clinical applications (Kadoma 2010). Derivatives of BisGMA containing fluorinated diluent monomers may be promising as they have shown to have greater hydrophobicity and lower water sorption and solubility in comparison to nonfluorinated diluents, with no significant effect on tensile strength (Li and Craig 1996).

5.6.1.3 Reducing the Rate of Collagen Degradation by MMPs and Cysteine Cathepsins

Collagen degradation by MMPs and cysteine cathepsins can be reduced by either inhibiting the activity of these enzymes or sealing the dentin matrix from its action (Delaviz et al. 2014; Serkies et al. 2016). This can be accomplished by overcoming the over-activation of MMPs and cysteine

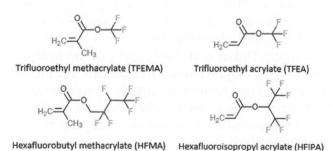

Trifluoroethyl methacrylate (TFEMA)   Trifluoroethyl acrylate (TFEA)

Hexafluorobutyl methacrylate (HFMA)   Hexafluoroisopropyl acrylate (HFIPA)

Figure 5.7   Chemical structure of various fluorinated monomers.

cathepsins during acid etching or by superior monomer infiltration during bonding (Hashimoto et al. 2000). MMP inhibitors such as chlorhexidine (CHX) (Almahdy et al. 2012; Gendron et al. 1999) and galardin (Breschi et al. 2010; Serkies et al. 2016) can be added into dental adhesives to improve the long-term stability of the resin-dentin interface (Delaviz et al. 2014).

Chlorhexidine is a broad-spectrum antimicrobial agent that has been shown to be effective in inhibiting the proteolytic activities of both MMP and cysteine cathepsins in dentin (Carrilho et al. 2007; Gendron et al. 1999; Scaffa et al. 2012), although these positive results may only be short term (Osorio et al. 2011). Galardin is a specific synthetic inhibitor that acts primarily on the major dentinal MMPs (MMP-2, -3, -8, and -9) (Breschi et al. 2010), by chelating with the zinc atom residing in the active site of the enzyme and preventing its catalytic activation. Galardin has been shown to be just as effective as CHX in preserving the integrity of resin-bonded interfaces (Breschi et al. 2010).

5.6.2 Reducing Bacterial Adherence by Imparting Resin Composites with Antimicrobial Properties

Resin composite restorations have a shorter lifespan, higher replacement rate, and higher rate of failure in comparison to amalgam restorations, predominately due to interfacial biofilm formation and formation of recurrent caries around the margin of dental restorations (Huang, Siqueira et al. 2018; Li et al. 2014). This can be attributed to the increased accumulation of bacteria on resin-based materials, which subsequently leads to recurrent caries in the surrounding tooth structure (Huang, Siqueiraet al. 2018; Li et al. 2014).

Although many restorative materials used today possess antimicrobial properties, their clinical use is limited due to poorer esthetic or mechanical properties (Chen et al. 2012). For example, amalgam has shown to release ions that are bactericidal to adhering bacteria (Netuschil et al. 1996), glass ionomers are designed to release fluoride ions that interfere with bacterial acid production (van Dijken et al. 1997), and calcium hydroxide releases hydroxyl ions, which are highly oxidant free radicals, and provides a highly alkaline environment that bacteria are unable to survive in (Siqueira and Lopes 1999). Resin composites, on the other hand, are aesthetically acceptable materials, but possess little to no antibacterial properties in long term (Matalon et al. 2004, 2009).

In fact, freshly polymerized composites, unreacted monomers, and some resin degradation by-products have been shown to support bacterial growth by altering gene expression and related proteins, thus increasing virulence of the bacteria in close proximity and within the restoration-tooth interface, and providing a potential explanation to the increase rate of recurrent caries around these restorations (Delaviz et al. 2014; Matalon et al. 2004; Sadeghinejad et al. 2016, 2017). Therefore, in the early 1980s, resin-based materials with antimicrobial properties were introduced to prevent recurrent caries and ultimately improve the longevity of these restorations (Chen et al. 2012).

Bacterial accumulation and proliferation at the resin-dentin interface can be controlled by either a passive or active approach. The passive approach prevents bacterial adhesion at the marginal interface through the incorporation of non-released antimicrobial monomers into the restorative material, which exerts its antibacterial effect by contact (Imazato et al. 2003). The active approach, on the other hand, involves the release of antimicrobial agents that kill bacteria. Examples of these antimicrobial agents include silver ions, fluoride ions, and CHX (Delaviz et al. 2014). These additive agents modify either the resin matrix or the filler particles within it (Hamouda 2012; Pereira-Cenci et al. 2013).

5.6.2.1 Released Antimicrobial Agents

In general, released soluble antimicrobial agents exert their effect upon gradual release into the surrounding environment. Initial attempts were to add antimicrobial compounds directly to the resin matrix by mixing in powdered antimicrobial agents. However, these antimicrobial agents leave voids in the matrix as they diffuse and penetrate through cell walls and membranes of neighboring bacteria, compromising the structural integrity of the restoration (Stewart et al. 2018).

Besides, this release is an uncontrollable process with limited antibacterial activity following an initial burst of release, inhibiting long-term efficacy against bacterial growth (Beyth et al. 2014; Stewart et al. 2018). Examples of these agents include CHX, silver ions, antibiotics, iodine, quaternary ammonium compounds, and fluoride (Beyth et al. 2014).

Fluoride is commonly added to resin matrix and filler particles as an antimicrobial-releasing agent for its ability to interfere with biofilm formation, reduce bacterial acid production and enhance remineralization (Wiegand et al. 2007). However, it has been shown that fluoride possesses limited long-lasting effects due to its short-term and predominant release during the setting reaction (Beyth et al. 2014; Huang, Cvitkovitch et al. 2018).

To overcome this drawback, the desirable physical and esthetic qualities of resin composites were combined with the fluoride-releasing ability of glass-ionomer cement to create a new antimicrobial resin-based dental material known as polyacid modified composite resins (PMCR or compomers) (Nicholson 2007).

Compomers contain reactive fluoro-aluminosilicate glass particles that are vulnerable to acid attack and provide a maintained level of fluoride ion release over time, without an initial fluoride "burst" effect (Attar and Turgut 2003; Shaw et al. 1998; Wiegand et al. 2007; Yap et al. 2002). However, the effect of compomers on recurrent caries is dependent on the type of caries present, the brand of material used, and how the study was conducted and therefore needs to be further investigated (van Dijken et al. 1997; Welbury et al. 2000; Wiegand et al. 2007).

The incorporation of antimicrobial agents into the polymeric matrix for long-term antibacterial activity is still under investigation. The antibiotic ciprofloxacin has been used to synthesize a dimethacrylate monomer via condensation-type bonds that are susceptible to hydrolysis (Delaviz et al. 2014). These antimicrobial agents are inactive when bound to a polymer but can be released when the ester groups within the resin composite are hydrolyzed, providing an antibacterial effect (Delaviz et al. 2014). However, the mechanical and clinical performance of these released antibacterial agents, along with their long-term efficacy, have yet to be fully investigated (Delaviz et al. 2014).

5.6.2.1.1 *Mesoporous Silica Nanoparticles (MSNs)*

Drug-loaded particles for dental restorative materials ideally should have an inert, non-degradable scaffold that can maintain structural integrity following the release of the drug so as not to compromise the mechanical properties of the restoration and have predictable drug release rates (Zilberman and Elsner 2008). Porous silica structures have been proposed to store antimicrobial at the site of action and release the drug over extended periods of time.

Highly ordered nanoporous inorganic scaffolds, such as mesoporous silica nanoparticles (MSNs), are ideal because they have ordered channels, are structurally and chemically stable, biocompatible, highly porous, and remain intact after drug release (Angelos et al. 2008; Faustini et al. 2014; Beltran-Osuna and Perilla 2016; Yamamoto and Kuroda 2016). Examples of MSNs loaded with drugs for diffusional release include antimicrobials such as chlorhexidine, peptides, and biosurfactants (Zhang et al. 2014; Izquierdo-Barba et al. 2009; Fontecave et al. 2013). Ordered mesoporous silica is formed through the condensation of a silica precursor in co-assembly with an organic surfactant template to form a porous mesostructure following the removal of the template by calcination (Lu et al. 2007;

Hatton et al. 2005; Angelos et al. 2008; Nooney et al. 2002; Yamamoto and Kuroda 2016). MSNs have sufficient mechanical strength for antimicrobial applications as filler particles for composites (Samuel et al. 2009). The templating agent may be a molecule that forms micelles and presents a hydrophilic interface for silica to condense around, such as surfactants and block copolymers (Zhao et al. 1998; Huo et al. 1996).

MSNs can be loaded by long-term suspension in a drug solution through diffusion, through the evaporation of a drug solution (incipient wetness technique), or through suspension in a melted liquid drug, when the drug chemistry will allow (Limnell et al. 2011). However, the usefulness of MSNs for antimicrobial release is limited by their low drug loading due to the utilization of concentration gradients to load pores resulting in 15% w/w drug to silica at most to a more typical sub-1% w/w, or unpredictable and short-term release profiles due to the adsorption of a drug on the external surface when loaded through solvent evaporation (Izquierdo-Barba et al. 2009; Lu et al. 2007; Han et al. 2015; He et al. 2010, 2011; Izquierdo-Barba et al. 2005). These traditionally loaded MSNs have been added to dental materials in several studies to impart the materials with antimicrobial activities, however, with a limited effective time frame of release (Carpenter et al. 2013; Lee et al. 2016; Zhang et al. 2014). These latter approaches demonstrate the weaknesses of inadequate longevity for clinical application and discounting of the complex oral biodegradative environment outlined above.

To overcome the above limitations, Stewart et al. (2018) have developed a novel, self-assembly approach to incorporate an antimicrobial drug into silica, by using the drug itself as the templating agent to synthesize drug-silica co-assembled particle (DSPs) (Figure 5.8b). By one-step self-assembly, these DSPs are very highly loaded with the drug, to levels of about 50 vol%, much higher than conventional drug-loading methods (about 1–3 vol%) (Izquierdo-Barba et al. 2009; Lu et al. 2007; Han et al. 2015; He et al. 2010, 2011; Izquierdo-Barba et al. 2005; Zhang et al. 2014). This bottom-up, tailored design of DSPs greatly extends the release timeframe, while also simplifying synthesis (Stewart et al. 2018). These advantages are made possible by the amphiphilic, self-assembling properties of several drug molecules. These drugs form micelles in solutions, creating a charged catalytic site at the micelle water-facing surface where silica precursors may hydrolyze and condense. This results in the formation of a stabilizing silica structure permeated by ordered drug channels, with a very high weight ratio of a drug (>30 wt%). The antimicrobial drug, in this case, octenidine dihydrochloride (OCT), is a highly biocompatible cationic surfactant antiseptic that shows broad efficacy against Gram-positive and Gram-negative bacteria with no known bacterial resistance (Hübner et al. 2010; Dogan et al. 2008; Rohrer et al. 2010).

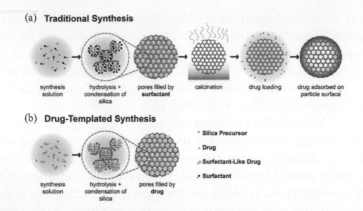

Figure 5.8 Traditional concentration-gradient (a) vs. drug-templated (b) synthesis of MSNs. (Used with permission from Stewart et al. (2018). This work is licensed under the Creative Commons Attribution 4.0 International License. To view a copy of this license, visit http://creativecommons.org/licenses/by/4.0/ or send a letter to Creative Commons, PO Box 1866, Mountain View, CA 94042, USA.)

OCT is not as easily solvated as a free drug, or drug adsorbed only to the outer surface of MSNs. In fact, it is released at much slower speeds than traditional MSNs. Incorporation of these particles into dental adhesive has been shown to exhibit slow and extended drug release, with increases in activity in response to enzymes produced by cariogenic bacteria and saliva, resulting in on-demand drug release that would be sufficient for the life of the restoration (Stewart et al. 2018). These advances in the long-term release have the potential to produce long-term anti-infective materials.

5.6.2.2 Non-Released Antimicrobial Agents
Non-released insoluble antimicrobial agents inhibit bacterial growth by inactivating target microorganisms through direct contact, without releasing any compounds from the carrier material (Beyth et al. 2014). This is achieved by the incorporation of immobilized bactericides, such as silver supported fillers, 12-methacryloyloxydodecylpyridinium bromide (MDPB), and triclosan, which are advantageous due to their nonvolatility, chemical stability, and potential for long-term bacterial inhibition (Yoshida et al, 1999; Imazato et al. 2003; Wicht et al. 2005; Beyth et al. 2014). However, some limitations do exist, such as the limited vicinity of action of these non-released agents, and therefore further studies are warranted to optimize the initiator system and test mechanical properties to produce a material that can effectively prevent secondary caries (Beyth et al. 2014; Fan et al. 2011; Imazato et al. 2003). Nevertheless, these

non-released agents highlight a means for controlling biofilm formation at the margins of restorations, in order to improve the longevity of resin composite materials.

5.6.2.2.1 Antibacterial Polycations in Resin Composites

Cations or polymers that retain positive charges on their surfaces can act as contact disinfectants to negatively charged bacterial cell membranes. These antibacterial polycations include but are not limited to ion exchange fibers, alkoxysilanes, insoluble pyridinium-type polymers, and immobilized N-alkylated polyethyleneimine (Beyth et al. 2014).

5.6.2.2.1.1 Polyethyleneimine Cationic polymers containing quaternary ammonium groups have demonstrated to be effective antimicrobial agents (Tiller et al. 2002). The mechanism of action of antibacterial quaternary ammonium compounds is primarily through interactions and disruption of bacterial cell membranes (Kawabata and Nishiguchi 1988). Quaternary ammonium polyethyleneimine (QPEI), whose chemical structure is illustrated in Figure 5.9, has shown to be highly potent (Gao et al. 2007). This can be attributed to the numerous quaternary ammonium groups along its backbone, and a high surface density of active groups (Beyth et al. 2014). In addition, N-alkylated polyethyleneimine has shown to be effective against various Gram-positive and Gram-negative bacteria due to its hydrophobic, positively charged, and immobilized long polymeric chains (Lin et al. 2002, 2003).

5.6.2.2.1.2 Polyethyleneimine Nanoparticles Antibacterial activity in polycations can also be achieved by using nanoparticles as active antimicrobial

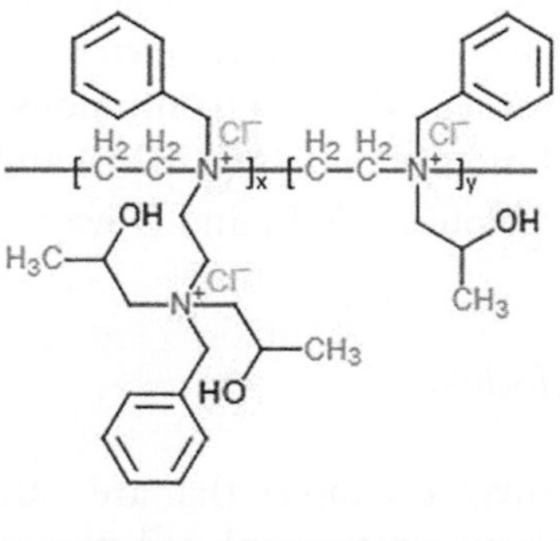

Quaternary ammonium polyethyleneimine (QPEI)

Figure 5.9 Chemical structure of QPEI.

agents (Gao et al. 2007). Nanoparticles are advantageous as only a small number of particles are necessary for high biological activity, an important attribute when dealing with resin composites (Beyth et al. 2014). Polycationic nanoparticles with quaternary ammonium groups (QPEI particles) exhibit strong antimicrobial activity and are desirable candidates as antibacterial additives (Beyth et al. 2014).

The incorporation of QPEI particles within resin composites has been found to effectively inhibit bacterial growth. This activity is primarily dependent on the hydrophobic nature of hydrophilic QPEI upon alkylation and the quantity of positively charged quaternary ammonium groups present (Beyth et al. 2014). Insoluble nanoparticles incorporated into restorative composites can withstand exposure to wet environments, and do not need to be released in order to produce an antibacterial effect. This results in improved mechanical properties and stability in aqueous conditions, compared to water-soluble and leachable antimicrobial agents (Beyth et al. 2014).

5.7 Bacterial Biofilm Caries Models

In vivo studies concerning caries formation have many ethical limitations. Therefore, different in vitro methods have been developed in order to improve our techniques in replicating the clinical condition and producing findings that are applicable to the actual caries process (Salli and Ouwehand 2015). Although an in vitro model cannot capture all aspects of caries formation in the oral cavity, it provides a means to perform experiments under controlled and reproducible conditions (Salli and Ouwehand 2015).

In vitro models differ depending on the desired nature of the biofilm (Rudney et al. 2012). Caries models that utilize bacterial biofilms can be divided into the closed batch culture and open continuous culture models (Table 5.1) (Salli and Ouwehand 2015). Continuous models can be further classified into artificial mouth models (AMMs) and flow cells with either single- or multi-species biofilms (Salli and Ouwehand 2015).

5.7.1 Batch Biofilm Models

Batch biofilm models involve samples that are immersed in a closed system; unless the growth media are replaced, the environment inside the well only changes with the consumption of nutrients and the accumulation of metabolic by-products (Coenye and Nelis 2010). The biofilm within

TABLE 5.1   Advantages and Disadvantages between Batch and Continuous Caries Models

		Continuous	
	Batch	AMM	Flow Cell
Advantages	Multiple compounds tested simultaneously Multiple conditions tested simultaneously Small volumes of reagents Easy to perform Simple equipment	Flow conditions Conditions closely mimicking in vivo situation Product and nutrient concentration stable during biofilm formation Perfect mixing	Flow conditions Possibility to analyze biofilm formation in real time Intermediate complex equipment
Disadvantages	Closed system No flow	Requires larger volumes of reagents Only one condition/run can be tested Complex equipment More expensive Usually less replicates	Conditions vary at different sites in the reactor Only one condition/ run can be tested Usually less replicates

the well can be formed on a plate wall, on the surface of discs, coupons, or pegs or on human or bovine enamel (Salli and Ouwehand 2015).

5.7.2 Continuous Biofilm Models

5.7.2.1 Artificial Mouth Model (AMM)

The AMM is an open system that has continuous, open-surface film fluid flow (Shu et al. 2000). The AMM can be designed to provide the biofilm with an intermittent or continuous supply of nutrients, and factors such as temperature, humidity, sucrose supply, pH, and nutrient/saliva flow rate can be controlled, in order to mimic the oral condition as closely as possible (Salli and Ouwehand 2015; Tang et al. 2003).

5.7.2.2 Flow Cell Biofilm Models

In flow cell systems, the media moves in one direction and mixing occurs by diffusion, creating varying conditions at different sites within the reactor

(Salli and Ouwehand 2015). Sequential colonization can be detected in real time under microscopy within this model, and therefore, it can be useful for studying biofilm formation and morphology (Coenye and Nelis 2010).

5.7.3 Single vs. Multi-Species Models

Both batch and continuous culture models can be used to grow a mono-culture biofilm (single species), a defined consortium biofilm (two to ten species), or a microcosm biofilm (from saliva or plaque samples) (Salli and Ouwehand 2015).

5.7.3.1 Monoculture Biofilm

Many investigators use single-species biofilms to simplify and standardize their models. *S. mutans* is considered the chief etiologic agent of dental caries (Smith and Spatafora 2012) and is commonly chosen as the single species (Rudney et al. 2012). *S. mutans* is acidogenic (produce acid) and facilitates the demineralization of enamel and dentin by producing lactic acid as a by-product of fermentable carbohydrate metabolism (Sansone et al. 1993). Nevertheless, *S. mutans* biofilm models are limited since single-species biofilms do not exist in the mouth. In fact, *S. mutans* may not even be the majority species in some individuals with active caries (Aas et al. 2008).

5.7.3.2 Defined Consortium Biofilm

An alternative model, also known as a defined multi-species biofilm model, includes a consortium of up to ten species, which can comprise commensal species, putative pathogens, or both (Rudney et al. 2012). Single- and multi-species models have been compared when studying enamel and root caries, using an AMM with four species (*S. mutans*, *S. sobrinus*, *Actinomyces naeslundii*, and *Lactobacillus rhamnosus*) (Shu et al. 2000). It was found that compared to monospecies biofilms, biofilms with defined consortium biofilms tended to be larger and were able to cause more enamel demineralization (Shu et al. 2000). In terms of bacterial strain selection to form defined-species consortia biofilms, a random selection of available strains is a common approach, but to obtain a highly cariogenic biofilm, screening and selection of strains with desired cariogenic properties may be the best strategy (Shu et al. 2000).

A modified model with a different group of bacterial species (*S. mutans*, *S. sobrinus*, and *S. gordonii*) was developed to evaluate biofilm-induced secondary caries (Hayati et al. 2011). Artificial biofilms were formed on specimens with resin composite restorations in a continuous flow reactor for 20h, and then incubated for 7 or 30days (Hayati et al. 2011). Using defined multi-species biofilms, this study established an artificial secondary caries model for in vitro studies, as well as verified the significance of using an adhesive bonding system (Hayati et al. 2011). Another AMM, using a five-species (*S. mutans*, *S. sobrinus*, *Lactobacillus acidophilus*, *L. rhamnosus*, and *A. naeslundii*) system, looked at the mechanism of action of silver diamine fluoride (SDF) on the biofilm (Mei et al. 2013). SDF was found to inhibit the formation of the biofilm and reduce demineralization (Mei et al. 2013). This study also determined the arrangement of bacteria within the biofilm and found that *Lactobacilli* and *Streptococci* mostly inhabited the upper and lower layers of the biofilm, respectively (Mei et al. 2013).

Furthermore, the effects of carbohydrate pulses and pH within oral microbial communities were tested using a continuous-culture chemostat system with the following nine oral bacteria: *Neisseria subflava* A1 078, *Veillonella dispar* ATCC 17748, *Lactobacillus casei* AC 41 3, *Fusobacterium nucleatum* ATCC 10953, *Actinomyces viscosus* WVU 627, *Porphyromonas gingivalis* W 50, *Streptococcus oralis* EF 186, *Streptococcus gordonii* NCTC 7865, and *Streptococcus mutans* R9 (Bradshaw et al. 1989). It was found that when the pH was not controlled, the composition of the microflora altered drastically as the pH dropped after each glucose pulse (Bradshaw et al. 1989).

Successive glucose pulses lead to amplified changes in the microflora, and a progressively greater degree and rate of acid production. The findings from this study suggest that the shifts in the metabolism and composition of the microflora in the oral cavity may result from the pH generated from carbohydrate metabolism, rather than carbohydrate availability (Bradshaw et al. 1989). Another nine-membered community of oral bacteria that has been used to investigate biofilm formation using a constant-depth film fermenter consisted of *Neisseria subflava* A1 078, *Veillonella dispar* ATCC 17748, *Lactobacillus casei* AC 413, *Fusobacterium nucleatum* ATCC 10953, *Actinomyces viscosus* WVU 627, *Porphyromonas gingivalis* W 50, *Streptococcus oralis* EF 186, *Streptococcus gordonii* NCTC 7865, and *Streptococcus mutans* R9 (Kinniment et al. 1996).

Currently, greater than 700 species have been reported in the oral biofilm (Dewhirst et al. 2010), and therefore the major limitation with defined multi-species models is that the consortia may still underrepresent the actual flora in the oral cavity and may not be generalizable. However, these models provide more control over the individual species present in the biofilm, as well as the study of their properties, allowing for more detailed and easier analysis of the bacteria compared to plaque microcosms, described in the next section (Marsh 1995; Shu et al. 2000).

5.7.3.3 Microcosm Biofilm

Samples from oral inoculum, most typically obtained from single or pooled donors, can be used as yet another alternative model (Rudney et al. 2012). Microcosm models can generate a complex microcosm in vitro that comes closest to replicating in vivo conditions in the oral cavity (Salli and Ouwehand 2015). However, the resultant consortium of bacterial species may be so diverse that it becomes difficult to determine its composition (Marsh 1995). Difficulties are also encountered in the interpretation of findings, standardization of the plaque inoculum for replication and comparison of results, and in the manipulation of the biofilm composition for experimental purposes (Marsh 1995; Rudney et al. 2012; Salli and Ouwehand 2015). Nonetheless, artificial mouth microcosm models prove to be a valuable method in studying the structure and function of dental biofilms (Salli and Ouwehand 2015).

5.8 Concluding Remarks

Resin composite is the most commonly used restorative material in dentistry today, but its longevity is often challenged by host and microbial interactions in the oral cavity. One of the main reasons for the high failure rates of resin composite restorations is the development of bacterial biofilm along the compromised restoration margins and subsequent recurrent caries due to bacterial acid and enzymes, and host activities.

Resin composite can also undergo a significant amount of biological breakdown, catalyzed by salivary and salivary-like enzymes and bacterial esterases and proteases, further degrading the tooth-restoration interface. Resin BBPs increase the virulence of cariogenic bacterium, in a positive feedback manner that accelerates the above processes. Strategies have been implemented to improve the longevity of resin composite restorations by enhancing the biostability of resin composites. This can be achieved by reducing polymerization shrinkage, shielding unprotected bonds, or using matrix-metalloproteinase and cathepsin inhibitors.

Incorporation of antimicrobial agents into resin composites or adhesive bonding systems is another strategy to improve the lifespan of restorations through the inhibition of bacterial adherence and enzymatic degradation. Recent developments in the latter strategy show great promise in developing materials that are more resistant to host and microbial degradation. New resin composite restorative systems should address these degradative challenges in order to prolong the service life of dental restorations and improve patient outcomes.

References

Aas, J.A., A.L. Griffen, S.R. Dardis, A.M. Lee, I. Olsen, F.E. Dewhirst, E.J. Leys, and B.J. Paster. 2008. "Bacteria of Dental Caries in Primary and Permanent Teeth in Children and Young Adults." *Journal of Clinical Microbiology* 46 (4): 1407–17. doi:10.1128/JCM.01410–07.

Almahdy, A., G. Koller, S. Sauro, J.W. Bartsch, M. Sherriff, T.F. Watson, and A. Banerjee. 2012. "Effects of MMP Inhibitors Incorporated within Dental Adhesives." *Journal of Dental Research* 91 (6): 605–11. doi:10.1177/0022034512446339.

Angelos, S., M. Liong, E. Choi, and J.I. Zink. 2008. "Mesoporous Silicate Materials as Substrates for Molecular Machines and Drug Delivery." *Chemical Engineering Journal* 137 (1): 4–13. doi:10.1016/j.cej.2007.07.074.

Attar, N., and M.D. Turgut. 2003. "Fluoride Release and Uptake Capacities of Fluoride-Releasing Restorative Materials." *Operative Dentistry* 28 (4): 395–402. http://www.ncbi.nlm.nih.gov/pubmed/12877430.

Beltran-Osuna, A.A., and J.E. Perilla. 2016. "Colloidal and Spherical Mesoporous Silica Particles: Synthesis and New Technologies for Delivery Applications." *Journal of Sol–Gel Science and Technology* 77 (45): 480–96. doi:10.1007/s10971-015-3874-2.

Bernardo, M., H. Luis, M.D. Martin, B.G. Leroux, T. Rue, J. Leitão, and T.A. Derouen. 2007. "Survival and Reasons for Failure of Amalgam versus Composite Posterior Restorations Placed in a Randomized Clinical Trial." *Journal of the American Dental Association* 138 (6): 775–83.

Beyth, N., S. Farah, A.J. Domb, and E.I. Weiss. 2014. "Antibacterial Dental Resin Composites." *Reactive and Functional Polymers* 75 (1). 81–8. doi:10.1016/j.reactfunctpolym.2013.11.011.

Bowen, R. L. 1956. "Use of Epoxy Resins in Restorative Materials." *Journal of Dental Research* 35 (3): 360–69. doi:10.1177/00220345560350030501.

Bortolotto, T., M. Ferrari, A. Susin, and I. Krejci. 2009. "Morphology of the Smear Layer after the Application of Simplified Self-Etch Adhesives on Enamel and Dentin Surfaces Created with Different Preparation Methods." *Clinical Oral Investigations* 13 (4): 409–17. doi:10.1007/s00784-008-0242-4.

Bouillaguet, S. 2004. "Biological Risks of Resin-Based Materials to the Dentin-Pulp Complex." *Critical Reviews in Oral Biology & Medicine* 15 (1): 47–60. doi:10.1146/annurev.physchem.50.1.347.

Boukpessi, T., S. Menashi, L. Camoin, J.M. TenCate, M. Goldberg, and C. Chaussain-Miller. 2008. "The Effect of Stromelysin-1 (MMP-3) on Non-Collagenous Extracellular Matrix Proteins of Demineralized Dentin and the Adhesive Properties of Restorative Resins." *Biomaterials* 29 (33): 4367–73. doi:10.1016/j.biomaterials.2008.07.035.

Bourbia, M., D. Ma, D.G. Cvitkovitch, J.P. Santerre, and Y. Finer. 2013. "Cariogenic Bacteria Degrade Dental Resin Composites and Adhesives." *Journal of Dental Research* 92 (11): 989–94. doi:10.1177/0022034513504436.

Bradshaw, D.J., A.S. McKee, and P.D. Marsh. 1989. "Effects of Carbohydrate Pulses and pH on Population Shifts within Oral Microbial Communities

In Vitro." *Journal of Dental Research* 68 (9): 1298–302. doi:10.117 7/00220345890680090101.

Breschi, L., A. Mazzoni, A. Ruggeri, M. Cadenaro, R.D. Lenarda, and E.D.S. Dorigo. 2008. "Dental Adhesion Review: Aging and Stability of the Bonded Interface." *Dental Materials* 24 (1): 90–101. doi:10.1016/j.dental.2007.02.009.

Breschi, L., P. Martin, A. Mazzoni, F. Nato, M. Carrilho, L. Tjäderhane, E. Visintini, et al. 2010. "Use of a Specific MMP-Inhibitor (Galardin) for Preservation of Hybrid Layer." *Dental Materials* 26 (6): 571–8. doi:10.1016/j. dental.2010.02.007.

Buchmann, G., W. Klimm, A. Gabert, and J. Edelmann. 1990. "Detection of Microecological Phenomena in Filled Teeth I. Phenomena in Gap Between Restoration and Cavity." *Microbial Ecology in Health and Disease* 3: 51–7.

Carpenter, A.W., K.P. Reighard, J.E. Saavedra, and M.H. Schoenfisch. 2013. "O_2-Protected Diazeniumdiolate-Modified Silica Nanoparticles for Extended Nitric Oxide Release from Dental Composites." *Biomaterials Science* 1 (5): 456–9. doi:10.1039/c3bm00153a.

Carrilho, M., S. Geraldeli, F. Tay, M.F. de Goes, R.M. Carvalho, L. Tjäderhane, A.F. Reis, et al. 2007. "In Vivo Preservation of the Hybrid Layer by Chlorhexidine." *Journal of Dental Research* 86 (6): 529–33. doi:10.1177/154405910708600608.

Chaussain-Miller, C., F. Fioretti, M. Goldberg, and S. Menashi. 2006. "The Role of Matrix Metalloproteinases (MMPs) in Human Caries." *Journal of Dental Research* 85 (1): 22–32. doi:10.1177/154405910608500104.

Chen, L., H. Shen, and B.I. Suh. 2012. "Antibacterial Dental Restorative Materials: A State-of-the-Art Review." *American Journal of Dentistry* 25 (6): 337–46.

Coenye, T., and H.J. Nelis. 2010. "In Vitro and In Vivo Model Systems to Study Microbial Biofilm Formation." *Journal of Microbiological Methods* 83 (2): 89–105. doi:10.1016/j.mimet.2010.08.018.

Deb, S. 1998. "Polymers in Dentistry." *Proceedings of the Institution of Mechanical Engineers, Part H* 212 (6): 453–64.

Delaviz, Y., Y. Finer, and J.P. Santerre. 2014. "Biodegradation of Resin Composites and Adhesives by Oral Bacteria and Saliva: A Rationale for New Material Designs That Consider the Clinical Environment and Treatment Challenges." *Dental Materials* 30 (1): 16–32. doi:10.1016/j.dental.2013.08.201.

Derouen, T.A., M.D. Martin, B.G. Leroux, B.D. Townes, J.S. Woods, H. Luis, M. Bernardo, G. Rosenbaum, and I.P. Martins. 2016. "Neurobehavioral Effects of Dental Amalgam in Children." *The Journal of the American Medical Association* 295 (15): 1784–92. doi:10.1001/jama.295.15.1784.

Dewhirst, F.E., T. Chen, J. Izard, B.J. Paster, A.C.R. Tanner, W.H. Yu, A. Lakshmanan, and W.G. Wade. 2010. "The Human Oral Microbiome." *Journal of Bacteriology* 192 (19): 5002–17. doi:10.1128/JB.00542–10.

Dogan, A.A., A.K. Adiloglu, S. Onal, E.S. Cetin, E. Polat, E. Uskun, and F. Koksal. 2008. "Short-Term Relative Antibacterial Effect of Octenidine Dihydrochloride on the Oral Microflora in Orthodontically Treated Patients." *International Journal of Infectious Diseases* 12 (6). doi:10.1016/j. ijid.2008.03.013.

Dogon, L. 1990. "Present and Future Value of Dental Composite Materials and Sealants." *International Journal of Technology Assessment in Health Care* 6: 369–77.

Fan, C., L. Chu, H. Ralph Rawls, B.K. Norling, H.L. Cardenas, and K. Whang. 2011. "Development of an Antimicrobial Resin—A Pilot Study." *Dental Materials* 27 (4): 322–8. doi:10.1016/j.dental.2010.11.008.

Faustini, M., D. Grosso, C. Boissière, R. Backov, and C. Sanchez. 2014. "'Integrative Sol-Gel Chemistry': A Nanofoundry for Materials Science." *Journal of Sol–Gel Science and Technology* 70 (2): 216–26. doi:10.1007/s10971-014-3321-9.

Ferracane, J.L. 2006. "Hygroscopic and Hydrolytic Effects in Dental Polymer Networks." *Dental Materials* 22 (3): 211–22. doi:10.1016/j.dental.2005.05.005.

Ferracane, J.L. 2011. "Resin Composite—State of the Art." *Dental Materials* 27 (1): 29–38. doi:10.1016/j.dental.2010.10.020.

Finer, Y., F. Jaffer, and J.P. Santerre. 2004. "Mutual Influence of Cholesterol Esterase and Pseudocholinesterase on the Biodegradation of Dental Composites." *Biomaterials* 25 (10): 1787–93. doi:10.1016/j.biomaterials.2003.08.029.

Finer, Y., and J.P. Santerre. 2004. "Salivary Esterase Activity and Its Association with the Biodegradation of Dental Composites." *Journal of Dental Research* 83 (1): 22–6. doi:10.1177/154405910408300105.

Fontecave, T., C. Boissiere, N. Baccile, F.J. Plou, and C. Sanchez. 2013. "Using Evaporation-Induced Self-Assembly for the Direct Drug Templating of Therapeutic Vectors with High Loading Fractions, Tunable Drug Release, and Controlled Degradation." *Chemistry of Materials* 25 (23): 4671–8. doi:10.1021/cm401807m.

Gao, B., X. Zhang, and Y. Zhu. 2007. "Studies on the Preparation and Antibacterial Properties of Quaternized Polyethyleneimine." *Journal of Biomaterials Science* (5): 531–44. doi:10.1163/156856207780852523.

Gendron, R., D. Grenier, T. Sorsa, and D. Mayrand. 1999. "Inhibition of the Activities of Matrix Metalloproteinases 2, 8, and 9 by Chlorhexidine." *Clinical and Diagnostic Laboratory Immunology* 6 (3): 437–9. http://www.pubmedcentral.nih.gov/articlerender.fcgi?artid=103739&tool=pmcentrez&rendertype=abstract.

Hamouda, I.M. 2012. "Current Perspectives of Nanoparticles in Medical and Dental Biomaterials." *Journal of Biomedical Research* 26 (3): 143–51. doi:10.7555/JBR.26.20120027.

Han, N., Q. Zhao, L. Wan, Y. Wang, Y. Gao, P. Wang, Z. Wang, J. Zhang, T. Jiang, and S. Wang. 2015. "Hybrid Lipid-Capped Mesoporous Silica for Stimuli-Responsive Drug Release and Overcoming Multidrug Resistance." *ACS Applied Materials and Interfaces* 7 (5): 3342–51. doi:10.1021/am5082793.

Hashimoto, M., H. Ohno, K. Endo, M. Kaga, H. Sano, and H. Oguchi. 2000. "The Effect of Hybrid Layer Thickness on Bond Strength: Demineralized Dentin Zone of the Hybrid Layer." *Dental Materials: Official Publication of the Academy of Dental Materials* 16: 406–11. doi:10.1016/S0109-5641(00)00035-5.

Hashimoto, M., S. Fujita, M. Kaga, and Y. Yawaka. 2008. "Effect of Water on Bonding of One-Bottle Self-Etching Adhesives." *Dental Materials Journal* 27 (2): 172–8. doi:10.4012/dmj.27.172.

Hatton, B., K. Landskron, W. Whitnall, D. Perovic, and G.A. Ozin. 2005. "Past, Present, and Future of Periodic Mesoporous Organosilicas—The PMOs." *Accounts of Chemical Research* 38 (4): 305–12. doi:10.1021/ar040164a.

Hayati, F., A. Okada, Y. Kitasako, J. Tagami, and K. Matin. 2011. "An Artificial Biofilm Induced Secondary Caries Model for In Vitro Studies." *Australian Dental Journal* 56 (1): 40–7. doi:10.1111/j.1834–7819.2010.01284.5.

He, Q., J. Shi, F. Chen, M. Zhu, and L. Zhang. 2010. "An Anticancer Drug Delivery System Based on Surfactant-Templated Mesoporous Silica Nanoparticles." *Biomaterials* 31 (12): 3335–46. doi:10.1016/j.biomaterials.2010.01.015.

He, Q., Y. Gao, L. Zhang, Z. Zhang, F. Gao, X. Ji, Y. Li, and J. Shi. 2011. "A pH-Responsive Mesoporous Silica Nanoparticles-Based Multi-Drug Delivery System for Overcoming Multi-Drug Resistance." *Biomaterials* 32 (30): 7711–20. doi:10.1016/j.biomaterials.2011.06.066.

Huang, B., D.G. Cvitkovitch, J.P. Santerre, and Y. Finer. 2018. "Biodegradation of Resin-Dentin Interfaces Is Dependent on the Restorative Material, Mode of Adhesion and a Combined Effects of Esterase and MMP Inhibition." *Dental Materials* 34 (9): 1253–62.

Huang, B., L. Sadeghinejad, O.I.A. Adebayo, D. Ma, Y. Xiao, W.L. Siqueira, D.G. Cvitkovitch, and Y. Finer. 2018. "Gene Expression and Protein Synthesis of Esterase from *Streptococcus mutans* Are Affected by Biodegradation By-Product from Methacrylate Resin Composites and Adhesives." *Acta Biomaterialia* 81: 158–68. doi:10.1016/j.actbio.2018.09.050.

Huang, B., W.L. Siqueira, D.G. Cvitkovitch, and Y. Finer. 2018. "Esterase from a Cariogenic Bacterium Hydrolyzes Dental Resins." *Acta Biomaterialia* 71: 330–8. doi:10.1016/j.actbio.2018.02.020.

Hübner, N.O., J. Siebert, and A. Kramer. 2010. "Octenidine Dihydrochloride, a Modern Antiseptic for Skin, Mucous Membranes and Wounds." *Skin Pharmacology and Physiology* 23 (5): 244–58. doi:10.1159/000314699.

Huo, Q., D.I. Margolese, and G.D. Stucky. 1996. "Surfactant Control of Phases in the Synthesis of Mesoporous Silica-Based Materials." *Chemistry of Materials* 8 (5): 1147–60. doi:10.1021/cm960137h.

Imazato, S., N. Ebi, Y. Takahashi, T. Kaneko, S. Ebisu, and R.R.B. Russell. 2003. "Antibacterial Activity of Bactericide-Immobilized Filler for Resin-Based Restoratives." *Biomaterials* 24 (20): 3605–9. doi:10.1016/S0142–9612(03)00217–5.

Izquierdo-Barba, I., Á. Martinez, A.L. Doadrio, J. Pérez-Pariente, and M. Vallet-Regí. 2005. "Release Evaluation of Drugs from Ordered Three-Dimensional Silica Structures." *European Journal of Pharmaceutical Sciences* 26 (5): 365–73. doi:10.1016/j.ejps.2005.06.009.

Izquierdo-Barba, I., M. Vallet-Regí, N. Kupferschmidt, O. Terasaki, A. Schmidtchen, and M. Malmsten. 2009. "Incorporation of Antimicrobial Compounds in Mesoporous Silica Film Monolith." *Biomaterials* 30 (29): 5729–36. doi:10.1016/j.biomaterials.2009.07.003.

Jaffer, F., Y. Finer, and J.P. Santerre. 2002. "Interactions between Resin Monomers and Commercial Composite Resins with Human Saliva Derived Esterases." *Biomaterials* 23 (7): 1707–19. doi:10.1016/S0142-9612(01)00298-8.

Jefferson, K.K. 2004. "What Drives Bacteria to Produce a Biofilm?" *FEMS Microbiology Letters* 236 (2): 163–73. doi:10.1016/j.femsle.2004.06.005.

Kadoma, Y. 2010. "Kinetic Polymerization Behavior of Fluorinated Monomers for Dental Use." *Dental Materials Journal* 29 (5): 602–8. doi:10.4012/dmj. 2010-054.

Kawabata, N., and M. Nishiguchi. 1988. "Antibacterial Activity of Soluble Pyridinium-Type Polymers." *Applied and Environmental Microbiology* 54 (10): 2532–5.

Kawai, K., and Y. Tsuchitani. 2000. "Effects of Resin Composite Components on Glucosyltransferase of Cariogenic Bacterium." *Journal of Biomedical Materials Research* 51 (1): 123–7. doi:10.1002/(SICI)1097-4636(200007)51:1<123::AID-JBM16>3.0.CO;2-7 [pii].

Kermanshahi, S., J.P. Santerre, D.G. Cvitkovitch, and Y. Finer. 2010. "Biodegradation of Resin-Dentin Interfaces Increases Bacterial Microleakage." *Journal of Dental Research* 89 (9): 996–1001. doi:10.1177/0022034510372885.

Khalichi, P., D.G. Cvitkovitch, and J.P. Santerre. 2004. "Effect of Composite Resin Biodegradation Products on Oral Streptococcal Growth." *Biomaterials* 25 (24): 5467–72. doi:10.1016/j.biomaterials.2003.12.056.

Khalichi, P., J. Singh, D.G. Cvitkovitch, and J.P. Santerre. 2009. "The Influence of Triethylene Glycol Derived from Dental Composite Resins on the Regulation of *Streptococcus mutans* Gene Expression." *Biomaterials* 30 (4): 452–9. doi:10.1016/j.biomaterials.2008.09.053.

Kinniment, S.L., J.W.T. Wimpenny, D. Adams, and P.D. Marsh. 1996. "Development of a Steady-State Oral Microbial Biofilm Community Using the Constant-Depth Film Fermenter." *Microbiology* 142 (3): 631–8. doi:10.1099/13500872-142-3-631.

Lee, J.H., A. El-Fiqi, J.K. Jo, D.A. Kim, S.C. Kim, S.K. Jun, H.W. Kim, and H.H. Lee. 2016. "Development of Long-Term Antimicrobial Poly(Methyl Methacrylate) by Incorporating Mesoporous Silica Nanocarriers." *Dental Materials* 32 (12): 1564–74. doi:10.1016/j.dental.2016.09.001.

Li, T., and R.G. Craig. 1996. "Synthesis of Fluorinated Bis-GMA and Its Use with Other Fluorinated Monomers to Formulate Hydrophobic Composites." *Journal of Oral Rehabilitation* 23 (3): 158–62. doi:10.1111/j.1365-2842.1996.tb01227.5.

Li, Y., C. Carrera, R. Chen, J. Li, P. Lenton, J.D. Rudney, R.S. Jones, C. Aparicio, and A. Fok. 2014. "Degradation in the Dentin-Composite Interface Subjected to Multi-Species Biofilm Challenges." *Acta Biomaterialia* 10 (1): 375–83. doi:10.1016/j.actbio.2013.08.034.

Limnell, T., H.A. Santos, E. Mäkilä, T. Heikkilä, J. Salonen, D.Y. Murzin, N. Kumar, T. Laaksonen, L. Peltonen, and J. Hirvonen. 2011. "Drug Delivery Formulations of Ordered and Nonordered Mesoporous Silica: Comparison of Three Drug Loading Methods." *Journal of Pharmaceutical Sciences* 100 (8): 3294–306. doi:10.1002/jps.22577.

Lin, J., S. Qiu, K. Lewis, and A.M. Klibanov. 2002. "Bactericidal Properties of Flat Surfaces and Nanoparticles Derivatized with Alkylated Polyethylenimines." *Biotechnology Progress* 18 (5): 1082–6. doi:10.1021/bp025597w.

Lin, J., S. Qiu, K. Lewis, and A.M. Klibanov. 2003. "Mechanism of Bactericidal and Fungicidal Activities of Textiles Covalently Modified with Alkylated Polyethylenimine." *Biotechnology and Bioengineering* 83 (2): 168–72. doi:10. 1002/bit.10651.

Liu, Y., L. Tjäderhane, L. Breschi, A. Mazzoni, N. Li, J. Mao, D.H. Pashley, and F.R. Tay. 2011. "Limitations in Bonding to Dentin and Experimental Strategies to Prevent Bond Degradation." *Journal of Dental Research* 90: 953–68. doi:10.1177/0022034510391799.

Lu, J., M. Liong, J.I. Zink, and F. Tamanoi. 2007. "Mesoporous Silica Nanoparticles as a Delivery System for Hydrophobic Anticancer Drugs." *Small* 3 (8): 1341–46. doi:10.1002/smll.200700005.

Mackert, J.R., and A. Berglund. 1997. "Mercury Exposure from Dental Amalgam Fillings: Absorbed Dose and the Potential for Adverse Health Effects." *Critical Reviews in Oral Biology & Medicine* 8 (4): 410–36. doi:10.117 7/10454411970080040401.

Marashdeh, M.Q., R. Gitalis, C. Levesque, and Y. Finer. 2018. "Enterococcus faecalis Hydrolyzes Dental Resin Composites and Adhesives." *Journal of Endodontics* 44 (4): 609–13. doi:10.1016/j.joen.2017.12.014.

Marsh, P.D. 1995. "The Role of Microbiology in Models of Dental Caries." *Advances in Dental Research* 9 (3): 244–54. doi:10.1177/08959374950090030901.

Martin-De Las Heras, S., A. Valenzuela, and C.M. Overall. 2000. "The Matrix Metalloproteinase Gelatinase A in Human Dentine." *Archives of Oral Biology* 45 (9): 757–65. doi:10.1016/S0003–9969(00)00052–2.

Matalon, S., E.I. Weiss, C. Gorfil, D. Noy, and H. Slutzky. 2009. "In Vitro Antibacterial Evaluation of Flowable Restorative Materials." *Quintessence International (Berlin, Germany: 1985)* 40 (4): 327–32.

Matalon, S., H. Slutzky, and E.I. Weiss. 2004. "Surface Antibacterial Properties of Packable Resin Composites: Part I." *Quintessence International* 35 (3): 189–93.

Mazzoni, A., F. Mannello, F.R. Tay, G.A.M. Tonti, S. Papa, G. Mazzotti, R. Di Lenarda, D.H. Pashley, and L. Breschi. 2007. "Zymographic Analysis and Characterization of MMP-2 and -9 Forms in Human Sound Dentin." *Journal of Dental Research* 86: 436–40. doi:10.1177/154405910708600509.

Mei, M., Q.-L. Li, C.-H. Chu, E. Chin-Man Lo, and L. Samaranayake. 2013. "Antibacterial Effects of Silver Diamine Fluoride on Multi-Species Cariogenic Biofilm on Caries." *Annals of Clinical Microbiology and Antimicrobials* 12 (1): 4. doi:10.1186/1476–0711–12–4.

Murray, P.E., L.J. Windsor, T.W. Smyth, A.A. Hafez, and C.F. Cox. 2002. "Analysis of Pulpal Reactions to Restorative Procedures, Materials, Pulp Capping, and Future Therapies." *Critical Reviews in Oral Biology & Medicine* 13 (6): 509–20. doi:10.1177/154411130201300607.

Nakabayashi, N., M. Nakamura, and N. Yasuda. 1991. "Hybrid Layer as a Dentin-Bonding Mechanism." *Journal of Esthetic and Restorative Dentistry* 3 (4): 133–8. doi:10.1111/j.1708–8240.1991.tb00985.5.

Nascimento, F.D., C.L. Minciotti, S. Geraldeli, M.R. Carrilho, D.H. Pashley, F.R. Tay, H.B. Nader, T. Salo, L. Tjäderhane, and I.L.S. Tersariol. 2011. "Cysteine Cathepsins in Human Carious Dentin." *Journal of Dental Research* 90 (4): 506–11. doi:10.1177/0022034510391906.

Netuschil, L., K.G. Vohrer, P. Riethe, Z. Kasioff, and M. Brecx. 1996. "Antibacterial Effects of Amalgam on Mutans Streptococci in an In Vitro Biofilm Test Procedure." *Acta Neurologica Belgica* 93 (2): 73–8.

Nicholson, J.W. 2007. "Polyacid-Modified Composite Resins ('Compomers') and Their Use in Clinical Dentistry." *Dental Materials* 23 (5): 615–22. doi:10.1016/j.dental.2006.05.002.

Nooney, R.I., D. Thirunavukkarasu, C. Yimei, R. Josephs, and A.E. Ostafin. 2002. "Synthesis of Nanoscale Mesoporous Silica Spheres with Controlled Particle Size." *Chemistry of Materials* 14 (11): 4721–8. doi:10.1021/cm0204371.

Osorio, R., M. Yamauti, E. Osorio, M.E. Ruiz-Requena, D. Pashley, F. Tay, and M. Toledano. 2011. "Effect of Dentin Etching and Chlorhexidine Application on Metalloproteinase-Mediated Collagen Degradation." *European Journal of Oral Sciences* 119 (1): 79–85. doi:10.1111/j.1600–0722.2010.00789.5.

Pereira-Cenci, T., S.C. Maximiliano, Z. Fedorowicz, and M. Azevedo. 2013. "Antibacterial Agents in Composite Restorations for the Prevention of Dental Caries." *Cochrane Database of Systematic Reviews*, 12. doi:10.1002/14651858.CD007819.pub3.

Popoff, D.A.V., T.T.A. Santa Rosa, R.C. Ferreira, C.S. Magalhães, A.N. Moreira, and I.A. Mjör. 2012. "Repair of Dimethacrylate-Based Composite Restorations by a Silorane-Based Composite: A One-Year Randomized Clinical Trial." *Operative Dentistry* 37 (5): E13–22. doi:10.2341/11–121–C.

Rohrer, N., A.F. Widmer, T. Waltimo, E.M. Kulik, R. Weiger, E. Filipuzzi-Jenny, and C. Walter. 2010. "Antimicrobial Efficacy of 3 Oral Antiseptics Containing Octenidine, Polyhexamethylene Biguanide, or Citroxx: Can Chlorhexidine Be Replaced?" *Infection Control & Hospital Epidemiology* 31 (07): 733–9. doi:10.1086/653822.

Rudney, J.D., R. Chen, P. Lenton, J. Li, Y. Li, R.S. Jones, C. Reilly, A.S. Fok, and C. Aparicio. 2012. "A Reproducible Oral Microcosm Biofilm Model for Testing Dental Materials." *Journal of Applied Microbiology* 113 (6): 1540–53. doi:10.1086/498510.Parasitic.

Sadeghinejad, L., D.G. Cvitkovitch, W.L. Siqueira, J. Merritt, J.P. Santerre, and Y. Finer. 2017. "Mechanistic, Genomic and Proteomic Study on the Effects of BisGMA-Derived Biodegradation Product on Cariogenic Bacteria." *Dental Materials* 33 (2): 175–90. doi:10.1016/j.dental.2016.11.007.

Sadeghinejad, L., D.G. Cvitkovitch, W.L. Siqueira, J.P. Santerre, and Y. Finer. 2016. "Triethylene Glycol Up-Regulates Virulence-Associated Genes and

Proteins in *Streptococcus mutans.*" *PLoS One* 11 (11): 1–22. doi:10.1371/-journal.pone.0165760.

Salli, K.M., and A.C. Ouwehand. 2015. "The Use of *In Vitro* Model Systems to Study Dental Biofilms Associated with Caries: A Short Review." *Journal of Oral Microbiology* 7 (1): 26149. doi:10.3402/jom.v7.26149.

Samuel, S.P., S. Li, I. Mukherjee, Y. Guo, A.C. Patel, G. Baran, and Y. Wei. 2009. "Mechanical Properties of Experimental Dental Composites Containing a Combination of Mesoporous and Nonporous Spherical Silica as Fillers." *Dental Materials* 25 (3): 296–301. doi:10.1016/j.dental.2008.07.012.

Sansone, C., J. Van Houte, K. Joshipura, R. Kent, and H.C. Margolis. 1993. "The Association of Mutans Streptococci and Non-Mutans Streptococci Capable of Acidogenesis at a Low pH with Dental Caries on Enamel and Root Surfaces." *Journal of Dental Research* 72 (2): 508–16. doi:10.117 7/00220345930720020701.

Santerre, J.P., L. Shajii, and B.W. Leung. 2001. "Relation of Dental Composite Formulations to Their Degradation and the Release of Hydrolyzed Polymeric-Resin-Derived Products." *Critical Reviews in Oral Biology & Medicine* 12 (2): 136–51. doi:10.1177/10454411010120020401.

Sayali, K., P. Sadichha, and S. Surekha. 2013. "Microbial Esterases: An Overview." *International Journal of Current Microbiology and Applied Sciences* 2 (7): 135–46.

Scaffa, P.M.C., C.M.P. Vidal, N. Barros, T.F. Gesteira, A.K. Carmona, L. Breschi, D.H. Pashley, et al. 2012. "Chlorhexidine Inhibits the Activity of Dental Cysteine Cathepsins." *Journal of Dental Research* 91 (4): 420–5. doi:10.1177/0022034511435329.

Serkies, K.B., R. Garcha, L.E. Tam, G.M. De Souza, and Y. Finer. 2016. "Matrix Metalloproteinase Inhibitor Modulates Esterase-Catalyzed Degradation of Resin–Dentin Interfaces." *Dental Materials* 32 (12): 1513–23. doi:10.1016/j. dental.2016.09.007.

Shaw, A.J., T. Carrick, and J.F. McCabe. 1998. "Fluoride Release from Glass-Ionomer and Compomer Restorative Materials: 6-Month Data." *Journal of Dentistry* 26 (4): 355–9. doi:10.1016/S0300–5712(97)00016–5.

Shokati, B., L.E. Tam, J.P. Santerre, and Y. Finer. 2010. "Effect of Salivary Esterase on the Integrity and Fracture Toughness of the Dentin-Resin Interface." *Journal of Biomedical Materials Research—Part B Applied Biomaterials* 94 (1): 230–7. doi:10.1002/jbm.b.31645.

Shu, M., L. Wong, J.H. Miller, and C.H. Sissons. 2000. "Development of Multi-Species Consortia Biofilms of Oral Bacteria as an Enamel and Root Caries Model System." *Archives of Oral Biology* 45 (1): 27–40. doi:10.1016/S0003–9969(99)00111–9.

Singh, J., P. Khalichi, D.G. Cvitkovitch, and J.P. Santerre. 2009. "Composite Resin Degradation Products from BisGMA Monomer Modulate the Expression of Genes Associated with Biofilm Formation and Other Virulence Factors in *Streptococcus mutans.*" *Journal of Biomedical Materials Research—Part A* 88 (2): 551–60. doi:10.1002/jbm.a.31879.

Siqueira, J.F., and H.P. Lopes. 1999. "Mechanisms of Antimicrobial Activity of Calcium Hydroxide: A Critical Review." *International Endodontic Journal* 32 (5): 361–9. doi:10.1046/j.1365-2591.1999.00275.5.

Smith, D.C. 1985. *Posterior Composite Resin Dental Restorative Materials*. The Netherlands: Peter Szulc Publishing Co.

Smith, E.G., and G.A. Spatafora. 2012. "Gene Regulation in *S. mutans*." *Journal of Dental Research* 91 (2): 133–41. doi:10.1177/0022034511415415.

Soncini, J.A., N.N. Maserejian, F. Trachtenberg, M. Tavares, and C. Hayes. 2007. "The Longevity of Amalgam versus Compomer/Composite Restorations in Posterior Primary and Permanent Teeth." *The Journal of the American Dental Association* 138 (6): 763–72. doi:10.14219/jada.archive.2007.0264.

Spencer, P., Q. Ye, J. Park, E.M. Topp, A. Misra, O. Marangos, Y. Wang, et al. 2010. "Adhesive/Dentin Interface: The Weak Link in the Composite Restoration." *Annals of Biomedical Engineering* 38 (6): 1989–2003. doi:10.1007/s10439-010-9969-6.

Stewart, C.A., J.H. Hong, B.D. Hatton, and Y. Finer. 2018. "Responsive Antimicrobial Dental Adhesive Based on Drug-Silica Co-Assembled Particles." *Acta Biomaterialia* 76: 283–94. doi:10.1016/j.actbio.2018.06.032.

Stewart, C.A., Y. Finer, and B.D. Hatton. 2018. "Drug Self-Assembly for Synthesis of Highly-Loaded Antimicrobial Drug-Silica Particles." *Scientific Reports* 8 (1): 1–12. doi:10.1038/s41598-018-19166-8.

Sulkala, M., T. Tervahartiala, T. Sorsa, M. Larmas, T. Salo, and L. Tjäderhane. 2007. "Matrix Metalloproteinase-8 (MMP-8) Is the Major Collagenase in Human Dentin." *Archives of Oral Biology* 52 (2): 121–7. doi:10.1016/j.archoralbio.2006.08.009.

Tang, G., H.K. Yip, T.W. Cutress, and L.P. Samaranayake. 2003. "Artificial Mouth Model Systems and Their Contribution to Caries Research: A Review." *Journal of Dentistry* 31 (3): 161–71. doi:10.1016/S0300-5712(03)00009-5.

Tay, F.R., and D.H. Pashley. 2003. "Have Dentin Adhesives Become Too Hydrophilic?" *Journal of the Canadian Dental Association* 69 (11): 726–31. doi:10.1016/S0109-5641(03)00110-6.

Tersariol, I.L., S. Geraldeli, C.L. Minciotti, F.D. Nascimento, V. Pääkkönen, M.T. Martins, M.R. Carrilho, et al. 2010. "Cysteine Cathepsins in Human Dentin-Pulp Complex." *Journal of Endodontics* 36 (3): 475–81. doi:10.1016/j.joen.2009.12.034.

Tiller, J.C., S.B. Lee, K. Lewis, and A.M. Klibanov. 2002. "Polymer Surfaces Derivatized with Poly(Vinyl-N-Hexylpyridinium) Kill Airborne and Waterborne Bacteria." *Biotechnology and Bioengineering* 79 (4): 465–71. doi:10.1002/bit.10299.

Tsumori, H., and H. Kuramitsu. 1997. "The Role of the *Streptococcus mutans* Glucosyltransferases in the Sucrose-Dependent Attachment to Smooth Surfaces: Essential Role of the GtfC Enzyme." *Oral Microbiology and Immunology* 12 (5): 274–80. doi:10.1111/j.1399-3025.1997.tb00391.5.

van Dijken, J.W.V., S. Kalfas, V. Litra, and A. Oliveby. 1997. "Fluoride and Mutans Streptococci Levels in Plaque on Aged Restorations of Resin-Modified Glass

Ionomer Cement, Compomer and Resin Composite." *Caries Research* 31 (5): 379–83. doi:10.1159/000262422.

Van Landuyt, K.L., J. Snauwaert, J.D. Munck, M. Peumans, Y. Yoshida, A. Poitevin, E. Coutinho, K. Suzuki, P. Lambrechts, and B.V. Meerbeek. 2007. "Systematic Review of the Chemical Composition of Contemporary Dental Adhesives." *Biomaterials* 28 (26): 3757–85. doi:10.1016/j.biomaterials.2007.04.044.

Verma, R.P., and C. Hansch. 2007. "Matrix Metalloproteinases (MMPs): Chemical-Biological Functions and (Q)SARs." *Bioorganic and Medicinal Chemistry* 15 (6): 2223–68. doi:10.1016/j.bmc.2007.01.011.

Wang, Y., and P. Spencer. 2003. "Hybridization Efficiency of the Adhesive/Dentin Interface with Wet Bonding." *Journal of Dental Research* 82 (2): 141–5. doi:1 0.1177/154405910308200213.

Wang, Y., P. Spencer, X. Yao, and B. Brenda. 2007. "Effect of Solvent Content on Resin Hybridization in Wet Dentin Bonding." *Journal of Biomedical Materials Research* 82 (4): 975–83. doi:10.1002/jbm.a.31232.Effect.

Welbury, R.R., A.J. Shaw, J.J. Murray, P.H. Gordon, and J.F. McCabe. 2000. "Clinical Evaluation of Paired Compomer and Glass Ionomer Restorations in Primary Molars: Final Results after 42 Months." *British Dental Journal* 189 (2): 93–7. doi:10.1038/sj.bdj.4800693.

Wicht, M.J., R. Haak, S. Kneist, and M.J. Noack. 2005. "A Triclosan-Containing Compomer Reduces *Lactobacillus* spp. Predominant in Advanced Carious Lesions." *Dental Materials* 21 (9): 831–6. doi:10.1016/j.dental.2004.09.011.

Wiegand, A., W. Buchalla, and T. Attin. 2007. "Review on Fluoride-Releasing Restorative Materials-Fluoride Release and Uptake Characteristics, Antibacterial Activity and Influence on Caries Formation." *Dental Materials* 23 (3): 343–62. doi:10.1016/j.dental.2006.01.022.

Yamamoto, E., and K. Kuroda. 2016. "Colloidal Mesoporous Silica Nanoparticles." *Bulletin of the Chemical Society of Japan* 89: 501–39. doi:10.1246/bcsj.20150420.

Yap, A., S. Tham, L. Zhu, and H. Lee. 2002. "Short-Term Fluoride Release from Various Aesthetic Restorative Materials." *Operative Dentistry* 27 (3): 259–65.

Yoshida, K., M. Tanagawa, and A. Mitsuru. 1999. "Characterization and Inhibitory Effect of Antibacterial Dental Resin Composites Incorporating Silver Supported Materials." *Journal of Biomedical Materials Research* 47: 516–22.

Zhang, J.F., R. Wu, Y. Fan, S. Liao, Y. Wang, Z.T. Wen, and X. Xu. 2014. "Antibacterial Dental Composites with Chlorhexidine and Mesoporous Silica." *Journal of Dental Research* 93 (12): 1283–9. doi:10.1177/0022034514555143.

Zhao, D., J. Feng, Q. Huo, N. Melosh, G.H. Fredrickson, B.F. Chmelka, and G.D. Stucky. 1998. "Triblock Copolymer Syntheses of Mesoporous Silica with Periodic 50 to 300 Angstrom Pores." *Science* 279 (5350): 548–52.

Zilberman, M., and J.J. Elsner. 2008. "Antibiotic-Eluting Medical Devices for Various Applications." *Journal of Controlled Release* 130 (3): 202–15. doi:10.1016/j.jconrel.2008.05.020.

6

Advances in the Development of Antibacterial Composites

Suping Wang, Haohao Wang, Xuedong Zhou, Jiyao Li, Libang He, and Lei Cheng
Sichuan University

Contents

6.1 Introduction

Modern resin-based dental composites have evolved significantly since early resin composites were first introduced in the late 1950s (Bowen 1963). Composite restorative materials stand out as one of the most successful cases in modern dental biomaterials research since they replace biological tissue in both appearance and function (Maktabi et al. 2018). Clinical evidence reported that composite restorations are currently used in 50% of all posterior direct restorations (Sadowsky 2006). Despite the widespread use of resin composites, numerous literature reviews stated that many disadvantages still remain in clinical applications, such as restoration fracture, recurrent caries, tooth sensitivity, side effects due to monomer release, etc., which significantly contribute to the failure of restorations (Balhaddad, Kansara et al. 2019; Chan et al. 2010).

Clinical studies suggest that nearly 70% of resin composite restorations were replacements for failed restorations (Murray et al. 2002), and replacement of failed restorations consumes 60% of the average dentist's practice time (NIDCR 13-DE-102). Recurrent or secondary caries at the tooth/composite interfaces was identified as one of the major reasons for composite restoration replacement, since the acid production or esterase from acidogenic bacteria could dissolve tooth minerals and degrade composite restorations and adhesive materials, leading to the decreased longevity of restorations (Delaviz et al. 2014; Bourbia et al. 2013; Kopperud et al. 2012). Therefore, restorative materials with antimicrobial functions are advantageous in order to prevent the spread of caries after completing the restoration, to inhibit recurrent decay and reduce restoration failure rates.

Resin composite restorations require the application of resin adhesives to bond efficiently to the tooth structure. Since Buonocore first described bonding acrylic resin to etched enamel in 1955 (Buonocore 1955), materials and techniques have developed to allow adhesive dentistry to become indispensable as it helped maintain a functional interface between composite restorations and tooth structure. With changing technologies, dental adhesives have evolved from no-etch to total-etch (fourth- and fifth-generation) to self-etch (sixth-, seventh-, and eighth-generation) systems (Sofan et al. 2017).

Over the past several decades, many studies have contributed to the improvements in bond strength, interface durability, and chemical compositions of bonding agents. However, many challenges still face adhesives in clinical applications such as residual bacteria continuing to reside in the prepared tooth cavity, as well as microleakage occurring once the bond between tooth/restoration degrades, and bacteria invade the tooth-restoration margins. These downfalls are the leading cause of secondary caries and pulp damage (Bourbia et al. 2013). Therefore, it is very important to develop a new generation of antibacterial adhesive that can effectively hinder bacterial invasion and combat biofilms and recurrent caries at the tooth-composite interfaces (Cocco et al. 2015). In addition to adhesives, primers with antibacterial efficacy are highly desirable, because primers directly contact the tooth structure and flow into dentinal tubules, and hence could serve as a carrier for antibacterial agents.

In this chapter, a brief review of the current stage and advanced development of antibacterial resin composites and adhesive systems in restorative dentistry is provided. Potential problems and possible future strategies for the development of dental materials with anti-biofilm properties will also be discussed.

6.2 Antibacterial Resin Composite

While adhesive systems containing antibacterial agents have been on the market for several years, studies on resin-based restorative composites with antibacterial activity are still at the stage of laboratory, although a number of studies have examined the antibacterial activity of commercial composites and their constituents since 1970s (Tobias et al. 1988; Orstavik and Hensten-Pettersen 1978; Imazato 2003; Kawai et al. 1988). The attempts to provide composites with antibacterial properties involve alterations to the resin components and filler components, and the trials can be subsequently classified into two groups based on the release profile of antibacterial components: agent-releasing or non-agent-releasing materials (Imazato 2003); the same situation applied to adhesive systems (to be mentioned in the following part).

Developing novel antibacterial composites in modern dentistry requires balancing a number of requirements (Maas et al. 2017). The primary requirements lie in the functional antibacterial capability that could cover a broad bacterial spectrum, optimize microorganisms' structure, and maintain long-lasting effects. At the same time, good biocompatibility without eliciting any undesirable local or systemic effects is required. Also, it is very important that incorporation of antibacterial agents does not compromise the mechanical, physical, or aesthetic properties of the restorative materials. In addition, the ideal antibacterial composites would not induce drug resistance in bacteria after long-term clinical service (Zhang et al. 2018; Ibrahim et al. 2018). To fulfill the above-mentioned properties, large numbers of investigations focused on the antibacterial improvements of current resin composites by incorporating different kinds of antimicrobial agents.

6.2.1 Antibacterial Efficacy Evaluation

To inhibit oral biofilm, many traditional antimicrobial agents such as silver (Ag), zinc oxide (ZnO) particles, and chlorhexidine (CHX) have been incorporated into a wide range of dental material applications (Niu et al. 2010; Noronha et al. 2017; Kim and Shin 2013). With broad-spectrum antibacterial activity, the addition of CHX has been proven to increase the antibacterial activity of dental composites (Leung et al. 2005; Jedrychowski et al. 1983), while such approach may suffer from the short-lived effectiveness with the release of CHX.

Another important antibacterial agent is Ag, which could inactivate the vital enzymes of bacteria, causing DNA replication failure and leading to cell death (Rai et al. 2009). Other studies synthesized antibacterial resins based on the release of Ag displayed long-lasting inhibitory effect against *Streptococcus mutans* and favorable mechanical properties (Yoshida et al. 1999). Also, new nanotechnology has brought out advance than traditional antibacterial agents, for example, nanoparticulate silver (NAg) become more favorable ones, because of their small particle size and the associated high specific surface area, which yielded superior bactericidal activity (Cheng, Weir, Xu et al. 2012).

Similarly, incorporation of ZnO nanoparticles has been found to impart dental composites with antibacterial activity because they may produce different active oxygen species that inhibit the growth of viable microbes (Tavassoli Hojati et al. 2013). However, the resins containing soluble antibacterial agents showed a release pattern in which a large amount of the agent leached out of mass within a few days and resulted in a dramatic decrease in the concentration (Wilson and Wilson 1993).

Compared to these releasing antibacterial agents reported, non-releasing monomers seem to be more advantageous. The use of antibacterial monomers is suggested to overcome the limitation associated with released antibacterial fillers and the concern related to the short-term effects of these fillers, which may affect the long-term effect of such materials. Antibacterial monomers can polymerize with the other incorporated monomers providing a long-term contact-killing mechanism against caries-related pathogens (Zhang et al. 2018). To inhibit caries, antibacterial resin composites containing quaternary ammonium salts (QAMs) were developed, including 12-methacryloyloxydodecyl pyridinium bromide (MDPB), quaternary ammonium dimethacrylate (QADM) (Cheng, Weir, Zhang et al. 2012), quaternary ammonium polyethyleneimine (QPEI) (Shvero et al. 2015), dimethylaminododecyl methacrylate (DMADDM) (Zhou, Weir et al. 2013), dimethylaminohexadecyl methacrylate (DMAHDM) (Balhaddad, Ibrahim et al. 2019; Zhang et al. 2017), and so on.

The anti-biofilm mechanism of QAMs is that quaternary ammonium can lead to bacterial lysis by adhering to the cell membrane to produce cytoplasmic leakage (Beyth et al. 2006; Namba et al. 2009). Novel resin composites with QAMs were demonstrated to effectively hinder bacterial and biofilm growth, in that QAMs are covalently bonded with the resin polymer structure and immobilized in the resin, exerting contact inhibition against adherent bacteria (Imazato et al. 2012; Liu et al. 2016). Quaternary ammonium polyethyleneimine (QPEI) nanoparticles immobilized in resin-based materials were proven to have a strong antibacterial activity upon contact, without leaching-out of the nanoparticles and without compromising the mechanical properties (Beyth et al. 2006). QPEI incorporation resulted in 70% viable bacterial reduction in vivo. Furanone-containing composites revealed an increased antibacterial function against *S. mutans* viability when 5%–30% of furanone derivatives were added (Weng et al. 2012).

Novel QAMs with a carbon chain length (CL) of 3–18 were synthesized and incorporated into an amorphous calcium phosphate (NACP) nano-composite to simultaneously endow the material with antibacterial and remineralization capabilities, where the results showed that increasing the CL reduced the metabolic activity and acid production of biofilms without compromising the mechanical properties (Zhou, Li et al. 2013).

Another study has attempted to develop a resin with a cationic bactericide, cetylpyridinium chloride (CPC), which was able to desorb and readsorb CPC by the ion-exchange mechanism and could show an inhibitory effect on *S. mutans* growth and plaque formation (Ehara et al. 2000). Among them, DMAHDM resin composite could not only effectively inhibit multi-species biofilm growth and cariogenic virulence, and decrease the proportion of *S. mutans* in multi-species biofilm, but also promote the biofilm bacterial composition to be a healthy one, thus further enhancing the anti-caries effects of resin composite (Wang, Wang et al. 2019).

Different from the synthetic QAMs with a double bond used for the polymerization with a resin matrix, recently, one new antibacterial agent derived deep eutectic solvent (DES) comprising benzalkonium chloride (BC) and acrylic acid (AA) was incorporated into a dental resin composite to develop an antibacterial dental composite, in which the vinyl group of AA contributes to the polymerization of DES into the composite matrix through covalent bonding, and the hydrogen bonding of BC is responsible for imparting antibacterial activity (Wang, Dong et al. 2017).

6.2.2 Mechanical Behavior Investigation

Mechanical properties are closely related to the service life of dental composite restorations; thus, dental composites that can inhibit cariogenic biofilms while maintaining their mechanical properties are highly desirable. While as exogenous additions, antibacterial agents such as CHX and silver may have an impact on materials' polymerization shrinkage and the degree of conversion, so evaluations of related physical and mechanical properties are always included during the development of novel antibacterial dental materials. It was reported that the modification of resin composite with small amounts of ZnO microparticles significantly inhibited the *S. mutans* growth on resin surface without significant alterations of its mechanical strength (Dias et al. 2017).

While studies showed that the dissolution of CHX from dental composites could lead to the formation of porous surface and decreased mechanical strength of the composites. Taken this into consideration, some attempts have been made to maintain the mechanical strength, surface esthetics, and surface integrity of the material; for example, a new type of dental composite was created with CHX and mesoporous silica nanoparticles (MSNs), which could be the reservoirs to encapsulate or recharge CHX, largely retain mechanical properties, and have smooth surfaces (Zhang, Wu et al. 2014).

Compared to the disadvantages of releasing antibacterial agents incorporated in resin composites, the QAMs antibacterial monomer is copolymerized with the resin matrix by forming a covalent bond with the polymer network, and therefore, this copolymerization and immobilization method imparts a durable antibacterial capability to the dental resin without influencing the mechanical properties. For example, a series of antibacterial quaternary ammonium methacrylate monomers with different substituted alkyl chain lengths (from 10 to 18) were incorporated into the commonly used dental resin as immobilized antibacterial agents, with the results showing that there was no significant difference in double-bond conversion (DC), flexural strength (FS), and elastic modulus (EM), between resins with and without 5 wt.% QAM, and the substituted alkyl chain lengths of QAM had no influence on DC, FS, and EM (He et al. 2013). Another study reported that bioactive NACP composite containing QADM and NAg not only possessed long-lasting, strong antibacterial capability up to one year but could also maintain flexural strength and elastic modulus that matched those of a commercial control composite after 12 months of water-aging (Cheng et al. 2016).

6.2.3 Biocompatibility Assessment

The development of antibacterial dental materials must first satisfy the basic requirements of being safe, or safer and more effective than the existing products, without potential hazards to patient safety and public care. The application of CHX as chemical agents for mouthwashes or dentifrices has been accepted for many years. Thus, CHX-containing resins could keep good biocompatibility. Similarly, silver compounds have been used in dentistry for more than a century, and silver-impregnated restorative materials showed obviously antibacterial effects along with accepted biocompatibility (Peng et al. 2012). Another nontoxic, biocompatible, biodegradable, and naturally acquired antibacterial, chitosan, has been incorporated into resin composites for antibacterial properties and maintained inside the materials because of its insolubility in water without any toxicity risk (Kim and Shin 2013; Thaya et al. 2016).

As for the biocompatibility evaluation of QAMs modified dental materials, in vivo study investigated the influences of DMADDM- and NACP-containing composites on the dentin-pulp complex using a rat model, showing that the antibacterial and remineralizing nanocomposite and adhesive were more biocompatible exhibiting milder pulpal inflammation and much greater tertiary dentin formation than traditional adhesive and composite (Li, Wang et al. 2014). So far, the novel biocompatible dental materials with antibacterial potency are promising for future clinical applications.

6.2.4 Multifunctional Strategy

The development of a versatile strategy for antibacterial dental materials is of great scientific interest and practical significance. The previous study has reported that the dual addition of MDPB and NAg to primer imparted strong antibacterial activity, exerting MDPB-induced contact inhibition against adherent bacteria and long-distance antibacterial effects due to the sustained silver ion release, without compromising the dentin bond strength and adverse effects on cytotoxicity when compared to the commercial primer (Zhang, Cheng et al. 2013).

In another study, universal dentine adhesive containing antibacterial quaternary ammonium silanes and quaternary ammonium methacryloxy silane (QAMS) displayed dual antibacterial activity. The approach includes release-killing by the release of non-copolymerizable quaternary ammonium silane species and contact-killing by QAMS that are copolymerized with adhesive resin comonomers, and the contact-killing was retained after three-month water-aging treatment (Zhang, Luo et al. 2014). The reported DMADDM- and NAg-containing bonding agent could substantially reduce biofilm growth even with salivary pellicle coating on surfaces, indicating a promising usage in a saliva-rich environment (Li, Weir et al. 2014).

In a more recent investigation, a resin composite restoration containing 3% DMAHDM and 20% NACP was found to inhibit the growth and activities of multi-species saliva-derived biofilm (Figure 6.1) (Al-Dulaijan

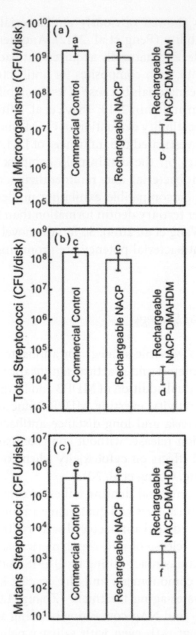

Figure 6.1 Colony-forming units (CFUs) of the multi-species biofilm were reduced in resin composites containing NACP and DMAHDM. The amount of reduction ranged between 3 and 4 log. (Adapted from Al-Dulaijan et al. (2018), with permission from © 2019 Elsevier.)

et al. 2018). The amount of reduction against total microorganisms, total *Streptococcus*, and S. *mutans* ranged between 3 and 4 log. This combination of DMAHDM and NACP also reduced the metabolic activities and lactic acid production, as well as the volume of viable microorganisms grown over the resin composite surface (Figure 6.2).

The main drawback of QAMs antibacterial monomers including DMAHDM is related to the ability of salivary protein coating to diminish the killing capability of QAMs as the contact between the resin composite and oral microorganisms could be reduced (Cheng et al. 2017). To

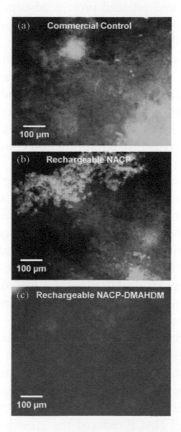

Figure 6.2 Live/dead staining illustrating 48 h biofilm grown over resin composite surfaces. (a and b) More viable microorganisms were found over the control and 20% NACP resin composites. (c) When the DMAHDM was added to the NACP in the formulation, more dead microorganisms and less biofilms were observed. (Adapted from Al-Dulaijan et al. (2018), with permission from © 2019 Elsevier.)

overcome this drawback, the incorporation of a protein-repellant agent into resin composites has been attempted.

The protein coating is an important stage for bacterial attachment and colonization. Thus, reducing the amount of protein coating over the resin composite surface may reduce the risk of dental caries. 2-Methacryloyloxyethyl phosphorylcholine (MPC) as a protein-repellant agent has been incorporated into resin composite formulation to reduce the bacterial attachment and enhance the contact-killing of QAMs. Incorporation of 0.75%, 1.5%, 2.25%, 3%, 4.5%, and 6% of MPC reveals that 3% of MPC has the greatest antibacterial function and reduced protein adsorption without compromising the mechanical properties of the resin composite compared to the other mass fractions (Zhang, Chen et al. 2015).

Combining MPC with DMAHDM in resin composite formulation demonstrated a better antibacterial function and a less amount of protein adsorption compared to DMAHDM alone and control. When only DMAHDM was incorporated into resin composites, the amount of protein adsorption was almost similar to control resin composites, while MPC alone revealed less antibacterial function compared to DMAHDM resin composites (Figure 6.3).

Combining MPC and DMAHDM in one formulation resulted in a resin composite with less protein adsorption and greater antibacterial function (Cao et al. 2018). Combining MPC and DMAHDM also resulted in lower biofilm growth of multi-species periodontal pathogens (Wang, Xie et al. 2019). In dental adhesives, the incorporation of agents such as CHX, fluoride, and silver was attempted (Cocco et al. 2015). The actions of these antibacterial monomers in dental adhesives include the suppression of caries-related pathogens' growth and the reduction of demineralization around orthodontic brackets (Cocco et al. 2015).

A novel adhesive with MPC, DMAHDM, and nanoparticles of NACP was developed for the prevention of tooth root caries and secondary caries, and the adhesive was showed to possess a combination of protein-repellent (by MPC), antibacterial (by DMAHDM), and remineralization (by NACP) capabilities (Zhang, Melo et al. 2015). The multifunctional combination of DMAHDM, MPC, and NACP reduced the growth of total microorganisms, total *Lactobacillus*, and *S. mutans* by around 4 log.

DMAHDM is also able to reduce the colony-forming unit (CFU) and polysaccharide production of the main periodontal and endodontic pathogens including *Porphyromonas gingivalis*, *Prevotella intermedia*, *Aggregatibacter actinomycetemcomitans*, *Fusobacterium nucleatum*, and *Enterococcus faecalis* (Xiao et al. 2019; Wang et al. 2016; Baras, Sun et al. 2019; Baras, Wang et al. 2019). In Figure 6.4, a novel bioactive resin

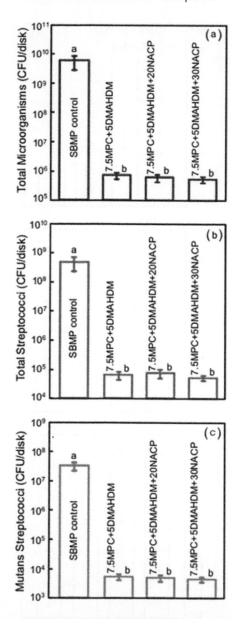

Figure 6.3 Dental adhesives containing 7.5% MPC and 5% DMAGDM were found effective in reducing the CFUs of total microorganisms (a), total *Lactobacillus* (b), and S. *mutans* (c) by around 4 log. Values with dissimilar letters are significantly different from each other ($p < 0.05$). (Adapted from Zhang, Melo et al. (2015), with permission from © 2019 Elsevier.)

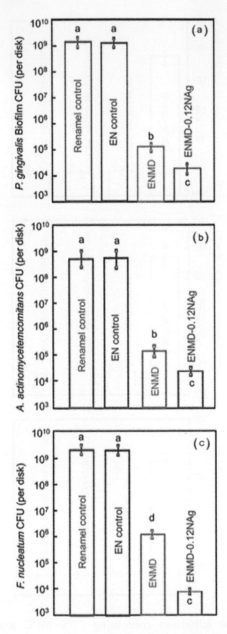

Figure 6.4 CFUs of the periodontal pathogens, *P. gingivalis* (a), *A. actinomycetemcomitans* (b), and *F. nucleatum* (c) were reduced by around 3–5 log when DMAHDM, MCP, and NACP were combined in the resin composite formulation. Values with dissimilar letters are significantly different from each other ($p < 0.05$). (Adapted from Xiao et al. (2019), with permission from © 2019 Elsevier.)

composite containing 30% NACP, 3% DMAHDM, and 3% MPC (ENMD) combined with silver nanoparticles was able to decrease the biofilm growth of *P. gingivalis, A. actinomycetemcomitans*, and *F. nucleatum* by around 3–5 log compared to the control resin composite.

6.3 Bioactivity in Commercially Available Materials for Caries Control

The construction of resin-based bioactive materials has increased the thoughts of applying the concept to other restorative materials such as pit and fissure sealants, and denture-base materials. The purpose of using pit and fissure sealants is to act as a physical barrier against food accumulation, especially at food-stagnating areas such as occlusal pits and fissures. The primary two materials used as sealants are glass ionomer and resin composite.

The advantages of glass ionomer sealant are related to the fluoride release, but the retention rate of glass ionomer sealants is found lower compared to resin composite sealants. On the other side, the retention rate of resin composite sealant is higher, but it is associated with more plaque accumulation and lack of bioactivity, making the sealant at risk of having microleakage and caries (Yu et al. 2016; Simonsen and Neal 2011). Therefore, introducing bioactivity in resin-based sealants can overcome the limitations that are found in conventional resin composite. 2-Methacryloxylethyl dodecyl methyl ammonium bromide (MAE-DB), an antibacterial monomer, was incorporated into resin composite formulation. MAE-DB reduced the activities of *S. mutans*, which may provide promising results about the ability of MAE-DB to diminish the risk of caries around the sealants (Yu et al. 2016). Methacryloxylethyl cetyl dimethyl ammonium chloride (DMAE-CB) containing sealant was found effective in reducing the growth of *S. mutans* without affecting the mechanical properties and the degree of conversion (Li et al. 2011).

Combining DMAHDM and NACP fillers in sealant formulation was attempted. The results showed that the DMAHDM-NACP sealant could reduce the growth and activities of *S. mutans*. Thinner *S. mutans* biofilm was observed over the sealant surface compared to the control samples where the *S. mutans* biofilm was reported as thick and more viable (Ibrahim, Ibrahim, Balhaddad, Weir, Lin et al. 2019; Ibrahim, Ibrahim, Balhaddad, Weir, Oates et al. 2019).

The adhesion of oral microorganisms to denture base materials are related to many oral health problems such as oral stomatitis, candidiasis, and dental caries in teeth-supported dentures. Acrylic polymethyl methacrylate resin

(PMMA) is considered one of the most commonly used materials as a denture base. Unfortunately, PMMA is highly susceptible to microbial adhesion and infiltration (Buergers et al. 2007).

Therefore, approaches with the capabilities to reduce the microbial complication in relation to denture materials are highly needed. It was found that phosphate incorporation into PMMA reduced the adhesion of *Candida albicans*. It was hypothesized that the phosphate content could decrease the contact angle and increase the hydrophilicity of the materials to reduce the fungal adhesion (Buergers et al. 2007; Dhir et al. 2007). Also, incorporating 10% of methacrylic acidic monomer reduces *C. albicans* adhesion (Park et al. 2003).

The utilization of MDPD and methacryloyloxy undecylpyridinium bromide (MUPB) monomers was found effective in reducing the growth of *S. mutans* and *C. albicans* over the denture base. Another monomer, 2-tert-butylaminoethyl methacrylate (TBAEMA), can effectively interact with the bacterial cell membrane via the charged amino groups causing cell lysis (Sivakumar et al. 2014). Denture base materials that contain silver, silver zeolites, or titanium dioxide nanoparticles showed antibacterial actions against several oral species (Sivakumar et al. 2014).

More recently, incorporating DMADDM into the acrylic resin denture base was effective in reducing the virulence factors of *C. albicans*. DMADDM belongs to QAM family with a positive charge surface that can interrupt the microbial cell wall. The use of 3.3% DMADDM in acrylic resin effectively reduced the growth and metabolic activities of *C. albicans* without compromising the biocompatibility of the material (Zhang et al. 2016).

6.4 Challenges of Antibacterial Products

In vitro trials on antibacterial modification of resin composite or adhesive system have showed great promise and advantages in inhibiting invading bacteria after the placement of restoration as well as residual bacteria in the cavity. However, these potential benefits should also be balanced against the risks. The main concern is on the potential oral hazards by these antibacterial agents in clinical applications. Although the lab data so far indicates that the toxicity is low, the oral reactions remain to be assessed. Specific researches need to done to see whether oral salivary or by-products from oral biofilm might weaken the anti-biofilm ability of antibacterial ingredients in dental materials. Furthermore, the transferred investigation from laboratory to clinical is needed to undergo.

Although antibacterial dental materials containing QAMs have promising clinical benefits, little attention has been paid to the potential drug resistance of oral microorganisms induced by QAMs. How to make rational use of antibacterial products, avoiding the development of drug resistance, is also a question to be considered. To date, there has been no report on any in vivo study on oral bacterial resistance to QAMs. A literature search revealed only two in vitro reports on the drug resistance of QAMs against oral microbes. One report showed that *Enterococcus faecalis* and *S. mutans* did not develop resistance to MDPB with ten repeated exposures (Kitagawa et al. 2016). The new study showed that eight common oral bacteria species did not develop resistance to DMAHDM, and only *Streptococcus gordonii* developed a mild resistance to DMADDM with ten passages (Wang, Wang et al. 2017).

6.5 Conclusions

There appears to be many potential benefits to restorative dentistry by developing new generations of antibacterial dental materials. The novel dental resin materials with antibacterial functions, like wearing protective clothing, could enhance their resistance ability to biofilm challenge in the oral environment. The antibacterial improvements of adhesive may reduce the bacterial invasion along with the tooth/restoration interface or penetration into dentin tubes, thus acting as a barrier to protect the dental pulp. Therefore, it's worthy of continuing attempts to develop bio-functional composites or adhesive with antibacterial and other therapeutic effects, which would undoubtedly contribute to preventing secondary caries and promote oral health.

References

Al-Dulaijan, Y. A., L. Cheng, M. D. Weir, M. A. S. Melo, H. Liu, T. W. Oates, L. Wang, and H. H. K. Xu. 2018. "Novel Rechargeable Calcium Phosphate Nanocomposite with Antibacterial Activity to Suppress Biofilm Acids and Dental Caries." *Journal of Dentistry* 72: 44–52. https://doi.org/10.1016/j.jdent.2018.03.003.

Balhaddad, A. A., A. A. Kansara, D. Hidan, M. D. Weir, H. H. K. Xu, and M. A. S. Melo. 2019. "Toward Dental Caries: Exploring Nanoparticle-Based Platforms and Calcium Phosphate Compounds for Dental Restorative

Materials." *Bioactive Materials* 4 (1): 43–55. https://doi.org/10.1016/j .bioactmat.2018.12.002.

Balhaddad, A. A., M. Ibrahim, M. D. Weir, H. H. K. Xu, and M. A. S. Melo. 2019. "Anti-Biofilm and Mechanically Stable Bioactive Composite for Root Caries Restorations." Dental Materials, Abstracts of the Academy of Dental Materials Annual Meeting, 02–05 October 2019—Jackson Hole, USA, 35 (January): e4–5. https://doi.org/10.1016/j.dental.2019.08.008.

Baras, B. H., J. Sun, M. A. S. Melo, F. R. Tay, T. W. Oates, K. Zhang, M. D. Weir, and H. H. K. Xu. 2019. "Novel Root Canal Sealer with Dimethylaminohexadecyl Methacrylate, Nano-Silver and Nano-Calcium Phosphate to Kill Bacteria Inside Root Dentin and Increase Dentin Hardness." *Dental Materials: Official Publication of the Academy of Dental Materials* 35 (10): 1479–89. https://doi.org/10.1016/j.dental.2019.07.014.

Baras, B.H., S. Wang, M. A. S. Melo, F. Tay, A. F. Fouad, D. D. Arola, M. D. Weir, and H. H. K. Xu. 2019. "Novel Bioactive Root Canal Sealer with Antibiofilm and Remineralization Properties." *Journal of Dentistry* 83: 67–76. https://doi .org/10.1016/j.jdent.2019.02.006.

Beyth, N., I. Yudovin-Farber, R. Bahir, A. J. Domb, and E. I. Weiss. 2006. "Antibacterial Activity of Dental Composites Containing Quaternary Ammonium Polyethylenimine Nanoparticles against Streptococcus Mutans." *Biomaterials* 27 (21): 3995–4002. https://doi.org/10.1016/j.biomaterials.2006 .03.003.

Bourbia, M., D. Ma, D. G. Cvitkovitch, J. P. Santerre, and Y. Finer. 2013. "Cariogenic Bacteria Degrade Dental Resin Composites and Adhesives." *Journal of Dental Research* 92 (11): 989–94. https://doi.org/10.1177/0022034513504436.

Bowen, R. L. 1963. "Properties of a Silica-Reinforced Polymer for Dental Restorations." *Journal of the American Dental Association (1939)* 66 (January): 57–64. https://doi.org/10.14219/jada.archive.1963.0010.

Buergers, R., M. Rosentritt, and G. Handel. 2007. "Bacterial Adhesion of Streptococcus Mutans to Provisional Fixed Prosthodontic Material." *The Journal of Prosthetic Dentistry* 98 (6): 461–69. https://doi.org/10.1016/S0022 –3913(07)60146–2.

Buonocore, M. G. 1955. "A Simple Method of Increasing the Adhesion of Acrylic Filling Materials to Enamel Surfaces." *Journal of Dental Research* 34 (6): 849–53. https://doi.org/10.1177/00220345550340060801.

Cao, L., X. Xie, B. Wang, M. D. Weir, T. W. Oates, H. H. K. Xu, N. Zhang, and Y. Bai. 2018. "Protein-Repellent and Antibacterial Effects of a Novel Polymethyl Methacrylate Resin." *Journal of Dentistry* 79: 39–45. https://doi .org/10.1016/j.jdent.2018.09.007.

Chan, K. H. S., Y. Mai, H. Kim, K. C. T. Tong, D. Ng, and J. C. M. Hsiao. 2010. "Review: Resin Composite Filling." *Materials* 3 (2): 1228–43. https://doi.org /10.3390/ma3021228.

Cheng, L., K. Zhang, C.-C. Zhou, M. D. Weir, X.-D. Zhou, and H. H. K. Xu. 2016. "One-Year Water-Ageing of Calcium Phosphate Composite Containing

Nano-Silver and Quaternary Ammonium to Inhibit Biofilms." *International Journal of Oral Science* 8 (3): 172–81. https://doi.org/10.1038/ijos.2016.13.

Cheng, L., K. Zhang, N. Zhang, M. A. S. Melo, M. D. Weir, X. D. Zhou, Y. X. Bai, M. A. Reynolds, and H. H. K. Xu. 2017. "Developing a New Generation of Antimicrobial and Bioactive Dental Resins." *Journal of Dental Research* 96 (8): 855–63. https://doi.org/10.1177/0022034517709739.

Cheng, L., M. D. Weir, H. H. K. Xu, J. M. Antonucci, N. J. Lin, S. Lin-Gibson, S. M. Xu, and X. Zhou. 2012. "Effect of Amorphous Calcium Phosphate and Silver Nanocomposites on Dental Plaque Microcosm Biofilms." *Journal of Biomedical Materials Research. Part B, Applied Biomaterials* 100 (5): 1378–86. https://doi.org/10.1002/jbm.b.32709.

Cheng, L., M. D. Weir, K. Zhang, E. J. Wu, S. M. Xu, X. Zhou, and H. H. K. Xu. 2012. "Dental Plaque Microcosm Biofilm Behavior on Calcium Phosphate Nanocomposite with Quaternary Ammonium." *Dental Materials: Official Publication of the Academy of Dental Materials* 28 (8): 853–62. https://doi.org/10.1016/j.dental.2012.04.024.

Cocco, A. R., W. L. de Oliveira da Rosa, A. F. da Silva, R. G. Lund, and E. Piva. 2015. "A Systematic Review About Antibacterial Monomers Used in Dental Adhesive Systems: Current Status and Further Prospects." *Dental Materials: Official Publication of the Academy of Dental Materials* 31 (11): 1345–62. https://doi.org/10.1016/j.dental.2015.08.155.

Delaviz, Y., Y. Finer, and J. P. Santerre. 2014. "Biodegradation of Resin Composites and Adhesives by Oral Bacteria and Saliva: A Rationale for New Material Designs That Consider the Clinical Environment and Treatment Challenges." *Dental Materials: Official Publication of the Academy of Dental Materials* 30 (1): 16–32. https://doi.org/10.1016/j.dental.2013.08.201.

Dhir, G., D. W. Berzins, V. B. Dhuru, A. Raj Periathamby, and A. Dentino. 2007. "Physical Properties of Denture Base Resins Potentially Resistant to Candida Adhesion." *Journal of Prosthodontics: Official Journal of the American College of Prosthodontists* 16 (6): 465–72. https://doi.org/10.1111/j.1532-849X.2007.00219.x.

Dias, H. B., M. I. B. Bernardi, M. A. Dos Santos Ramos, T. C. Trevisan, T. M. Bauab, A. C. Hernandes, and A. N. de Souza Rastelli. 2017. "Zinc Oxide 3D Microstructures as an Antimicrobial Filler Content for Composite Resins." *Microscopy Research and Technique* 80 (6): 634–43. https://doi.org/10.1002/jemt.22840.

Ehara, A., M. Torii, S. Imazato, and S. Ebisu. 2000. "Antibacterial Activities and Release Kinetics of a Newly Developed Recoverable Controlled Agent-Release System." *Journal of Dental Research* 79 (3): 824–28. https://doi.org/10.1177/00220345000790030701.

He, J., E. Söderling, P. K. Vallittu, and L. V. J. Lassila. 2013. "Investigation of Double Bond Conversion, Mechanical Properties, and Antibacterial Activity of Dental Resins with Different Alkyl Chain Length Quaternary Ammonium Methacrylate Monomers (QAM)." *Journal of Biomaterials Science. Polymer Edition* 24 (5): 565–73. https://doi.org/10.1080/09205063.2012.699709.

Ibrahim, M. S., A. S. Ibrahim, A. A. Balhaddad, M. D. Weir, N. J. Lin, F. R. Tay, T. W. Oates, H. H. K. Xu, and M. A. S. Melo. 2019. "A Novel Dental Sealant Containing Dimethylaminohexadecyl Methacrylate Suppresses the Cariogenic Pathogenicity of Streptococcus Mutans Biofilms." *International Journal of Molecular Sciences* 20 (14). https://doi.org/10.3390/ijms20143491.

Ibrahim, M. S., A. S. Ibrahim, A. A. Balhaddad, M. D. Weir, T. W. Oates, H. H. K. Xu, and M. A. S. Melo. 2019. "Rechargeable Dual Function Dental Sealant against Cariogencity of Streptococcus Mutans." Dental Materials, Abstracts of the Academy of Dental Materials Annual Meeting, 02–05 October 2019— Jackson Hole, USA, 35 (January): e45. https://doi.org/10.1016/j.dental.2019.08.091.

Ibrahim, M. S., F. D. AlQarni, Y. A. Al-Dulaijan, M. D. Weir, T. W. Oates, H. H. K. Xu, and M. A. S. Melo. 2018. "Tuning Nano-Amorphous Calcium Phosphate Content in Novel Rechargeable Antibacterial Dental Sealant." *Materials (Basel, Switzerland)* 11 (9). https://doi.org/10.3390/ma11091544.

Imazato, S. 2003. "Antibacterial Properties of Resin Composites and Dentin Bonding Systems." *Dental Materials: Official Publication of the Academy of Dental Materials* 19 (6): 449–57. https://doi.org/10.1016/s0109-5641(02)00102-1.

Imazato, S., J.-H. Chen, S. Ma, N. Izutani, and F. Li. 2012. "Antibacterial Resin Monomers Based on Quaternary Ammonium and Their Benefits in Restorative Dentistry." *Japanese Dental Science Review* 48 (2): 115–25. https://doi.org/10.1016/j.jdsr.2012.02.003.

Jedrychowski, J. R., A. A. Caputo, and S. Kerper. 1983. "Antibacterial and Mechanical Properties of Restorative Materials Combined with Chlorhexidines." *Journal of Oral Rehabilitation* 10 (5): 373–81. https://doi.org/10.1111/j.1365-2842.1983.tb00133.x.

Kawai, K., M. Torii, and Y. Tuschitani. 1988. "Effect of Resin Components on the Growth of Streptococcus Mutans." *The Journal of Osaka University Dental School* 28 (December): 161–70.

Kim, J.-S., and D.-H. Shin. 2013. "Inhibitory Effect on Streptococcus Mutans and Mechanical Properties of the Chitosan Containing Composite Resin." *Restorative Dentistry & Endodontics* 38 (1): 36–42. https://doi.org/10.5395/rde.2013.38.1.36.

Kitagawa, H., N. Izutani, R. Kitagawa, H. Maezono, M. Yamaguchi, and S. Imazato. 2016. "Evolution of Resistance to Cationic Biocides in Streptococcus Mutans and Enterococcus Faecalis." *Journal of Dentistry* 47 (April): 18–22. https://doi.org/10.1016/j.jdent.2016.02.008.

Kopperud, S. E., A. B. Tveit, T. Gaarden, L. Sandvik, and I. Espelid. 2012. "Longevity of Posterior Dental Restorations and Reasons for Failure." *European Journal of Oral Sciences* 120 (6): 539–48. https://doi.org/10.1111/eos.12004.

Leung, D., D. A. Spratt, J. Pratten, K. Gulabivala, N. J. Mordan, and A. M. Young. 2005. "Chlorhexidine-Releasing Methacrylate Dental Composite Materials." *Biomaterials* 26 (34): 7145–53. https://doi.org/10.1016/j.biomaterials.2005.05.014.

Li, F., F. Li, D. Wu, S. Ma, J. Gao, Y. Li, Y. Xiao, and J. Chen. 2011. "The Effect of an Antibacterial Monomer on the Antibacterial Activity and Mechanical Properties of a Pit-and-Fissure Sealant." *Journal of the American Dental Association (1939)* 142 (2): 184–93. https://doi.org/10.14219/jada.archive .2011.0062.

Li, F., M.D. Weir, A. F. Fouad, and H. H. K. Xu. 2014. "Effect of Salivary Pellicle on Antibacterial Activity of Novel Antibacterial Dental Adhesives Using a Dental Plaque Microcosm Biofilm Model." *Dental Materials: Official Publication of the Academy of Dental Materials* 30 (2): 182–91. https://doi .org/10.1016/j.dental.2013.11.004.

Li, F., P. Wang, M. D. Weir, A. F. Fouad, and H. H. K. Xu. 2014. "Evaluation of Antibacterial and Remineralizing Nanocomposite and Adhesive in Rat Tooth Cavity Model." *Acta Biomaterialia* 10 (6): 2804–13. https://doi.org/10 .1016/j.actbio.2014.02.033.

Liu, S.-Y., L. Tonggu, L.-N. Niu, S.-Q. Gong, B. Fan, L. Wang, J.-H. Zhao, C. Huang, D. H. Pashley, and F. R. Tay. 2016. "Antimicrobial Activity of a Quaternary Ammonium Methacryloxy Silicate-Containing Acrylic Resin: A Randomised Clinical Trial." *Scientific Reports* 6 (February): 21882. https:// doi.org/10.1038/srep21882.

Maas, M. S., Y. Alania, L. C. Natale, M. C. Rodrigues, D. C. Watts, and R. R. Braga. 2017. "Trends in Restorative Composites Research: What Is in the Future?" *Brazilian Oral Research* 31 (Suppl 1): e55. https://doi.org/10.1590 /1807-3107BOR-2017.vol31.0055.

Maktabi, H., A. A. Balhaddad, Q. Alkhubaizi, H. Strassler, and M. A. S. Melo. 2018. "Factors Influencing Success of Radiant Exposure in Light-Curing Posterior Dental Composite in the Clinical Setting." *American Journal of Dentistry* 31 (6): 320–28.

Murray, P. E., L. J. Windsor, T. W. Smyth, A. A. Hafez, and C. F. Cox. 2002. "Analysis of Pulpal Reactions to Restorative Procedures, Materials, Pulp Capping, and Future Therapies." *Critical Reviews in Oral Biology and Medicine: An Official Publication of the American Association of Oral Biologists* 13 (6): 509–20. https://doi.org/10.1177/154411130201300607.

Namba, N., Y. Yoshida, N. Nagaoka, S. Takashima, K. Matsuura-Yoshimoto, H. Maeda, B. Van Meerbeek, K. Suzuki, and S. Takashiba. 2009. "Antibacterial Effect of Bactericide Immobilized in Resin Matrix." *Dental Materials: Official Publication of the Academy of Dental Materials* 25 (4): 424–30. https://doi.org/10.1016/j.dental.2008.08.012.

Niu, L. N., M. Fang, K. Jiao, L. H. Tang, Y. H. Xiao, L. J. Shen, and J. H. Chen. 2010. "Tetrapod-Like Zinc Oxide Whisker Enhancement of Resin Composite." *Journal of Dental Research* 89 (7): 746–50. https://doi.org/10.1177 /0022034510366682.

Noronha, V. T., A. J. Paula, G. Durán, A. Galembeck, K. Cogo-Müller, M. Franz-Montan, and N. Durán. 2017. "Silver Nanoparticles in Dentistry." *Dental Materials: Official Publication of the Academy of Dental Materials* 33 (10): 1110–26. https://doi.org/10.1016/j.dental.2017.07.002.

Orstavik, D., and A. Hensten-Pettersen. 1978. "Antibacterial Activity of Tooth-Colored Dental Restorative Materials." *Journal of Dental Research* 57 (2): 171–74. https://doi.org/10.1177/00220345780570020101.

Park, S. E., A. R. Periathamby, and J. C. Loza. 2003. "Effect of Surface-Charged Poly(Methyl Methacrylate) on the Adhesion of Candida Albicans." *Journal of Prosthodontics: Official Journal of the American College of Prosthodontists* 12 (4): 249–54. https://doi.org/10.1016/s1059-941x(03)00107-4.

Peng, J. J.-Y., M. G. Botelho, and J. P. Matinlinna. 2012. "Silver Compounds Used in Dentistry for Caries Management: A Review." *Journal of Dentistry* 40 (7): 531–41. https://doi.org/10.1016/j.jdent.2012.03.009.

Rai, M., A. Yadav, and A. Gade. 2009. "Silver Nanoparticles as a New Generation of Antimicrobials." *Biotechnology Advances* 27 (1): 76–83. https://doi.org/10.1016/j.biotechadv.2008.09.002.

Sadowsky, S. J. 2006. "An Overview of Treatment Considerations for Esthetic Restorations: A Review of the Literature." *The Journal of Prosthetic Dentistry* 96 (6): 433–42. https://doi.org/10.1016/j.prosdent.2006.09.018.

Shvero, D. K., N. Zatlsman, R. Hazan, E. I. Weiss, and N. Beyth. 2015. "Characterisation of the Antibacterial Effect of Polyethyleneimine Nanoparticles in Relation to Particle Distribution in Resin Composite." *Journal of Dentistry* 43 (2): 287–94. https://doi.org/10.1016/j.jdent.2014.05.003.

Simonsen, R. J., and R. C. Neal. 2011. "A Review of the Clinical Application and Performance of Pit and Fissure Sealants." *Australian Dental Journal* 56 (Suppl 1 (June)): 45–58. https://doi.org/10.1111/j.1834-7819.2010.01295.x.

Sivakumar, I., K. S. Arunachalam, S. Sajjan, A. V. Ramaraju, B. Rao, and B. Kamaraj. 2014. "Incorporation of Antimicrobial Macromolecules in Acrylic Denture Base Resins: A Research Composition and Update." *Journal of Prosthodontics: Official Journal of the American College of Prosthodontists* 23 (4): 284–90. https://doi.org/10.1111/jopr.12105.

Sofan, E., A. Sofan, G. Palaia, G. Tenore, U. Romeo, and G. Migliau. 2017. "Classification Review of Dental Adhesive Systems: From the IV Generation to the Universal Type." *Annali Di Stomatologia* 8 (1): 1–17. https://doi.org/10.11138/ads/2017.8.1.001.

Tavassoli Hojati, S., H. Alaghemand, F. Hamze, F. A. Babaki, R. Rajab-Nia, M. B. Rezvani, M. Kaviani, and M. Atai. 2013. "Antibacterial, Physical and Mechanical Properties of Flowable Resin Composites Containing Zinc Oxide Nanoparticles." *Dental Materials: Official Publication of the Academy of Dental Materials* 29 (5): 495–505. https://doi.org/10.1016/j.dental.2013.03.011.

Thaya, R., B. Malaikozhundan, S. Vijayakumar, J. Sivakamavalli, R. Jeyasekar, S. Shanthi, B. Vaseeharan, P. Ramasamy, and A. Sonawane. 2016. "Chitosan Coated Ag/ZnO Nanocomposite and Their Antibiofilm, Antifungal and Cytotoxic Effects on Murine Macrophages." *Microbial Pathogenesis* 100 (November): 124–32. https://doi.org/10.1016/j.micpath.2016.09.010.

Tobias, R. S., J. W. Rippin, R. M. Browne, and C. A. Wilson. 1988. "A Further Study of the Antibacterial Properties of Dental Restorative Materials."

International Endodontic Journal 21 (6): 381–92. https://doi.org/10.1111/j
.1365-2591.1988.tb00905.x.

Wang, H., S. Wang, L. Cheng, Y. Jiang, M. A. S. Melo, M. D. Weir, T. W. Oates,
X. Zhou, and H. H. K. Xu. 2019. "Novel Dental Composite with Capability
to Suppress Cariogenic Species and Promote Non-Cariogenic Species in
Oral Biofilms." *Materials Science and Engineering: C* 94 (January): 587–96.
https://doi.org/10.1016/j.msec.2018.10.004.

Wang, J., X. Dong, Q. Yu, S. N. Baker, H. Li, N. E. Larm, G. A. Baker, L. Chen,
J. Tan, and M. Chen. 2017. "Incorporation of Antibacterial Agent Derived
Deep Eutectic Solvent into an Active Dental Composite." *Dental Materials:
Official Publication of the Academy of Dental Materials* 33 (12): 1445–55.
https://doi.org/10.1016/j.dental.2017.09.014.

Wang, L., Mary A. S. Melo, M. D. Weir, X. Xie, M. A. Reynolds, and H. H. K. Xu.
2016. "Novel Bioactive Nanocomposite for Class-V Restorations to Inhibit
Periodontitis-Related Pathogens." *Dental Materials: Official Publication of
the Academy of Dental Materials* 32 (12): e351–61. https://doi.org/10.1016/j
.dental.2016.09.023.

Wang, L., X. Xie, M. Qi, M. D. Weir, M. A. Reynolds, C. Li, C. Zhou, and H. H. K.
Xu. 2019. "Effects of Single Species versus Multispecies Periodontal Biofilms
on the Antibacterial Efficacy of a Novel Bioactive Class-V Nanocomposite."
Dental Materials: Official Publication of the Academy of Dental Materials 35
(6): 847–61. https://doi.org/10.1016/j.dental.2019.02.030.

Wang, S., H. Wang, B. Ren, H. Li, M. D. Weir, X. Zhou, T. W. Oates, L. Cheng, and
H. H. K. Xu. 2017. "Do Quaternary Ammonium Monomers Induce Drug
Resistance in Cariogenic, Endodontic and Periodontal Bacterial Species?"
Dental Materials: Official Publication of the Academy of Dental Materials 33
(10): 1127–38. https://doi.org/10.1016/j.dental.2017.07.001.

Weng, Y., L. Howard, X. Guo, V. J. Chong, R. L. Gregory, and D. Xie. 2012. "A
Novel Antibacterial Resin Composite for Improved Dental Restoratives."
Journal of Materials Science. Materials in Medicine 23 (6): 1553–61. https://
doi.org/10.1007/s10856-012-4629-z.

Wilson, S. J., and H. J. Wilson. 1993. "The Release of Chlorhexidine from Modified
Dental Acrylic Resin." *Journal of Oral Rehabilitation* 20 (3): 311–19. https://
doi.org/10.1111/j.1365-2842.1993.tb01613.x.

Xiao, S., H. Wang, K. Liang, F. Tay, M. D. Weir, M. A. S. Melo, L. Wang, et al.
2019. "Novel Multifunctional Nanocomposite for Root Caries Restorations
to Inhibit Periodontitis-Related Pathogens." *Journal of Dentistry* 81: 17–26.
https://doi.org/10.1016/j.jdent.2018.12.001.

Yoshida, K., M. Tanagawa, and M. Atsuta. 1999. "Characterization and Inhibitory
Effect of Antibacterial Dental Resin Composites Incorporating Silver-Supported
Materials." *Journal of Biomedical Materials Research* 47 (4): 516–22. https://doi
.org/10.1002/(sici)1097-4636(19991215)47:4<516::aid-jbm7>3.0.co;2-e.

Yu, F., H. Yu, P. Lin, Y. Dong, L. Zhang, X. Sun, Z. Liu, H. Guo, L. Huang, and
J. Chen. 2016. "Effect of an Antibacterial Monomer on the Antibacterial

Activity of a Pit-and-Fissure Sealant." *PLoS One* 11 (9): e0162281. https://doi
.org/10.1371/journal.pone.0162281.

Zhang, J. F., R. Wu, Y. Fan, S. Liao, Y. Wang, Z. T. Wen, and X. Xu. 2014. "Antibacterial
Dental Composites with Chlorhexidine and Mesoporous Silica." *Journal of
Dental Research* 93 (12): 1283–89. https://doi.org/10.1177/0022034514555143.

Zhang, K., B. Baras, C. D. Lynch, M. D. Weir, M. A. S. Melo, Y. Li, M. A. Reynolds,
et al. 2018. "Developing a New Generation of Therapeutic Dental Polymers
to Inhibit Oral Biofilms and Protect Teeth." *Materials (Basel, Switzerland)*
11 (9). https://doi.org/10.3390/ma11091747.

Zhang, K., B. Ren, X. Zhou, H. H. K. Xu, Y. Chen, Q. Han, B. Li, et al. 2016. "Effect
of Antimicrobial Denture Base Resin on Multi-Species Biofilm Formation."
International Journal of Molecular Sciences 17 (7). https://doi.org/10.3390
/ijms17071033.

Zhang, K., L. Cheng, S. Imazato, J. M. Antonucci, N. J. Lin, S. Lin-Gibson, Y. Bai,
and H. H. K. Xu. 2013. "Effects of Dual Antibacterial Agents MDPB and
Nano-Silver in Primer on Microcosm Biofilm, Cytotoxicity and Dentine
Bond Properties." *Journal of Dentistry* 41 (5): 464–74. https://doi.org/10.1016
/j.jdent.2013.02.001.

Zhang, N., C. Chen, M. A. Melo, Y.-X. Bai, L. Cheng, and H. H. Xu. 2015. "A Novel
Protein-Repellent Dental Composite Containing 2-Methacryloyloxyethyl
Phosphorylcholine." *International Journal of Oral Science* 7 (2): 103–9.
https://doi.org/10.1038/ijos.2014.77.

Zhang, N., K. Zhang, M. A. S. Melo, M. D. Weir, D. J. Xu, Y. Bai, and H. H. K.
Xu. 2017. "Effects of Long-Term Water-Aging on Novel Anti-Biofilm and
Protein-Repellent Dental Composite." *International Journal of Molecular
Sciences* 18 (1). https://doi.org/10.3390/ijms18010186.

Zhang, N., M. A. S. Melo, C. Chen, J. Liu, M. D. Weir, Y. Bai, and H. H. K. Xu.
2015. "Development of a Multifunctional Adhesive System for Prevention of
Root Caries and Secondary Caries." *Dental Materials: Official Publication
of the Academy of Dental Materials* 31 (9): 1119–31. https://doi.org/10.1016/j
.dental.2015.06.010.

Zhang, W., X.-J. Luo, L.-N. Niu, S.-Y. Liu, W.-C. Zhu, J. Epasinghe, L. Chen, et al.
2014. "One-Pot Synthesis of Antibacterial Monomers with Dual Biocidal
Modes." *Journal of Dentistry* 42 (9): 1078–95. https://doi.org/10.1016/j.jdent
.2014.06.001.

Zhou, C., M. D. Weir, K. Zhang, D. Deng, L. Cheng, and H. H. K. Xu. 2013.
"Synthesis of New Antibacterial Quaternary Ammonium Monomer
for Incorporation into CaP Nanocomposite." *Dental Materials: Official
Publication of the Academy of Dental Materials* 29 (8): 859–70. https://doi
.org/10.1016/j.dental.2013.05.005.

Zhou, H., F. Li, M. D. Weir, and H. H. K. Xu. 2013. "Dental Plaque Microcosm Response
to Bonding Agents Containing Quaternary Ammonium Methacrylates with
Different Chain Lengths and Charge Densities." *Journal of Dentistry* 41 (11):
1122–31. https://doi.org/10.1016/j.jdent.2013.08.003.

7

Nanotechnology and Delivery System for Bioactive Antibiofilm Dental Materials

Jin Xiao

University of Rochester Medical Center

Yuan Liu

University of Pennsylvania

Marlise I. Klein

São Paulo State University

Anna Nikikova and Yanfang Ren

University of Rochester Medical Center

Contents

7.1 Applications of Biomaterials to Prevent Oral Biofilm Formation

Many oral diseases are considered as chronic bacterial infectious diseases, such as dental caries, periodontitis, and peri-implantitis (Kolenbrander et al. 2006, Petersen et al. 2010, Ruby et al. 2002; Figure 7.1). Some microorganisms, such as *Streptococcus mutans*, *Lactobacillus acidophilus*, and *Actinomyces viscosus*, can colonize and form pathogenic plaques/biofilms on tooth surfaces and have been proven to be major contributors to oral infectious diseases (Kolenbrander et al. 2006, Ruby et al. 2002, Selwitz et al. 2007). Effectively inhibiting the growth of oral pathogens and biofilm formation is fundamental to the prevention and treatment of these oral diseases (Padmanaban et al. 1989).

Current antimicrobial modalities for biofilm control are limited. Chlorhexidine (CHX) has been considered as a long-term "gold standard" for oral antimicrobial therapy, but it has adverse side effects including tooth staining and calculus formation, and is not recommended for daily therapeutic use (Autio-Gold 2008). In addition, some antimicrobial agents can only provide short-term antimicrobial efficacy due to the dilution and degradation effect of the human saliva (Huang et al. 2016). Therefore, there is great need to explore other novel antibiofilm materials for controlling biofilm-associated oral diseases.

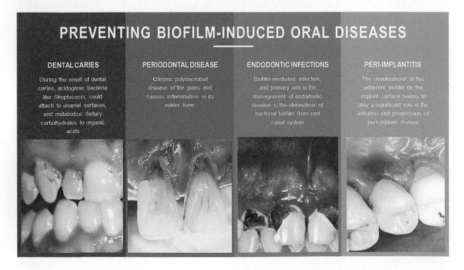

Figure 7.1   Prevention of biofilm-induced oral diseases.

7.1.1 Preventing Cariogenic Biofilm Formation

Dental caries is a dietary carbohydrate-modified bacterial infectious disease caused by biofilms and is one of the most prevalent chronic diseases in people worldwide (Paes Leme et al. 2006, Selwitz et al. 2007, Takahashi and Nyvad 2008). During the onset of dental caries, acidogenic bacteria like *Streptococci* could attach to enamel surfaces and metabolize dietary carbohydrates to organic acids. The frequent acidification favors the demineralization of enamel and selects for more aciduric species, like *S. mutans*, that further lower the environmental pH. Demineralization of enamel and degradation of the organic matrix in dentin lead to cavity formation and expansion (Takahashi and Nyvad 2011, 2016). It is the main cause of oral pain and tooth loss, affecting the oral health of human beings seriously and also creating a heavy financial burden; meanwhile, it has been associated with some systemic diseases as well (Fejerskov Ole 2003, Hu et al. 2011).

Antimicrobial therapies for dental caries have been used for centuries; although antibiotics are very effective in preventing caries in vivo and in vitro, their excessive use can lead to alterations of the oral and intestinal flora (Goldin and Gorbach 1984). Besides, undesirable side effects such as the development of bacteria to tolerance, vomiting, diarrhea, and teeth stains limited their use (Dickinson and Surawicz 2014, Gopinath et al. 2014, Vennila et al. 2014). As an alternative, several antimicrobial peptides (AMPs) have emerged with potential antibiofilm effects against caries-causing oral pathogens, including *S. mutans* (da Silva et al. 2012, Guo et al. 2015).

When compared with conventional antibiotics, AMPs provide additional advantages for oral antimicrobial therapy. For example, AMPs possess not only bactericidal activity but also to have other biological functions like immunomodulation by activating mast cells and wound healing (Gupta et al. 2015), while playing a critical role in angiogenesis (Koczulla et al. 2003). Furthermore, they are potently active against bacteria (particularly Gram-positive), fungi, and viruses and can be tailored to target specific pathogens by fusion with their surface antigens (Gupta et al. 2015, Lee et al. 2011, DeGray et al. 2001). AMPs can kill and restrict microbial infection by multiple mechanisms, including altered cell surface charge, disruption of membrane integrity, and pore formation while also neutralizing lipopolysaccharides-induced endotoxin shock (DeGray et al. 2001, Gupta et al. 2015, Lee et al. 2011; Figure 7.2).

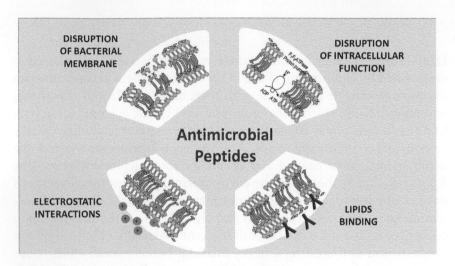

Figure 7.2   The mechanism of antimicrobial peptides.

In previous studies, a few AMPs have been identified as a potent killer of cariogenic bacteria. Liu et al. (2011) found that KSL (KKVVFKVKFK-NH$_2$) showed antimicrobial activity against several major cariogenic bacteria, including *S. mutans* and *L. acidophilus*. KSL also inhibited *S. mutans* biofilm formation and reduced one-day-old developed biofilm (Liu et al. 2011). In their study, Guo et al. (2015) have developed a specifically targeted antimicrobial peptide-C16G2, which is able to selectively kill cariogenic pathogen *S. mutans* with high efficacy within a human saliva-derived in vitro oral multispecies community.

Meanwhile, C16G2 rinse usage was associated with reductions in plaque and salivary *S. mutans*, lactic acid production, and enamel demineralization (Sullivan et al. 2011). However, the high cost of producing sufficient amounts of AMPs usually is a major barrier to their clinical development and commercialization. Liu, Kamesh et al. (2016) developed an exciting low-cost approach using plant-made AMPs protegrin with complex secondary structures for topical use to control biofilms. The plant-made protegrin rapidly killed the pathogen *S. mutans* and impaired biofilm formation following a single topical application of the tooth-mimetic surface. Furthermore, a synergistic approach using AMPs combined with matrix-degrading enzymes can facilitate the peptide's access into biofilms and kill the embedded bacteria (Liu, Kamesh, et al. 2016).

Dental caries is a multifactorial disease, but demineralization of susceptible dental hard tissues resulting from acidic by-products from bacterial fermentation of dietary carbohydrates is considered to be the fundamental mechanisms. Numerous clinical and laboratory papers in the past decades have indicated the anticaries effect of fluoride, which exerts its caries-preventive effect by shifting de-/remineralization balance favorably. However, there is still a need to seek products complementary to fluoride. There has been a rising interest in biologically active compounds derived from natural products that may have potential therapeutic uses in dentistry (Groppo et al. 2008, Newman 2008). In several previous studies, galla chinensis extracts (GCE) have been found to be effective in inhibiting demineralization and enhancing remineralization (Chu et al. 2007, Cheng et al. 2008). Cheng et al. (2008) found that GCE had enhanced the efficacy of fluoride in shifting the de-/remineralization of dental enamel. In the study of Huang et al. (2010), there was a significant synergistic effect of combined nanohydroxyapatite and galla chinensis treatments on the remineralization. Besides its potential effects in shifting the de-/remineralization balance, GCE has been proven to be able to inhibit dental biofilms.

In an in vitro experiment, Cheng et al. (2010) investigated the effects of GCE at different stages of biofilms formed with saliva as inoculum. The results demonstrated that GCE treatments inhibited growth and acid metabolism of both nascent and mature microcosm biofilms. Xie et al. (2008) designed an experiment to investigate the antibiofilm effect of GCE using a four-organism bacterial consortium (*Streptococcus sanguis*, *Streptococcus mutans*, *Actinomyces naeslundii*, and *Lactobacillus rhamnosus*). GCE were able to inhibit the growth of multiple-species biofilms on enamel blocks and reduced the demineralization of dental enamel.

Although employed widely in the remineralization of carious dentin, such an ion-based strategy cannot be effective in locations where the crystallites are totally destroyed (Frencken et al. 2012). Another promising class of mineralization materials is the biomineralization agents. Inspired from the function of noncollagenous proteins (NCPs) in the biomineralization process of natural teeth, using biomimetic templates to remineralize the demineralized dentin is of great interest in the recent years as NCPs, the natural nucleation templates, lose their abilities to induce in situ remineralization in the mature dentin (Chen, Liang et al. 2013). Poly(amino amine) (PAMAM)-type dendrimer is widely studied in dental biomineralization. It is a class of monodispersed polymeric nanomaterials with plenty of branches radiating from one central core and highly ordered architecture. It has been referred to as "artificial protein" due to its biomimetic properties and well-defined/easily tailored structure, such as its functional group, generation, and spatial structure. Previous studies have clearly demonstrated that PAMAM and its derivatives could induce

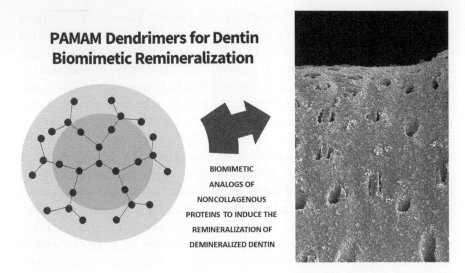

Figure 7.3 Poly(amino amine) (PAMAM)-type dendrimers for dental biomineralization.

biomineralization of demineralized dentin (Chen, Liang et al. 2013, Wu et al. 2013). PAMAM combined with antibacterial agents also obtained double effects of mineralization, and antibacterial and needlelike crystals can precipitate both on the dentin surface and in the dentinal tubules (Lei Cheng et al. 2016; Figure 7.3).

7.1.2 Preventing Periodontal Biofilm Formations

Periodontal diseases are a major public health concern due to their high prevalence in the general population. According to the National Health Service, it was estimated that more than 50% of the US adult population is affected by periodontal disease to a certain degree, and approximately 15% of UK population have been diagnosed with severe periodontitis (Hussain et al. 2015). Periodontitis is a chronic polymicrobial disease of the gums and causes inflammation in its milder form. As the disease worsens, periodontal tissues become severely inflamed and can eventually progress to tooth loss. Microbial biofilms formation is the major etiological agent for periodontitis.

The biofilm bacteria and their toxins perturb gingival epithelial cells as the first stage in a cascade of inflammatory and immune processes that lead to the destruction of gingival tissues and ultimately, in susceptible patients, alveolar bone loss and tooth loss as a result of periodontal disease (Gorr and Abdolhosseini 2011). Mixed biofilms are communities of bacteria that communicate by quorum sensing to change the bacteria's physiology. The biofilm contains channels to aid nutrient transport and is typically encapsulated by an extracellular polysaccharide matrix (ten Cate 2006). These features combine to make antibiotic treatment difficult. Traditional antibiotics were often selected against metabolically active bacteria in a planktonic state and are therefore less effective against the physiologically dormant bacteria encapsulated in a biofilm (ten Cate 2006). Meanwhile, the abuse of antibiotics in recent years has led to the emerging of drug-resistant bacterial strains (Chastre 2008). Currently, the first-line treatment for periodontitis is metronidazole. However, the beneficial effects of metronidazole are accompanied by undesirable side effects, including diarrhea, vomiting, metallic taste, headache, and dizziness. CHX is another potent antiplaque chemical agent, but its clinical application is limited by bitter taste and teeth stain (Eley 1999, Addy and Moran 1997).

AMPs are emerging as promising antimicrobial agents due to their rapid bactericidal activities. However, a potential confounding problem with the use of AMP as therapeutic agents is their susceptibility to proteolytic degradation and high-salt conditions (Jang et al. 2008). *Porphyromonas gingivalis*, which is considered to play a major role causing periodontitis, is known as a highly proteolytic organism. In order to improve the protease resistance of AMP, Wang et al. have designed a second generation of Nal-P-113 by replacing the histidine 4, 5, and 12 with β-naphthylalanines. In this case, the new Nal-P-113 was shown to have the ability to resist proteolytic degradation and high-salt conditions(Wang et al. 2015). In their study, comparing the sterilized abilities of Nal-P-113 with CHX, penicillin, and metronidazole, Nal-P-113 was found to be effectively inhibiting the exponential growth of oral bacteria. Besides, its antibacterial effect on *P. gingivalis* is more potent than penicillin and metronidazole (Wang et al. 2015). Importantly, Nal-P-113 could inhibit the formation of biofilms in the early stage, which was very important to control periodontal infection. Once the early biofilms were inhibited, the mature biofilms might, in turn, be prevented. The inhibition of Nal-P-113 on biofilm formation might be due to its inhibition of the growth of planktonic bacteria and bacterial colonization at the early stage of biofilm formation (Wang et al. 2015).

Recently, some new molecules are designed for efficient intraoral delivery of antimicrobials to prevent and treat the periodontal infection. The salivary statherin fragment, which has a high affinity for the tooth surfaces, was used as a carrier peptide. This was linked through the side chain of the N-terminal residue to the C-terminus of a defensive-like 12-residue peptide to generate two bifunctional hybrid molecules: one with an ester linkage, and the other with an anhydride bond between the carrier and the antimicrobial components. The bifunctional hybrid molecules could adhere to the tooth and pellicle surfaces uniformly and inhibit microbial accumulation. In addition, these bifunctional molecules would decrease the limitations and discomfort associated with the currently available local drug-delivery devices (Raj et al. 2008).

7.1.3 Preventing Endodontic-Related Biofilms

Endodontic disease is also a biofilm-mediated infection, and the primary aim in the management of the endodontic disease is the elimination of bacterial biofilm from the root canal system. The most common endodontic infection is caused by the surface-associated growth of microorganisms (Jhajharia et al. 2015). To the best of our knowledge, among different clinical bacterial isolates recovered from endodontic infections, *Enterococcus faecalis* is the only species that has been widely studied for its capacity to form biofilms (Duggan and Sedgley 2007). Being an opportunistic pathogen, it causes nosocomial infections and is frequently isolated from the failed root canals undergoing retreatment. *E. faecalis* in dentinal tubules can resist intracanal dressings of calcium hydroxide for over ten days by forming a biofilm that helps it resist destruction by enabling the bacteria to become 1,000 times more resistant to phagocytosis, antibodies, and antimicrobials than non-biofilm-producing organisms (Jhajharia et al. 2015). It should also be kept in mind that the complex anatomy of the root canal poses further difficulties for treatment because biofilms of persistent microorganisms within the root canals may also be located on the walls of ramifications and isthmuses (Jhajharia et al. 2015).

Antimicrobial irrigating solutions and other locally used disinfecting agents and medications play a key role in the eradication of microbes. Ideal root canal irrigants should have high efficacy against microorganisms in biofilms while being systemically non-toxic and non-caustic to periodontal tissues (Penick and Osetek 1970). Although current irrigation regimens using sodium hypochlorite (NaOCl) exhibit excellent antimicrobial activity, caustic and toxic effects to vital tissues are often noted. Calcium hydroxide and CHX have also been widely used for root canal therapy due to their excellent biological and antimicrobial activities. However, previous studies have demonstrated that the antimicrobial efficacy of calcium hydroxide varies depending on its location in the root canal and is compromised by the buffering effect of dentin, the resistance of *E. faecalis* to the hydroxyl ion, and its low solubility and diffusibility (Evans et al. 2002, Haapasalo et al. 2007). The fact that CHX is inactivated by physiological salts and has limited ability to penetrate the deep layers of biofilms also limits its use as an intracanal medicament (Portenier et al. 2002).

N-acetylcysteine (NAC), a derivative of the amino acid L-cysteine, is a potent thiol-containing antioxidant and mucolytic agent that disrupts disulfide bonds in mucus and reduces the viscosity of secretions (Zhao and Liu 2010). NAC is considered a nonantibiotic compound possessing antimicrobial properties that decrease biofilm formation by a variety of medically important bacteria, including *Pseudomonas aeruginosa*, *Escherichia coli*, *Staphylococcus epidermidis*, and *Streptococcus pneumonia* (Zhao and Liu 2010, Moon et al. 2016). Recently, it was shown that NAC inhibits the growth of *E. faecalis* at concentrations of 0.78–1.56 mg/mL. Notably, the mature biofilms, which are reported to be more resistant than planktonic bacteria and young biofilms, were disrupted within 10 min by NAC (>25 mg/mL), and the viability of mature biofilms was reduced by 99% compared to control. Moreover, treatment with NAC for 24 h was significantly more effective than 2% CHX. Furthermore, even a 10 min exposure to higher concentrations of NAC (100–200 mg/mL) almost completely removed mature biofilms (Moon et al. 2016).

Another alternative is AMPs, and the main advantage of AMPs resides in the mechanism of their action, which is different from that of conventional antibiotics currently used in endodontic treatment (Winfred et al. 2014). Recently, researchers showed that designed AMPs (VSL and VS2) exhibited activity against *E. faecalis* and could reduce biofilm formation (Winfred et al. 2014). Ex vivo study on the dentinal tubule model demonstrated a drastic reduction in microbial load at different depths in the root canal. Moreover, the AMPs needed to be in place for only 12 h, beyond which permanent dentures could be affixed, showing high efficacy and fast response for the medicament. Meanwhile, these peptides were found to be non-cytotoxic to human cell lines (Winfred et al. 2014).

7.1.4 Preventing Peri-Implant Biofilm Formation

Just as the subgingival microflora associated with periodontitis becomes established around the exposed surfaces of natural teeth, dental implants become contaminated soon after installation into the oral cavity. The development of this adherent biofilm on the implant surface seems to play a significant role in the initiation and progression of peri-implant disease.

This process mimics the establishment of subgingival microflora around the exposed surface of natural teeth, a process that has been associated with periodontitis (Quirynen et al. 2006). Furthermore, peri-implant diseases have been associated with predominantly Gram-negative anaerobic bacteria, similar to those found around natural teeth in patients with advanced periodontitis (Leonhardt et al. 1999). As for periodontitis, peri-implantitis can be aggressive with suppuration and bone loss and may lead to the loss of "implant tooth." As a result, elimination of the established biofilm from the implant surface is the main objective in the treatment of peri-implantitis.

Antimicrobial features can be introduced to implant surfaces by different surface modifications and coating techniques, including direct impregnation with antibiotics and coating with antimicrobial metals such as copper and silver (Tasman et al. 2000, Bosetti et al. 2002). However, the local application of antimicrobial agents (antibiotics or antiseptics) rapidly induces the growth of multidrug-resistant pathogens (Darouiche 2003). It has been demonstrated by animal studies that the accumulation of silver granules in the eyes, heart enlargement, anemia, and pathological changes to the liver and kidneys may be caused by the prolonged administration of silver ions in low doses (Drake and Hazelwood 2005). Copper ion implantation leads to the compromises of the physical properties of titanium (Ti), such as corrosion resistance (Wan et al. 2007).

Therefore, it is necessary to develop an alternative method for antimicrobial modifying dental implant surfaces for biofilm control. Natural AMPs have become a promising candidate due to their minimal side effects and the unlikely acquisition of resistance by sensitive microbial strains (Zasloff 2002). Liu et al. (2011) constructed chimeric peptides by connecting JH 8194 and minTBP-1 to modify Ti surfaces. It was shown that *Streptococcus gordonii* and *Streptococcus sanguinis*, which are primary pathogens of the early biofilm stage on Ti plants, were damaged on the Ti surfaces treated with peptides (Liu, Ma et al. 2016). Titanium coated with hLf1–11 peptide displayed a remarkable inhibitory effect on *S. sanguinis* and *L. salivarius* adhesion with modest antibacterial activity. It is interesting that the antibacterial effect displayed at early adhesion times was also maintained after 24 h of incubation (Godoy-Gallardo et al. 2014).

7.2 Nanotechnology and Delivery System of Biomaterials

Most infectious diseases in humans, including those occurring within the mouth, are caused by virulent biofilms. The development of therapeutic approaches against biofilm-related diseases in the mouth is difficult due to the following factors: (1) lack of retention of exogenously introduced agents through topical application, (2) rapid clearance by oral environment buffering, and (3) poor penetration through complex oral biofilm structure. Thus, drugs often fail to reach or kill bacterial clusters within the extracellular matrix (EPS) encased microcolonies (Xiao et al. 2012, Xiao and Koo 2010).

Ideal topical antimicrobial agents should target disease-specific microorganisms, without disrupting the complex oral (commensal) flora. Moreover, it should not form complexes with salivary proteins that lead to rapid clearance from the mouth. These challenges could be addressed by using them as an incentive to design successful approaches. Several strategies have been developed including (1) materials with inherent antimicrobial properties such as cationic liposomes and silver particles (Allaker 2010, Besinis et al. 2015, Cottenye et al. 2013, del Pozo and Patel 2007, Jones et al. 1993, Radovic-Moreno et al. 2012), (2) drug delivery systems that bind to tooth surfaces (Chen, Jia, et al. 2013, Chen et al. 2010), and (3) delivery systems that exploit the presence of extracellular matrix substances and the pH microenvironments to enhance retention and controlled release of drugs (Gao et al. 2016, Horev et al. 2015, Zhou et al. 2016).

In the past decade, the development of antibiofilm nanoparticles and drug-delivery systems has shown great promises in preventing and treating biofilm-associated oral diseases (Chen et al. 2010, Chen, Jia et al. 2013, Gao et al. 2016, Horev et al. 2015, Zhou et al. 2016). Nanoparticle delivery systems usually first bind or adsorb to microorganisms or salivary pellicle-coated and glucan-coated surfaces, and then release active reagents when the local pH drops. Meanwhile, nanoparticles are designed to have a deleterious effect on biofilms in an acidic environment. Although researches have evolved in the past decades to improve biofilm control with topically applied agents, challenges still exist, which include incorporating nanoparticles into dental biomaterials, persevering their activity, and further fulfilling the antibiofilm function in the complex oral environment. In this section, we will discuss the current advances and challenges in utilizing nanotechnology to prevent and treat dental biofilms (Figure 7.4).

7.2.1 Tooth-Binding Micelles

Initial strategy to achieve localized and prolonged antimicrobials retention at tooth surface was using gels and varnishes containing CHX and/or fluoride (Emilson 1981, Kohler et al. 1982, Schwendicke and Gostemeyer 2017). However, both gels and varnishes need to be applied by clinical

NANO DRUG-DELIVERY SYSTEMS

in preventing and treating biofilm associated oral diseases

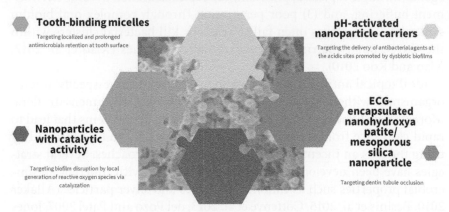

Tooth-binding micelles

Targeting localized and prolonged
antimicrobials retention at tooth surface

**pH-activated
nanoparticle carriers**

Targeting the delivery of antibacterial agents at
the acidic sites promoted by dysbiotic biofilms

**Nanoparticles
with catalytic
activity**

Targeting biofilm disruption by local
generation of reactive oxygen species via
catalyzation

**ECG-
encapsulated
nanohydroxya
patite/
mesoporous
silica
nanoparticle**

Targeting dentin tubule occlusion

Figure 7.4   Nano drug-delivery systems in preventing and treating biofilm associated oral diseases.

professionals, which limited the applications within broad populations. With the advent of nanotechnology, novel approaches emerged. At the beginning, most approaches focused on the tooth-binding ability of localized delivery systems to maintain higher drug concentration on the tooth surface [i.e., designed to bind to hydroxyapatite (Chen et al. 2009)], but not at or within biofilms (del Pozo and Patel 2007).

Nevertheless, it was groundbreaking having tooth-binding micelles that were developed by covalently attaching a prototype biomineral-binding moiety (alendronate) to the chain termini of biocompatible pluronic copolymers (Chen et al. 2009). These micelles were predicted to bind to hydroxyapatite immediately upon exposure and immobilized as a drug reservoir that steadily releases the pre-loaded antimicrobial (i.e., farnesol, as a model drug for encapsulation) (Chen et al. 2009). These farnesol-loaded micelles were negatively charged and could bind to hydroxyapatite discs before the incubation with *S. mutans*, enabling the release of farnesol over time, thereby effectively reducing the bacteria population by 4 logs (Chen et al. 2009). In follow-up work, these micelles and modified micelles were loaded with triclosan (Chen et al. 2010) and used to treat (1) hydroxyapatite discs before the incubation with *S. mutans* and (2) pre-formed *S. mutans* biofilms at 48, 72, and 96 h for 5 min.

The reduction in *S. mutans* viability was approximately 6 and 4 logs for the initial hydroxyapatite and pre-formed biofilms treatment, indicating that the tooth-binding micelles are effective in preventing preventing biofilm accumulation once they are bound to hydroxyapatite surface, and to control pre-formed biofilms by potential binding to biofilm components. However, a drawback of these two important studies aswas insufficient reporting on the ability of these micelles adhering to salivary-coated hydroxyapatite or biofilm/extracellular matrix, as well as the effect of saliva per se.

Thus, an additional study was performed to answer whether saliva and/or its components could influence these tooth-binding micelles drug-releasing capability, tooth-binding potential and binding stability, and *S. mutans* population in biofilms (Chen, Jia et al. 2013). These tooth-binding micelles (Pluronic P123 with and without tricolsan) were conjugated with a diphosphoserine peptide via "click" chemistry, while pyrophosphate was attached to P123 through an ester bond. It was found that saliva did not affect triclosan release from these micelles. However, saliva did affect the binding capacity of micelles to hydroxyapatite, allowing binding of more than 60% of micelles (thus a reduction of ~40%). However However, the retention of these bound micelles on surfaces was not compromised. These influences of saliva on drug-loaded micelles may explain why the population of *S. mutans* was lowered by 2 log compared to the negative control, which was still significant but not as pronounced as when saliva was not present (Chen et al. 2010).

7.2.2 pH-Activated Nanoparticle Carriers (NPCs)

These tooth-binding micelles approaches were designed to target hydroxy-apatite, not other important components of the mouth, such as salivary pellicles or biofilm extracellular matrix. Other than bactericidal, additional approaches attenuating microorganism virulence traits, especially extracellular matrix formation, presents challenges and opportunities. One example is dental caries, which initiated from the virulent biofilms attached to tooth surfaces. Cariogenic bacteria such as *S. mutans* formed an acidic environment within intricate biofilm microcolonies, and further triggered tooth structure demineralization (Xiao and Koo 2010, Xiao et al. 2012, 2017). Inspired by the research in cancer filed that delivers drugs at the acidic sites inside tumors (Benoit et al. 2010), novel delivery systems such as pH-activated nanoparticle carriers (NPCs) were developed in dental biomaterials (Horev et al. 2015, Zhou et al. 2016).

To address these challenges, NPCs were designed to (1) bind avidly to pellicle and EPS surfaces, enhancing retention at sites, where virulent biofilm actively develops, and (2) contain pH-responsive moieties that expedite release of bioactive agents at acidic pH found within cariogenic biofilms, when the agents are most needed (Horev et al. 2015). The drug-loaded NPCs are intact at pH 7.2. As the pH becomes acidic, NPC disassembles, and active drugs are released.

NPCs with cationic poly(dimethylaminoethyl methacrylate) [p(DMAEMA)] coronas and hydrophobic cores were synthesized via reversible addition-fragmentation chain transfer polymerization (Horev et al. 2015). These diblock copolymers self-assemble into micelle-based nanoparticle carriers in aqueous solutions via sonication. The NPC is non-toxic in vivo.

To check the NPC binding to dental surfaces mimetics, three surfaces were prepared to test NPC binding: hydroxyapatite beads or HA, saliva-coated HA (or pellicle), and glucan-coated sHA (or EPS matrix). These surfaces were treated with NPC and controls. After incubation, the supernatant was used to verify the amount of unbound NPC or controls. Still, the beads were washed three times before using confocal microscopy to verify the pattern of NPC binding. *S. mutans* biofilms were also prepared to test the binding of NPC. Remarkably, NPC bond with high avidity to HA, sHA (pellicle), and glucan-sHA (exopolysaccharide) surfaces because of its cationic corona. Furthermore, NPC effectively penetrated and bonded to EPS matrix and bacteria cluster within intact biofilms, despite short topical exposure. Thus, NPC enhances retention at sites where biofilms develop.

Furthermore, NPCs were loaded with farnesol. Farnesol is an antibacterial agent that is highly effective in disrupting acid tolerance and glucan synthesis of planktonic cells of *S. mutans*, and is more active at acidic pH (Koo et al. 2005). However, topically applied farnesol has demonstrated limited activity against *S. mutans* biofilms due to the suboptimal retention and poor aqueous solubility. Thus, farnesol is an ideal model agent to demonstrate NPC efficacy, as verified previously (Chen et al. 2009). NPC can load farnesol at ~22% wt, which shows a high loading capacity. Importantly, it increases the aqueous solubility 400 times more than free farnesol. NPC-encapsulated farnesol is completely water-soluble, which is crucial for formulation development. Moreover, the release of farnesol that encapsulated within NPC can be expedited in response to acidic pH. Specifically, the initial release rate, constant and half time was 2.5 times faster at pH 4.5 vs. pH 7.2.

In vitro *S. mutans* biofilms were formed on sHA surfaces with the presence of sucrose, and treated with either farnesol-loaded NPC (15% wt; 1.5 mg/mL NPC loaded with 0.5 mg/mL farnesol, in PBS, pH 7.0) or controls [free NPC (1.5 mg/mL in PBS, pH 7.0), NPC-farnesol, free-farnesol (0.5 mg/mL farnesol, in PBS, pH 7.0, 15% EtOH), vehicle control for free-farnesol (PBS, pH 7.0, 15% EtOH), or PBS (pH 7.0)], using a clinically relevant treatment regimen of two to three times treatment per day. The analyses of those biofilms included the determination of biomass, number of viable cells, and biofilm mechanical stability assessed by a shear-inducing device. Because of enhanced retention at sites (e.g., pellicle, matrix) and release at low pH, the antibiofilm effects were significantly enhanced. NPC-farnesol disrupted S. mutans biofilms four times more effective than the same amount of free farnesol, and also affected biofilm structural integrity, leading to a two-fold increase in biofilm removal (vs. free farnesol and controls).

To evaluate the in vivo efficacy of topical applications of farnesol-loaded NPC, the number (total lesions) and different stages of carious lesions severity were examined in a rodent caries model. The treatments were topical applications of NPC-farnesol or free farnesol (and controls), twice daily (for 60 s). The effects of NPC-mediated farnesol delivery on the onset of carious lesions were remarkable. Both the amount and severity of carious lesions were significantly reduced (compared to NPC control). In contrast, free farnesol only showed slight reductions of severity of lesions, but no effect on the incidence of the carious lesion.

In conclusion, NPC binds avidly to pellicle and EPS and enhances retention at sites where biofilms initiate and accumulate. NPC has a high capacity for drug loading, and robustly increases the aqueous solubility of farnesol. The nanocarrier is tuned to expedite farnesol release as the environment becomes acidic. As a result, NPC-mediated drug delivery converts farnesol, an antibacterial with poor retention and solubility, into an effective therapy against biofilms and dental caries disease. Altogether, NPCs have great potential to enhance the efficacy of bioactive agents to disrupt cariogenic biofilms, while facilitating formulation development for clinical use. Further optimization on corona: core molecular weight ratios improved the pH-response behavior of the cationic, pH-responsive p(DMAEMA)-b-p(DMAEMA-co-BMA-co-PAA) block copolymer micelles (Zhou et al. 2016), which could further enhance antibiofilm efficacy in situ.

7.2.3 Nanoparticles with Catalytic Activity

Equally important and innovative strategy is the development of nanoparticles with catalytic activity [i.e., catalytic nanoparticles or CAT-NP (Gao et al. 2014, 2007)] that also exhibit a pH-dependent property for degradation of S. mutans biofilm matrix, enhanced bacterial killing and reduction of apatite demineralization under acidic conditions, suppressing dental caries in vivo without damage to the oral mucosa (Gao et al. 2016). These CAT-NP contain biocompatible Fe_3O_4 were and catalyze hydrogen peroxide (H_2O_2) to generate free-radicals in situ, which affect the matrix structure by degrading glucans and inactivate bacteria living within it.

First, it was shown that S. mutans biofilm grown on sHA surface in the presence of sucrose retain CAT-NP within its structure following topical treatments (5 or 10 min). The maximum binding of CAT-NP to biofilms is of 0.5 mg/mL, and these nanoparticles were bound throughout the biofilm structure. These nanoparticles retained inside biofilms catalyzed the reaction of 3,30,5,50-tetramethylbenzidine or di-azo-aminobenzene (both are peroxidase substrates) in the presence of H_2O_2, demonstrating the generation of free radicals. This peroxidase-like activity occurred in CAT-NP treated biofilms was better in concentrations between 0.5 and 2.0 mg/mL. In addition, peroxidase-like activity of the nanoparticles that were bound to biofilm structures was tested by incubating biofilms in buffers with pHs from 4.5 to 6.5. The highest catalytic activity occurred at acidic pH. Additionally, "trace amounts of free iron leached from either CAT-NP in acidic pH buffer (pH 4.5) or in the soluble-fraction of the CAT-NP-treated biofilm" minimally affect the catalytic activity (Gao et al. 2016). However, the released iron ions even at trace amounts can hinder apatite acid-dissolution.

Next, to verify whether CAT-NP-mediated H_2O_2 catalysis and generation of free radicals in situ could affect residing bacteria and the EPS matrix, S. mutans biofilms were treated with CAT-NP (0.5 mg/mL) and instantly exposed to several concentrations of H_2O_2 (0.1%–1%, v/v). There was a remarkable biocidal effect on S. mutans cells within biofilms, with >99.9% killing in 5 min; with more than 5-log reduction in the presence of 1% H_2O_2, compared to control biofilms or CAT-NP-treated biofilms without H_2O_2. This effective outcome is more than 5,000-fold better than H_2O_2 alone and several-fold more than CHX at 0.12%. Moreover, the free radicals produced from H_2O_2 catalysis also degraded soluble and insoluble exopolysaccharides in vitro, as CAT-NP-treated biofilms exposed to H_2O_2 presented pronounced reduction of insoluble EPS, but not much for soluble EPS compared to control and either H_2O_2 or CAT-NP alone. Furthermore, topical treatments performed twice daily (for 5 or 1 min) of CAT-NP (at 0.5 mg/mL) immediately followed by H_2O_2 (at 1%, v/v) exposure (CAT-NP/H2O2), impaired both the formation of bacterial microcolonies and the assembly of EPS matrix (more extensively at 5 min). Thus, the combination of CAT-NP with H_2O_2 could effectively hinder S. mutans biofilm development.

Finally, to evaluate the in vivo efficacy of topical applications of the combination of CAT-NP with H_2O_2 and controls, the number (of total lesions) and different stages of carious lesions severity were determined in the rodent model of dental caries. The agents were topically applied twice daily for three weeks (100 µl per rat/for 1 min). CAT-NP/H_2O_2 significantly diminished both the number and severity of carious lesions (vs. vehicle control). However, treatments with H_2O_2 alone had a negligible effect, whereas CAT-NP slightly sreduced the severity of lesions (vs. vehicle control). Thus, CAT-NP may exert an additional pH-dependent mechanism to prevent caries, possibly by reducing demineralization at low pH. In addition, histopathology analysis demonstrated no toxic effects, but more work is needed.

To summarize, Cat-NP activates hydrogen peroxide to (1) efficiently disrupt biofilms, being 5,000 times more effective than hydrogen peroxide alone; (2) inhibit the development of biofilm by degrading matrix and killing bacteria; and (3) suppress dental caries in vivo, blocking cavitation in rat teeth. These outcomes demonstrated that these nanocatalysts with enzyme-like activity could be an alternative approach to control cariogenic biofilm.

7.2.4 Epigallocatechin-3-Gallate-Encapsulated Nanohydroxyapatite/Mesoporous Silica Nanoparticle

Another aspect that has been associated with biofilm control and prevention of dental caries is the management of exposed dentin surface and dentin hypersensitivity. A recent work combined information from natural product research and nanotechnology to develop a versatile biomaterial, epigallocatechin-3-gallate-encapsulated nanohydroxyapatite/mesoporous silica nanoparticle (EGCG@nHAp@MSN), for therapeutic management of the dentin surface (Yu et al. 2017). This study demonstrated that the topical application of a slurry of the novel biomaterial was effective for dentinal tubule occlusion, hindering treated dentin more resistant against acid and abrasion. Moreover, EGCG@nHAp@MSN can continuously release EGCG, Ca, and P, significantly inhibiting S. mutans biofilm development on the dentin surface, is a promising material for clinical testing.

Therefore, taking advantage of knowledge on biofilms assembly and virulence traits plus nanotechnology tools yielded improved anticaries effect of antimicrobials, leading to better ways to control pathogenicity.

7.3 Dental Material Modifications with Novel Antimicrobial/Antibiofilm Compounds

Novel dental material adhesives and composites have been developed to increase their biological activity while maintaining adequate mechanical properties. Common modifications include adding antimicrobial drugs (natural or synthetic) and combining with remineralization strategies (Cheng et al. 2017; Figure 7.5).

Quercetin, a naturally derived plant extract, was incorporated into a commercially developed adhesive using three different concentrations: 100, 500, and 1,000 μg/mL (Yang et al. 2017). Quercetin was dissolved with ethanol. An unmodified adhesive served as a control. The antibacterial ability on *S. mutans* biofilm, conversion degree, microtensile bond strength, failure modes, in situ zymography, nanoleakage expression, and cytotoxicity of quercetin-doped adhesive were comprehensively evaluated. The quercetin-doped adhesive (500 μg/mL) preserved its bonding properties against collagenase aging, suggesting that quercetin may work as a cross-linker of dentin collagen.

Moreover, the therapeutic adhesive inhibited the growth of *S. mutans* biofilm, on immediate and thermocycled specimens. Efficient bonding interface sealing ability, matrix metalloproteinase inhibition, and acceptable biocompatibility were also achieved. However, it is not clear from the type of quercetin from Sigma (which sells several formulations), whether ethanol is added to the control adhesive, whether this new adhesive is resistant to esterase activity, or if quercetin affects the color of the material.

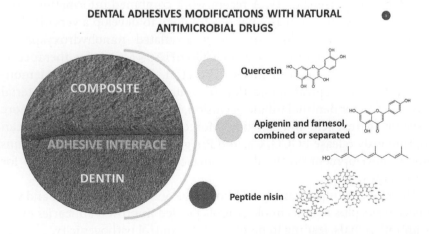

Figure 7.5   Modification of dental adhesives with natural antimicrobial agents.

Another study evaluated two naturally occurring agents (apigenin and farnesol) that have been tested as effective antibiofilm, and anticaries used isolated or in combination into the dental adhesive system (Andre et al. 2017). The new adhesives arecontaining the agents, combined or separated, affected *S. mutans* biofilm development by reducing total biomass and insoluble exopolysaccharide and intracellular polysaccharide, without changing the dentin bond strength and resin-dentin interfacial morphology. However, no information was available on the bioactivity of these agents after aging, and whether these agents were being released to the surrounding milieu.

The incorporation of the antibacterial peptide nisin at distinct concentrations into an etch-and-rinse dental adhesive inhibited the growth of *S. mutans*, and the inhibitory effect was concentration-dependent (Su et al. 2017). Moreover, the cured nisin-incorporated adhesive affected the adherence of *S. mutans* and the integrity of its biofilms. In addition, the use of 1% nisin did not interfere with microtensile bond strength, whereas 3% and 5% nisin decreased bond strength (vs. control group without nisin). However, as for the previous studies, it is unclear whether this peptide is released, and for how long it is active.

A novel antibacterial composite was developed by directly incorporating polymerizable imidazolium-containing resin (antibacterial a resin with carbonate linkage; ABR-C) into a methacrylate-based scaffold (ABR modified composite; ABR-MC) (Hwang et al. 2017). The addition of a low dose of non-leachable imidazolium moiety (~2% wt/wt) was bioactive with acceptable cytotoxicity while maintaining the mechanical integrity of the material. Moreover, the surface of ABR-MC yielded *S. mutans* biofilm with compromised 3D structural organization that detaches easily from the surface (compared to control resin), demonstrating antibiofilm activity. However, the "lifetime" of this new resin is unclear. Thus, it may require additional research to determine also whether this novel material is less degradable in the oral cavity environment (e.g., can salivary and microbial esterase activity degrade it?).

An innovative study has combined three agents into one multiagent anticaries dental material, capitalizing the properties of each of them shown previously: silver nanoparticles (NAg, releasable antibacterial agent), dimethylaminohexadecyl methacrylate (DMAHDM, non-releasable antibacterial macromolecule), and amorphous calcium phosphate nanoparticles (NACP, releasable acid neutralizer) (Melo et al. 2016). These agents were synthetized and incorporated into distinct combinations of materials needed for a composite restoration: dental primer, adhesive, and composite. The multiagent material hindered the impact of acid from oral biofilms derived from human saliva, which improved the strength and resistance to fatigue failure of the dentin-resin bonded interface. This new approach may yield better clinical outcomes, but needs to be tested further in animal model and clinical studies.

7.4 The Durability of Antibiofilm Biomaterials

The use of antimicrobial and antibiofilm agents (drugs) in the oral cavity brings the issues of drug resistance and tolerance. The products/strategies designed for short-term and topical applications, such as mouthwash or dentifrice, usually raise questions about drug resistance and tolerance, and more recently, about the generation of persisters (Lewis 2007). In addition, dental materials with modified antimicrobial activities are originally designed to hinder secondary caries and delay/avoid restoration replacement (or tooth loss), but can also alter the oral microorganisms and its host's reaction, especially those living as adherent biofilms. Until now, few studies have addressed these issues that are paramount for the safe implementation of these new-generation antimicrobial dental monomers/resins that capitalize on nanotechnology and delivery systems. Moreover, many pieces of research work assume that the incorporation of naturally occurring compounds into dental materials will not lead to antimicrobial resistance and tolerance, but few testing was performed to prove this hypothesis.

Regarding dental material with antimicrobial properties, only initial groundbreaking work has been done. However, these studies were performed with "free" non-light-cured adhesive systems, specifically with quaternary ammonium monomers (Wang, Wang et al. 2017, Wang, Zhou et al. 2017), which may be problematic. These quaternary ammonium monomers have shown good biological and mechanical properties.

The antimicrobial monomers dimethylaminohexadecyl methacrylate (DMAHDM) and dimethylaminododecyl methacrylate (DMADDM) were used to test on the induction of drug resistance in eight oral species: *Streptococcus mutans*, *Streptococcus sanguis*, *Streptococcus gordonii*, *Enterococcus faecalis*, *Aggregatibacter actinomycetemcomitans*, *Fusobacterium nucleatum*, *Porphyromonas gingivalis*, and *Prevotella intermedia* (Wang, Wang et al. 2017). The methodology included minimum inhibitory concentration (MIC), minimal bactericidal concentration (MBC), bacterial growth, and membrane permeability properties, using CHX as control. After ten passages, DMAHDM did not induce any resistance, while DMADDM induced drug resistance in *S. gordonii* (at passage 4, the MIC changed from 12.5 to 25 µg/mL). *S. gordonii* is considered an earlier colonizer linked to a noncariogenic microbiota, but also an accessory pathogen for periodontal disease (Whitmore and Lamont 2011).

The permeabilization of cell membranes eliminated the resistance of *S. gordonii* to DMADDM. In addition, the control CHX induced drug resistance in *S. gordonii*, *E. faecalis*, *F. nucleatum*, and *P. gingivalis*, which indicates that biomaterials and/or mouthwash containing CHX should be used only when indicated clinically. Moreover, the DMADDM- and CHX-resistant *S. gordonii* had the same MIC and MBC values as *S. gordonii* parental strain against DMAHDM, which effectively inhibited the resistant strains. The authors concluded that DMAHDM is promising for applications in restorative, periodontal, and endodontic treatments with no drug resistance in eight species.

Next, the generation of *S. mutans* persisters cells by DMAHDM was investigated using planktonic culture and biofilms, using CHX as control (Wang, Zhou et al. 2017). To evaluate drug persistence, dose- and time-dependent killing curves of *S. mutans* planktonic cultures and biofilms were obtained. The characteristics of persisters cells were investigated by inheritability assay, MIC, and live/dead biofilm assay. DMAHDM and the control CHX generated persistence in *S. mutans* biofilms (grown for 24 h, and treated for additional 24 h) but not in planktonic bacteria. DMAHDM matched the killing potency of the gold-standard CHX against *S. mutans* biofilms. *S. mutans* biofilm persistence to DMAHDM or CHX was not transferrable because the tolerance of the persisters in the initial population was not transferred to subsequent generations. "The MIC of *S. mutans* parental strain and induced persisters remained the same," which differentiates from drug resistance. The induced persisters in *S. mutans* biofilms were eliminated by higher amounts of DMAHDM and CHX (300 µg/mL). However, additional studies using distinct oral microbial species should be performed.

From the microbiological point of view, the non-cured material is ready to use in standard tests for drug resistance and tolerance with distinct concentrations of solubilized tested agent. However, this may be an issue clinically, because these materials will be light-cured when applied for teeth restorations (even though a small fraction may not), and the number of agents with antimicrobial properties may be negligible, thereby deserving future studies. Both studies by Wang, Wang et al. (2017) used CHX as an antimicrobial gold-standard control and yielded additional information for this antimicrobial, demonstrating that it should be used carefully. Finally, these two studies did perform three independent experiments, in triplicate. However, many studies fail to test antimicrobial properties on distinct occasions, which can introduce bias to the outcomes.

Therefore, more studies are needed to pinpoint whether the newly generated monomers and/or strategies incorporating antimicrobials can indeed not elicit microbial tolerance in a clinical setting, in longitudinal well-controlled clinical studies.

7.5 Biological Safety of Biomaterials

The powerful antibacterial agents, such as sodium hypochlorite (NaOCl), are caustic to human tissues and thus have limited implications in the elimination of bacterial pathogens and cannot be routinely used on a daily basis for plaque control. Antibiotics, although very effective against pathogens, have systemic effects, bacterial resistance and usually have a wide range of antibacterial actions, which often causes overall dysbacteriosis of oral and intestinal microbiota.

Plant-derived flavonoids such as epigallocatechin-3-gallate (EGCG), farnesol, and quercetin are generally non-toxic and effective in use against oral pathogens; the latter has shown in high doses to be potentially toxic to mitochondria and could have mutagenic effect on human cells (Chen et al. 2014, Okamoto 2005, Zhang et al. 2009, Tyagi et al. 2017). Gallotanins, the major component of GCE studied for enhancing remineralization of dentin, in very high concentrations could have cytotoxic effects on eukaryotic cells in a rat model (Xiang et al. 2015); thus, the dosing of topical applications is important.

A very promising avenue is AMPs for their specific targeted action on the bacterial pathogen and potential of enhancing innate immune response; however, toxicity of these agents on eukaryotic system still remains unexplored (Gupta et al. 2014). It has been noted the toxic effect of antibacterial peptides toward the epithelia of a delicate mucosal surface (Gordon et al. 2005. AMPs can also have either or both pro- and anti-inflammatory functions (Koczulla and Bals 2003), which can modify the immune response to oral bacteria and potentially shift host response toward exacerbating periodontal inflammation. Although potential toxicity of antibacterial peptide nisin has been reported toward eukaryotic cells in selective apoptotic effect toward human melanoma cells (Lewies et al. 2018), is considered to be low toxic and continues to be widely used in the food industry preventing the growth of Gram-positive and pathogenic bacteria. Nisin presents as a promising antibacterial agent in the battle with oral biofilms without toxicity to oral epithelial cells (Gupta et al. 2008, Vaucher Rde et al. 2011, Gordon et al. 2005); nevertheless, it's imperative to continue to study its effects on human cells to guarantee its safe use.

In the human innate immune system, the AMPs are stored in granules, and their activation and deactivation involve mechanisms of enzymatic interaction of proteins (Gordon et al. 2005); , therefore, delivery systems for the AMPs are essential to avoid prolonged exposure of tissues and thus their adverse effects.

Nanoparticles are a promising delivery system currently widely studied as they have biocompatibility with human cells and oral epithelial cells. However, nanoparticles can pass through cell membranes, interact with biological systems, enter the bloodstream, and translocate to other organs (De Jong and Borm 2008). Catalytic nanoparticles CAT-NP contain iron oxides, which are commonly used as food additives and Feraheme, and currently approved by the FDA for chronic treatment. However, the current safety data available is based on in vitro studies only (Gao and Koo 2017), and in vivo studies are required to determine the adverse effects of lengthy-term daily application of CAT-NPs.

Poly(amino amine) (PAMAM)-type dendrimer, which is widely studied in various medical applications and dental biomineralization, have shown no toxicity and very low immunogenicity in earlier in vivo studies in mouse model (Roberts et al. 1996). However, later in vitro studies in human keratinocytes have shown that depending on dendrimer generation and dose, PAMAM being absorbed by the cells could cause harm to the cell's mitochondria and lead to cell death (Mukherjee and Byrne 2013).

N-acetylcysteine (NAC) is a powerful antioxidant widely used in medicine as micolytic and antidote in oxidative stress. The effect of NAC on the cells is generally protective, and the documented adverse effects of the drug are mostly from high-dose IV formulations and inhalation, including rash, urticarial, and stomatitis (Ahola et al. 1999). Toxicity to epithelial cells in the topical application of NAC in long-term therapeutic doses has not been reported.

Although antibiofilm biomaterials are exciting new avenues in the fight against dental diseases, the implementation of new materials presents essential challenges of establishing biosafety of such new materials. Most of the studies are conducted on the single-species biofilm model, and though the effect of the material might be evident in such a system, the oral ecosystem comprises the intricate balance of multiple species. Contact-killing capability of imidazolium-containing resin could leave a layer of dead bacteria and other cell components and could facilitate attachment and nutrition for new bacterial species (Hwang et al. 2017). Thus, it is crucial to determine the effect of the material on the multispecies biofilms to to implement it as a therapeutic or preventive measure safely. The imidazolium-containing resin could exert a cytotoxic effect and could be harmful to human cells (Raab and Hogl 1980). Although the goal of the researches is to create non-leachable incorporation of antibacterial agents into composite resins, inevitable contact of these materials with human tissues and long-term contact could potentially be damaging to oral cells (odontoblasts, epithelial cells, immune). Imidazolium has been reported to be corrosive to skin under occlusive conditions and have teratogenic effects (International Labour Organization 2004). The in vivo and animal studies are important in determining long-term effects of the presence of such materials in oral environment.

The subject of toxicity of new developing biomaterials has to be constantly studied and addressed to avoid low clinical efficacy, failure in clinical trials, and long-term complications.

7.6 Future Perspectives

One of the critical challenges in optimizing dental biomaterials is to maximize the antibiofilm activities against disease-related bacterial species, but maintain the population of beneficial microorganisms in the oral cavity, which means precision microorganisms were controlling. Strategies to achieve this goal should be developed to target specific disease-related bacteria, and/or factors that promote oral biofilm formation, such as saliva (glycol) proteins that select specific early-colonizing bacterial species, biofilm matrix formation, and acidic microenvironment.

Another challenge is to precisely measure the active antimicrobial compound releasing from dental biomaterials and the duration of the activity, particularly in human studies. Furthermore, other aspects that need to be considered in future researches in the context of applying antimicrobial dental materials to control oral biofilm formation include antimicrobial resistance to dental biomaterials, clinical waste management of newly developed materials, and cost-effective outcome of these newly proposed antibiofilm strategies.

References

Addy, M., and J. M. Moran. 1997. "Evaluation of oral hygiene products: science is true; do not be misled by the facts." *Periodontol* 2000 15:40–51.
Ahola, T., V. Fellman, R. Laaksonen, J. Laitila, R. Lapatto, P. J. Neuvonen, and K. O. Raivio. 1999. "Pharmacokinetics of intravenous N-acetylcysteine in pre-term new-born infants." *Eur J Clin Pharmacol* 55 (9):645–50.

Allaker, R. P. 2010. "The use of nanoparticles to control oral biofilm formation." *J Dent Res* 89 (11):1175–86. doi: 10.1177/0022034510377794.

Andre, C. B., P. L. Rosalen, L. C. C. Galvao, B. M. Fronza, G. M. B. Ambrosano, J. L. Ferracane, and M. Giannini. 2017. "Modulation of *Streptococcus mutans* virulence by dental adhesives containing anti-caries agents." *Dent Mater* 33 (10):1084–92. doi: 10.1016/j.dental.2017.07.006.

Autio-Gold, J. 2008. "The role of chlorhexidine in caries prevention." *Oper Dent* 33 (6):710–6. doi: 10.2341/08-3.

Benoit, D. S., S. M. Henry, A. D. Shubin, A. S. Hoffman, and P. S. Stayton. 2010. "pH-responsive polymeric sirna carriers sensitize multidrug resistant ovarian cancer cells to doxorubicin via knockdown of polo-like kinase 1." *Mol Pharm* 7 (2):442–55. doi: 10.1021/mp9002255.

Besinis, A., T. De Peralta, C. J. Tredwin, and R. D. Handy. 2015. "Review of nanomaterials in dentistry: interactions with the oral microenvironment, clinical applications, hazards, and benefits." *ACS Nano* 9 (3):2255–89. doi: 10.1021/nn505015e.

Bosetti, M., A. Masse, E. Tobin, and M. Cannas. 2002. "Silver coated materials for external fixation devices: in vitro biocompatibility and genotoxicity." *Biomaterials* 23 (3):887–92.

Chastre, J. 2008. "Evolving problems with resistant pathogens." *Clin Microbiol Infect* 14 (Suppl 3):3–14 doi: 10.1111/j.1469–0691.2008.01958.x.

Chen, F., K. C. Rice, X. M. Liu, R. A. Reinhardt, K. W. Bayles, and D. Wang. 2010. "Triclosan-loaded tooth-binding micelles for prevention and treatment of dental biofilm." *Pharm Res* 27 (11):2356–64. doi: 10.1007/s11095-010-0119-5.

Chen, F., X. M. Liu, K. C. Rice, X. Li, F. Yu, R. A. Reinhardt, K. W. Bayles, and D. Wang. 2009. "Tooth-binding micelles for dental caries prevention." *Antimicrob Agents Chemother* 53 (11):4898–902. doi: 10.1128/AAC.00387–09.

Chen, F., Z. Jia, K. C. Rice, R. A. Reinhardt, K. W. Bayles, and D. Wang. 2013. "The development of dentotropic micelles with biodegradable tooth-binding moieties." *Pharm Res* 30 (11):2808–17. doi: 10.1007/s11095-013-1105-5.

Chen, L., K. Liang, J. Li, D. Wu, X. Zhou, and J. Li. 2013. "Regeneration of biomimetic hydroxyapatite on etched human enamel by anionic PAMAM template in vitro." *Arch Oral Biol* 58 (8):975–80. doi: 10.1016/j.archoralbio.2013.03.008.

Chen, R., J. Lin, J. Hong, D. Han, A. D. Zhang, R. Lan, L. Fu, Z. Wu, J. Lin, W. Zhang, Z. Wang, W. Chen, C. Chen, and H. Zhang. 2014. "Potential toxicity of quercetin: the repression of mitochondrial copy number via decreased POLG expression and excessive TFAM expression in irradiated murine bone marrow." *Toxicol Rep* 1:450–8. doi: 10.1016/j.toxrep.2014.07.014.

Cheng, L., J. Li, Y. Hao, and X. Zhou. 2008. "Effect of compounds of Galla chinensis and their combined effects with fluoride on remineralization of initial enamel lesion in vitro." *J Dent* 36 (5):369–73. doi: 10.1016/j.jdent.2008.01.011.

Cheng, L., J. Li, Y. Hao, and X. Zhou. 2010. "Effect of compounds of Galla chinensis on remineralization of enamel surface in vitro." *Arch Oral Biol* 55 (6):435–40. doi: 10.1016/j.archoralbio.2010.03.014.

Cheng, L., K. Zhang, N. Zhang, M. A. S. Melo, M. D. Weir, X. D. Zhou, Y. X. Bai, M. A. Reynolds, and H. H. K. Xu. 2017. "Developing a new generation of antimicrobial and bioactive dental resins." *J Dent Res* 96 (8):855–63. doi: 10.1177/0022034517709739.

Chu, J. P., J. Y. Li, Y. Q. Hao, and X. D. Zhou. 2007. "Effect of compounds of Galla chinensis on remineralisation of initial enamel carious lesions in vitro." *J Dent* 35 (5):383–7. doi: 10.1016/j.jdent.2006.11.007.

Cottenye, N., Z. K. Cui, K. J. Wilkinson, J. Barbeau, and M. Lafleur. 2013. "Interactions between non-phospholipid liposomes containing cetyl-pyridinium chloride and biofilms of *Streptococcus mutans*: modulation of the adhesion and of the biodistribution." *Biofouling* 29 (7):817–27. doi: 10.1080/08927014.2013.807505.

da Silva, B. R., V. A. de Freitas, L. G. Nascimento-Neto, V. A. Carneiro, F. V. Arruda, A. S. de Aguiar, B. S. Cavada, and E. H. Teixeira. 2012. "Antimicrobial peptide control of pathogenic microorganisms of the oral cavity: a review of the literature." *Peptides* 36 (2):315–21. doi: 10.1016/j.peptides.2012.05.015.

Darouiche, R. O. 2003. "Antimicrobial approaches for preventing infections associated with surgical implants." *Clin Infect Dis* 36 (10):1284–9. doi: 10.1086/374842.

De Jong, W. H., and P. J. Borm. 2008. "Drug delivery and nanoparticles:applications and hazards." *Int J Nanomedicine* 3 (2):133–49.

DeGray, G., K. Rajasekaran, F. Smith, J. Sanford, and H. Daniell. 2001. "Expression of an antimicrobial peptide via the chloroplast genome to control phyto-pathogenic bacteria and fungi." *Plant Physiol* 127 (3):852–62.

del Pozo, J. L., and R. Patel. 2007. "The challenge of treating biofilm-associated bacterial infections." *Clin Pharmacol Ther* 82 (2):204–9. doi: 10.1038/sj.clpt.6100247.

Dickinson, B., and C. M. Surawicz. 2014. "Infectious diarrhea: an overview." *Curr Gastroenterol Rep* 16 (8):399. doi: 10.1007/s11894-014-0399-8.

Drake, P. L., and K. J. Hazelwood. 2005. "Exposure-related health effects of silver and silver compounds: a review." *Ann Occup Hyg* 49 (7):575–85. doi: 10.1093/annhyg/mei019.

Duggan, J. M., and C. M. Sedgley. 2007. "Biofilm formation of oral and endodontic Enterococcus faecalis." *J Endod* 33 (7):815–8. doi: 10.1016/j.joen.2007.02.016.

Eley, B. M. 1999. "Antibacterial agents in the control of supragingival plaque—a review." *Br Dent J* 186 (6):286–96.

Emilson, C. G. 1981. "Effect of chlorhexidine gel treatment on *Streptococcus mutans* population in human saliva and dental plaque." *Scand J Dent Res* 89 (3):239–46.

Evans, M., J. K. Davies, G. Sundqvist, and D. Figdor. 2002. "Mechanisms involved in the resistance of Enterococcus faecalis to calcium hydroxide." *Int Endod J* 35 (3):221–8.

Fejerskov Ole, N. B., K. Edwina. 2003. Dental *Caries: The Disease* and *Its Clinical Management.* 3rd edition: Wiley Blackwell, Hoboken, NJ. Reprint, 3rd edition.

Frencken, J. E., M. C. Peters, D. J. Manton, S. C. Leal, V. V. Gordan, and E. Eden. 2012. "Minimal intervention dentistry for managing dental caries— a review: report of a FDI task group." *Int Dent J* 62 (5):223–43. doi: 10.1111/idj.12007.

Gao, L., and H. Koo. 2017. "Do catalytic nanoparticles offer an improved therapeutic strategy to combat dental biofilms?" *Nanomedicine (Lond)* 12 (4):275–9. doi: 10.2217/nnm-2016-0400.

Gao, L., J. Zhuang, L. Nie, J. Zhang, Y. Zhang, N. Gu, T. Wang, J. Feng, D. Yang, S. Perrett, and X. Yan. 2007. "Intrinsic peroxidase-like activity of ferromagnetic nanoparticles." *Nat Nanotechnol* 2 (9):577–83. doi: 10.1038/nnano.2007.260.

Gao, L., K. M. Giglio, J. L. Nelson, H. Sondermann, and A. J. Travis. 2014. "Ferromagnetic nanoparticles with peroxidase-like activity enhance the cleavage of biological macromolecules for biofilm elimination." *Nanoscale* 6 (5):2588–93. doi: 10.1039/c3nr05422e.

Gao, L., Y. Liu, D. Kim, Y. Li, G. Hwang, P. C. Naha, D. P. Cormode, and H. Koo. 2016. "Nanocatalysts promote *Streptococcus mutans* biofilm matrix degradation and enhance bacterial killing to suppress dental caries in vivo." *Biomaterials* 101:272–84 doi: 10.1016/j.biomaterials.2016.05.051.

Godoy-Gallardo, M., C. Mas-Moruno, M. C. Fernandez-Calderon, C. Perez-Giraldo, J. M. Manero, F. Albericio, F. J. Gil, and D. Rodriguez. 2014. "Covalent immobilization of hLf1–11 peptide on a titanium surface reduces bacterial adhesion and biofilm formation." *Acta Biomater* 10 (8):3522–34. doi: 10.1016/j.actbio.2014.03.026.

Goldin, B. R., and S. L. Gorbach. 1984. "Alterations of the intestinal microflora by diet, oral antibiotics, and *Lactobacillus*: decreased production of free amines from aromatic nitro compounds, azo dyes, and glucuronides." *J Natl Cancer Inst* 73 (3):689–95.

Gopinath, S., J. S. Lichtman, D. M. Bouley, J. E. Elias, and D. M. Monack. 2014. "Role of disease-associated tolerance in infectious superspreaders." *Proc Natl Acad Sci U S A* 111 (44):15780–5. doi: 10.1073/pnas.1409968111.

Gordon, Y. J., E. G. Romanowski, and A. M. McDermott. 2005. "A review of antimicrobial peptides and their therapeutic potential as anti-infective drugs." *Curr Eye Res* 30 (7):505–15. doi: 10.1080/02713680590968637.

Gorr, S. U., and M. Abdolhosseini. 2011. "Antimicrobial peptides and periodontal disease." *J Clin Periodontol* 38 (Suppl 11):126–41 doi: 10.1111/j.1600-051X.2010.01664.x.

Groppo, F. C., C. Bergamaschi Cde, K. Cogo, M. Franz-Montan, R. H. Motta, and E. D. de Andrade. 2008. "Use of phytotherapy in dentistry." *Phytother Res* 22 (8):993–8. doi: 10.1002/ptr.2471.

Guo, L., J. S. McLean, Y. Yang, R. Eckert, C. W. Kaplan, P. Kyme, O. Sheikh, B. Varnum, R. Lux, W. Shi, and X. He. 2015. "Precision-guided antimicrobial peptide as a targeted modulator of human microbial ecology." *Proc Natl Acad Sci U S A* 112 (24):7569–74. doi: 10.1073/pnas.1506207112.

Gupta, K., A. Kotian, H. Subramanian, H. Daniell, and H. Ali. 2015. "Activation of human mast cells by retrocyclin and protegrin highlight their immuno-modulatory and antimicrobial properties." *Oncotarget* 6 (30):28573–87. doi: 10.18632/oncotarget.5611.

Gupta, R., S. Sarkar, and S. Srivastava. 2014. "In vivo toxicity assessment of antimi-crobial peptides (AMPs LR14) derived from *Lactobacillus plantarum* strain LR/14 in *Drosophila melanogaster.*" *Probiotics Antimicrob Proteins* 6 (1):59–67. doi: 10.1007/s12602-013-9154–y.

Gupta, S. M., C. C. Aranha, and K. V. Reddy. 2008. "Evaluation of developmental toxicity of microbicide Nisin in rats." *Food Chem Toxicol* 46 (2):598–603. doi: 10.1016/j.fct.2007.09.006.

Haapasalo, M., W. Qian, I. Portenier, and T. Waltimo. 2007. "Effects of dentin on the antimicrobial properties of endodontic medicaments." *J Endod* 33 (8):-917–25. doi: 10.1016/j.joen.2007.04.008.

Horev, B., M. I. Klein, G. Hwang, Y. Li, D. Kim, H. Koo, and D. S. Benoit. 2015. "pH-activated nanoparticles for controlled topical delivery of farnesol to disrupt oral biofilm virulence." *ACS Nano* 9 (3):2390–404. doi: 10.1021/nn507170s.

Hu, D. Y., X. Hong, and X. Li. 2011. "Oral health in China—trends and challenges." *Int J Oral Sci* 3 (1):7–12. doi: 10.4248/IJOS11006.

Huang, S., S. Gao, L. Cheng, and H. Yu. 2010. "Combined effects of nano-hydroxyapatite and Galla chinensis on remineralisation of initial enamel lesion in vitro." *J Dent* 38 (10):811–9. doi: 10.1016/j.jdent.2010.06.013.

Huang, Z. B., X. Shi, J. Mao, and S. Q. Gong. 2016. "Design of a hydroxyapatite-binding antimicrobial peptide with improved retention and antibacterial efficacy for oral pathogen control." *Sci Rep* 6:38410. doi: 10.1038/srep38410.

Hussain, M., C. M. Stover, and A. Dupont. 2015. "*P. gingivalis* in periodontal dis-ease and atherosclerosis—scenes of action for antimicrobial peptides and complement." *Front Immunol* 6:45. doi: 10.3389/fimmu.2015.00045.

Hwang, G., B. Koltisko, X. Jin, and H. Koo. 2017. "Nonleachable imidazolium-incorporated composite for disruption of bacterial clustering, exopolysaccharide-matrix assembly, and enhanced biofilm removal." *ACS Appl Mater Interfaces* 9 (44):38270–80. doi: 10.1021/acsami.7b11558.

International Labour Organization. 2004. "Imidazole. International Chemical Safety Cards (ICSC) are data sheets intended to provide essential safety and health information on chemicals in a clear and concise way." National Center for Biotechnology Information. *PubChem Compound Database; CID=795.*

Jang, W. S., X. S. Li, J. N. Sun, and M. Edgerton. 2008. "The P-113 fragment of histatin 5 requires a specific peptide sequence for intracellular translocation in *Candida albicans*, which is independent of cell wall binding." *Antimicrob Agents Chemother* 52 (2):497–504. doi: 10.1128/AAC.01199–07.

Jhajharia, K., A. Parolia, K. V. Shetty, and L. K. Mehta. 2015. "Biofilm in end-odontics: a review." *J Int Soc Prev Community Dent* 5 (1):1–12. doi: 10.4103/2231-0762.151956.

Jones, M. N., S. E. Francis, F. J. Hutchinson, P. S. Handley, and I. G. Lyle. 1993. "Targeting and delivery of bactericide to adsorbed oral bacteria by use of proteoliposomes." *Biochim Biophys Acta* 1147 (2):251–61.

Koczulla, A. R., and R. Bals. 2003. "Antimicrobial peptides: current status and therapeutic potential." *Drugs* 63 (4):389–406.

Koczulla, R., G. von Degenfeld, C. Kupatt, F. Krotz, S. Zahler, T. Gloe, K. Issbrucker, P. Unterberger, M. Zaiou, C. Lebherz, A. Karl, P. Raake, A. Pfosser, P. Boekstegers, U. Welsch, P. S. Hiemstra, C. Vogelmeier, R. L. Gallo, M. Clauss, and R. Bals. 2003. "An angiogenic role for the human peptide antibiotic LL-37/hCAP-18." *J Clin Invest* 111 (11):1665–72. doi: 10.1172/JCI17545.

Kohler, B., I. Andreen, B. Jonsson, and E. Hultqvist. 1982. "Effect of caries preventive measures on *Streptococcus mutans* and *lactobacilli* in selected mothers." *Scand J Dent Res* 90 (2):102–8.

Kolenbrander, P. E., R. J. Palmer, Jr., A. H. Rickard, N. S. Jakubovics, N. I. Chalmers, and P. I. Diaz. 2006. "Bacterial interactions and successions during plaque development." *Periodontol 2000* 42:47–79 doi: 10.1111/j.1600–0757.2006.00187.x.

Koo, H., B. Schobel, K. Scott-Anne, G. Watson, W. H. Bowen, J. A. Cury, P. L. Rosalen, and Y. K. Park. 2005. "Apigenin and tt-farnesol with fluoride effects on *S. mutans* biofilms and dental caries." *J Dent Res* 84 (11):1016–20. doi: 10.1177/154405910508401109.

Lee, S. B., B. Li, S. Jin, and H. Daniell. 2011. "Expression and characterization of antimicrobial peptides retrocyclin-101 and protegrin-1 in chloroplasts to control viral and bacterial infections." *Plant Biotechnol J* 9 (1):100–15. doi: 10.1111/j.1467–7652.2010.00538.x.

Lei Cheng, Y. J., Y. Hu, J. Li, H. H. K. Xu, L. He, B. Ren, X. Zhou. 2016. Biomaterials in caries prevention and treatment. *Interface Oral Health Science* 101–110. doi:10.1007/978-981-10-1560-1_9.

Leonhardt, A., S. Renvert, and G. Dahlen. 1999. "Microbial findings at failing implants." *Clin Oral Implants Res* 10 (5):339–45.

Lewies, A., J. F. Wentzel, H. C. Miller, and L. H. Du Plessis. 2018. "The antimicrobial peptide nisin Z induces selective toxicity and apoptotic cell death in cultured melanoma cells." *Biochimie* 144:28–40 doi: 10.1016/j.biochi.2017.10.009.

Lewis, K. 2007. "Persister cells, dormancy and infectious disease." *Nat Rev Microbiol* 5 (1):48–56. doi: 10.1038/nrmicro1557.

Liu, Y., A. C. Kamesh, Y. Xiao, V. Sun, M. Hayes, H. Daniell, and H. Koo. 2016. "Topical delivery of low-cost protein drug candidates made in chloroplasts for biofilm disruption and uptake by oral epithelial cells." *Biomaterials* 105:-156–66 doi: 10.1016/j.biomaterials.2016.07.042.

Liu, Y., L. Wang, X. Zhou, S. Hu, S. Zhang, and H. Wu. 2011. "Effect of the antimicrobial decapeptide KSL on the growth of oral pathogens and *Streptococcus mutans* biofilm." *Int J Antimicrob Agents* 37 (1):33–8. doi: 10.1016/j.ijantimicag.2010.08.014.

Liu, Z., S. Ma, S. Duan, D. Xuliang, Y. Sun, X. Zhang, X. Xu, B. Guan, C. Wang, M. Hu, X. Qi, X. Zhang, and P. Gao. 2016. "Modification of titanium substrates with chimeric peptides comprising antimicrobial and titanium-binding motifs connected by linkers to inhibit biofilm formation." *ACS Appl Mater Interfaces* 8 (8):5124–36. doi: 10.1021/acsami.5b11949.

Melo, M. A., S. Orrego, M. D. Weir, H. H. Xu, and D. D. Arola. 2016. "Designing multiagent dental materials for enhanced resistance to biofilm damage at the bonded interface." *ACS Appl Mater Interfaces* 8 (18):11779-87. doi: 10.1021/acsami.6b01923.

Moon, J. H., Y. S. Choi, H. W. Lee, J. S. Heo, S. W. Chang, and J. Y. Lee. 2016. "Antibacterial effects of N-acetylcysteine against endodontic pathogens." *J Microbiol* 54 (4):322-9. doi: 10.1007/s12275-016-5534-9.

Mukherjee, S. P., and H. J. Byrne. 2013. "Polyamidoamine dendrimer nanoparticle cytotoxicity, oxidative stress, caspase activation and inflammatory response: experimental observation and numerical simulation." *Nanomedicine* 9 (2):-202-11. doi: 10.1016/j.nano.2012.05.002.

Newman, D. J. 2008. "Natural products as leads to potential drugs: an old process or the new hope for drug discovery?" *J Med Chem* 51 (9):2589-99. doi: 10.1021/jm0704090.

Okamoto, T. 2005. "Safety of quercetin for clinical application (review)." *Int J Mol Med* 16 (2):275-8.

Padmanaban, G., V. Venkateswar, and P. N. Rangarajan. 1989. "Haem as a multifunctional regulator." *Trends Biochem Sci* 14 (12):492-6.

Paes Leme, A. F., H. Koo, C. M. Bellato, G. Bedi, and J. A. Cury. 2006. "The role of sucrose in cariogenic dental biofilm formation—new insight." *J Dent Res* 85 (10):878-87. doi: 10.1177/154405910608501002.

Penick, E. C., and E. M. Osetek. 1970. "Intracanal drugs and chemicals in endodontic therapy." *Dent Clin North Am* 14 (4):743-56.

Petersen, P. E., D. Kandelman, S. Arpin, and H. Ogawa. 2010. "Global oral health of older people—call for public health action." *Community Dent Health* 27 (4 Suppl 2):257-67.

Portenier, I., H. Haapasalo, D. Orstavik, M. Yamauchi, and M. Haapasalo. 2002. "Inactivation of the antibacterial activity of iodine potassium iodide and chlorhexidine digluconate against *Enterococcus faecalis* by dentin, dentin matrix, type-I collagen, and heat-killed microbial whole cells." *J Endod* 28 (9):634-7. doi: 10.1097/00004770-200209000-00002.

Quirynen, M., R. Vogels, W. Peeters, D. van Steenberghe, I. Naert, and A. Haffajee. 2006. "Dynamics of initial subgingival colonization of 'pristine' peri-implant pockets." *Clin Oral Implants Res* 17 (1):25-37. doi: 10.1111/j.1600-0501.2005 .01194.x.

Raab, W., and F. Hogl. 1980. "Effect of imidazole derivatives on various numbers of microbes to determine microbial sensitivity." *Z Hautkr* 55 (17):1116-22.

Radovic-Moreno, A. F., T. K. Lu, V. A. Puscasu, C. J. Yoon, R. Langer, and O. C. Farokhzad. 2012. "Surface charge-switching polymeric nanoparticles for bacterial cell wall-targeted delivery of antibiotics." *ACS Nano* 6 (5):4279-87. doi: 10.1021/nn3008383.

Raj, P. A., L. Rajkumar, and A. R. Dentino. 2008. "Novel molecules for intra-oral delivery of antimicrobials to prevent and treat oral infectious diseases." *Biochem J* 409 (2):601-9. doi: 10.1042/BJ20070810.

Roberts, J. C., M. K. Bhalgat, and R. T. Zera. 1996. "Preliminary biological evaluation of polyamidoamine (PAMAM) starburst dendrimers." *J Biomed Mater Res* 30 (1):53–65. doi: 10.1002/(SICI)1097-4636(199601)30:1<53::AID-JBM8>3.0.CO;2-Q.

Ruby, J. D., Y. Li, Y. Luo, and P. W. Caufield. 2002. "Genetic characterization of the oral *Actinomyces*." *Arch Oral Biol* 47 (6):457–63.

Schwendicke, F., and G. Gostemeyer. 2017. "Cost-effectiveness of root caries preventive treatments." *J Dent* 56:58–64 doi: 10.1016/j.jdent.2016.10.016.

Selwitz, R. H., A. I. Ismail, and N. B. Pitts. 2007. "Dental caries." *Lancet* 369 (9555):51–9. doi: 10.1016/S0140-6736(07)60031-2.

Su, M., S. Yao, L. Gu, Z. Huang, and S. Mai. 2017. "Antibacterial effect and bond strength of a modified dental adhesive containing the peptide nisin." *Peptides* 99:189–94 doi: 10.1016/j.peptides.2017.10.003.

Sullivan, R., P. Santarpia, S. Lavender, E. Gittins, Z. Liu, M. H. Anderson, J. He, W. Shi, and R. Eckert. 2011. "Clinical efficacy of a specifically targeted antimicrobial peptide mouth rinse: targeted elimination of *Streptococcus mutans* and prevention of demineralization." *Caries Res* 45 (5):415–28. doi: 10.1159/000330510.

Takahashi, N., and B. Nyvad. 2008. "Caries ecology revisited: microbial dynamics and the caries process." *Caries Res* 42 (6):409–18. doi: 10.1159/000159604.

Takahashi, N., and B. Nyvad. 2011. "The role of bacteria in the caries process: ecological perspectives." *J Dent Res* 90 (3):294–303. doi: 10.1177/0022034510379602.

Takahashi, N., and B. Nyvad. 2016. "Ecological hypothesis of dentin and root caries." *Caries Res* 50 (4):422–31. doi: 10.1159/000447309.

Tasman, A. J., F. Wallner, and R. Neumeier. 2000. "Antibiotic impregnation of cartilage implants: diffusion kinetics of fluoroquinolones." *Laryngorhinootologie* 79 (1):30–3. doi: 10.1055/s-2000-8778.

ten Cate, J. M. 2006. "Biofilms, a new approach to the microbiology of dental plaque." *Odontology* 94 (1):1–9. doi: 10.1007/s10266-006-0063-3.

Tyagi, N., R. De, J. Begun, and A. Popat. 2017. "Cancer therapeutics with epigallocatechin-3-gallate encapsulated in biopolymeric nanoparticles." *Int J Pharm* 518 (1–2):220–7. doi: 10.1016/j.ijpharm.2016.12.030.

Vaucher Rde, A., C. V. Gewehr Cde, A. P. Correa, V. Sant'Anna, J. Ferreira, and A. Brandelli. 2011. "Evaluation of the immunogenicity and in vivo toxicity of the antimicrobial peptide P34." *Int J Pharm* 421 (1):94–8. doi: 10.1016/j.ijpharm.2011.09.020.

Vennila, V., V. Madhu, R. Rajesh, K. K. Ealla, S. R. Velidandla, and S. Santoshi. 2014. "Tetracycline-induced discoloration of deciduous teeth: case series." *J Int Oral Health* 6 (3):115–9.

Wan, Y., S. Raman, F. He, Y. Huang. 2007. "Surface modification of medical metals by ion implantation of silver and copper." *Vacuum* 81:1114–8.

Wang, H. Y., J. W. Cheng, H. Y. Yu, L. Lin, Y. H. Chih, and Y. P. Pan. 2015. "Efficacy of a novel antimicrobial peptide against periodontal pathogens in both planktonic and polymicrobial biofilm states." *Acta Biomater* 25:150–61 doi: 10.1016/j.actbio.2015.07.031.

Wang, S., C. Zhou, B. Ren, X. Li, M. D. Weir, R. M. Masri, T. W. Oates, L. Cheng, and H. K. H. Xu. 2017. "Formation of persisters in *Streptococcus mutans* biofilms induced by antibacterial dental monomer." *J Mater Sci Mater Med* 28 (11):178. doi: 10.1007/s10856-017-5981-9.

Wang, S., H. Wang, B. Ren, H. Li, M. D. Weir, X. Zhou, T. W. Oates, L. Cheng, and H. H. K. Xu. 2017. "Do quaternary ammonium monomers induce drug resistance in cariogenic, endodontic and periodontal bacterial species?" *Dent Mater* 33 (10):1127–38. doi: 10.1016/j.dental.2017.07.001.

Whitmore, S.E., and R. J. Lamont. 2011. "The pathogenic persona of community-associated oral streptococci." *Mol Microbiol* 81 (2):305–14.

Winfred, S. B., G. Meiyazagan, J. J. Panda, V. Nagendrababu, K. Deivanayagam, V. S. Chauhan, and G. Venkatraman. 2014. "Antimicrobial activity of cationic peptides in endodontic procedures." *Eur J Dent* 8 (2):254–60. doi: 10.4103/1305-7456.130626.

Wu, D., J. Yang, J. Li, L. Chen, B. Tang, X. Chen, W. Wu, and J. Li. 2013. "Hydroxyapatite-anchored dendrimer for in situ remineralization of human tooth enamel." *Biomaterials* 34 (21):5036–47. doi: 10.1016/j.biomaterials.2013.03.053.

Xiang, F., L. Peng, Z. Yin, R. Jia, Z. Hu, Z. Li, X. Ni, X. Liang, L. Li, C. He, L. Yin, G. Su, and C. Lv. 2015. "Acute and subchronic toxicity as well as evaluation of safety pharmacology of Galla chinensis solution." *J Ethnopharmacol* 162: 181–90 doi: 10.1016/j.jep.2014.12.021.

Xiao, J., A. T. Hara, D. Kim, D. T. Zero, H. Koo, and G. Hwang. 2017. "Biofilm three-dimensional architecture influences in situ pH distribution pattern on the human enamel surface." *Int J Oral Sci* 9 (2):74–9. doi: 10.1038/ijos.2017.8.

Xiao, J., and H. Koo. 2010. "Structural organization and dynamics of exopolysaccharide matrix and microcolonies formation by *Streptococcus mutans* in biofilms." *J Appl Microbiol* 108 (6):2103–13. doi: 10.1111/j.1365-2672.2009.04616.x.

Xiao, J., M. I. Klein, M. L. Falsetta, B. Lu, C. M. Delahunty, J. R. Yates 3rd, A. Heydorn, and H. Koo. 2012. "The exopolysaccharide matrix modulates the interaction between 3D architecture and virulence of a mixed-species oral biofilm." *PLoS Pathog* 8 (4):e1002623. doi: 10.1371/journal.ppat.1002623.

Xie, Q., J. Li, and X. Zhou. 2008. "Anticaries effect of compounds extracted from Galla chinensis in a multispecies biofilm model." *Oral Microbiol Immunol* 23 (6):459–65. doi: 10.1111/j.1399-302X.2008.00450.x.

Yang, H., K. Li, H. Yan, S. Liu, Y. Wang, and C. Huang. 2017. "High-performance therapeutic quercetin-doped adhesive for adhesive-dentin interfaces." *Sci Rep* 7 (1):8189. doi: 10.1038/s41598-017-08633-3.

Yu, J., H. Yang, K. Li, H. Ren, J. Lei, and C. Huang. 2017. "Development of epigallocatechin-3-gallate-encapsulated nanohydroxyapatite/mesoporous silica for therapeutic management of dentin surface." *ACS Appl Mater Interfaces* 9 (31):25796–807. doi: 10.1021/acsami.7b06597.

Zasloff, M. 2002. "Antimicrobial peptides of multicellular organisms." *Nature* 415 (6870):389–95. doi: 10.1038/415389a.

Zhang, Q., X. H. Zhao, and Z. J. Wang. 2009. "Cytotoxicity of flavones and flavonols to a human esophageal squamous cell carcinoma cell line (KYSE-510) by induction of G2/M arrest and apoptosis." *Toxicol In Vitro* 23 (5):797–807. doi: 10.1016/j.tiv.2009.04.007.

Zhao, T., and Y. Liu. 2010. "N-acetylcysteine inhibit biofilms produced by *Pseudomonas aeruginosa.*" *BMC Microbiol* 10:140. doi: 10.1186/1471-2180-10-140.

Zhou, J., B. Horev, G. Hwang, M. I. Klein, H. Koo, and D. S. Benoit. 2016. "Characterization and optimization of pH-responsive polymer nanoparticles for drug delivery to oral biofilms." *J Mater Chem B Mater Biol Med* 4 (18):- 3075–85. doi: 10.1039/C5TB02054A.

8

Antibacterial, pH Neutralizing, and Remineralizing Fillers in Polymeric Restorative Materials

Abdulrahman A. Balhaddad and Maria S. Ibrahim
University of Maryland School of Dentistry
Imam Abdulrahman Bin Faisal University

Michael D. Weir and Hockin H.K. Xu
University of Maryland School of Dentistry

Contents

8.1 Limitations of the Available Resin-Based Materials

Dental caries is an infectious disease that affects most of the world population and compromises the quality of life. The tooth structure may undergo mineral detachment due to the acid attack by caries-related pathogens, causing demineralization and weakening of the enamel and dentin (Balhaddad et al. 2019c). One of targeting caries-related factor is the loss of mineral content due the acid attack. With this in mind, bioactive materials able to (1) deposit hydroxyapatite or fluorohydroxyapatite to remineralize the tooth surface, and (2) able to release ion in order to saturate the microenviroment and reduce the diffusion of calcium and phosphate have been extensively investigated in the last 20 years (Balhaddad et al. 2019b).

Remineralization therapy involves the use of particular approaches to arrest early and moderate carious lesions without the need for restorative intervention (Philip 2019). The most commonly used products in remineralization therapy are fluoride-containing products, such as fluoridated-toothpaste, mouthwashes gel, and varnish.

The purpose of the remineralization therapy is to arrest the demineralization attack and enhance the remineralization process by promoting mineral gain in the affected tooth structure (Philip 2019). The fluoride-containing products can provide fluoride ions in the oral environment, which facilitates the diffusion of calcium and phosphate ions to the tooth structure (Pitts et al. 2017). Also, the deposition of fluorohydroxyapatite to the tooth structure results in higher resistance to any future demineralization attack (Hamba et al. 2011; Reynolds et al. 2003; Kitasako et al. 2012).

The incorporation of calcium and fluoride ions to some of the commercially available sugar-free gums and varnishes has gained recognition within the last few years. Furthermore, casein phosphopeptide-amorphous calcium phosphate (CPP-ACP) products are hypothesized to bind the enamel through casein phosphopeptide (CPP), which can bind a considerable amount of calcium, phosphate, and fluoride ions to favor the process of remineralization. These products have the potential to keep the environments supersaturated with calcium and phosphate ions rendering the process of remineralization over demineralization (Hamba et al. 2011; Reynolds et al. 2003; Kitasako et al. 2012).

In more extensive carious lesions, the need for restorative intervention is recommended to remove the carious lesions and defective tooth structures, and then restore the form and function of the tooth using dental restorations (Zhang et al. 2017). The use of resin composites in the past two decades increased due to the significant improvement in the material properties and the esthetic appearance by matching the color of the bonded tooth (Maktabi et al. 2018). The two main reasons associated with resin composite failure are secondary caries around the restoration and restoration fracture. Subsequently, the replacement of dental restorations is a frequent procedure, consuming a high amount of time and money (AlShaafi 2017; Maktabi et al. 2018; Price et al. 2014). Therefore, increasing the longevity of resin composite restorations are necessary either by enhancing the mechanical properties of the materials or by developing approaches to prevent the bacterial attachment and invasion at the tooth/restoration interface.

Many factors are critical for the longevity of composite resin restoration, with special consideration to increasing dental plaque accumulation compared to other restorations (Zhang et al. 2017). Resin composites depend on the polymerization reaction activated by the light-curing unit to start the cross-linking of the resin matrix, which the monomers transform into polymers. The transformation of monomers to polymers is referred to as the degree of conversion, which represents the percentage of double C=C bonds in the monomers that transformed into single C–C bonds.

The degree of conversion is an essential factor to assure the quality of the placed resin composites, as a high amount of conversion is associated with excellent mechanical and physical properties (AlShaafi 2017; Maktabi et al. 2018; Price et al. 2014, 2015). In the dental literature, the amount of conversion was reported between 40% and 80% concerning the variation of the resin composite materials. Unreacted monomers inside the resin composite system can contribute to the secondary caries process by facilitating the plaque accumulation and increasing the cariogenicity of caries-related pathogens (AlShaafi 2017; Maktabi et al. 2018; Price et al. 2014, 2015).

In other scenarios where that resin composite monomeric conversion is far from the optimal, the release of unreacted monomers could be enhanced, favoring biofilm build-up over composites (Maktabi et al. 2018). Another limitation is related to the polymerization shrinkage of resin composite as a consequence of the polymerization reaction (Kaisarly and Gezawi 2016). While theoretically increasing the degree of conversion is beneficial to reduce the unreacted monomers, a high degree of conversion is associated with more shrinkage. The shrinkage of resin composites may create micro gaps at the tooth/restoration interface, which could eventually be a preferable target for the cariogenic bacteria to accumulate and invade the tooth structure (Maktabi et al. 2018; Kermanshahi et al. 2010). With these significant limitations in resin composite restorations, new approaches should be explored and investigated to reduce the growth and activities of caries-related pathogens over the surface of such restoration.

With the advancement of nanotechnology and polymer engineering, several approaches have been established to introduce bioactivity into resin composites. As the use of antibacterial monomer systems was discussed comprehensively in the previous chapter, this chapter focuses on the use of remineralizing, pH neutralizing, and antibacterial fillers to modulate oral biofilms.

8.2 Remineralizing Fillers in Restorative Dentistry

Early studies in this field focused on using antibacterial or remineralization fillers as a component in the resin composite system. Fluoride-containing restorations are the most popular restorations to be used as a remineralizing approach (Balhaddad et al. 2019b; Cheng et al. 2015). Glass ionomer and resin-modified glass ionomer (RMGI) restorations can release fluoride ions to neutralize the acidity produced by bacteria, and also remineralize the demineralized adjacent tooth structure. The burst release of fluoride can last only for three days, then the amount of release becomes very low, and so the material needs to be recharged (Cabral et al. 2015; Hasan et al. 2019). Likewise, solvent disinfectants were coordinated into composites, including chlorhexidine, triclosan, and antibacterial antibiotics. Their significant limitation is that a large amount of the material is released rapidly, rendering the effect of such material to be short. Also, the release of agents may compromise the mechanical properties of the resin composites (Balhaddad et al. 2019b; Cheng et al. 2015).

More recently, nano-sized amorphous calcium phosphate (NACP) fillers have shown good remineralizing and neutralizing ability. The main advantage of NACP is that it is composed of hydroxyapatite [$Ca_{10}(PO_4)_6(OH)_2$], the main component of human bone and teeth (Cheng, Weir, Limkangwalmongkol, et al. 2012). The incorporation of calcium and phosphate compounds into resin composites has undergone many phases of modifications, including dicalcium phosphate dihydrate (DCPD), dicalcium phosphate anhydrous (DCPA) and tetra-calcium phosphate (TTCP), tricalcium phosphate (TCP), and amorphous calcium phosphate (ACP) (Balhaddad et al. 2019b). Table 8.1 summarizes different calcium orthophosphate phases used in dental resin composites.

In the early stage, ACP fillers in a micro-sized level were synthesized. Despite the sustained release of ions and the remineralization ability, the mechanical properties were weak compared to the control (Skrtic et al. 1996). The other phases of DCPD, DCPA, and TTCP were synthesized, which demonstrated a good amount of ion release with good mechanical properties (Balhaddad et al. 2019b). To overcome the problem of weak mechanical properties associated with ACP, nanotechnology has been employed to synthesize the fillers in a nano-sized level.

NACP fillers produce a higher amount of calcium and phosphate ions and excellent mechanical properties compared to ACP fillers (Al-Dulaijan et al. 2018a,b). The vast amount of ion release produced by NACP can neutralize the acid and increase the pH. As a result, the number of attached S. mutans biofilm in NACP resin composite was less compared to resin composite with no NACP (Moreau et al. 2011). A study using in situ models revealed the ability of NACP resin composite to reduce the subsurface enamel lesions compared to control resin composite (Melo et al. 2013). Representative mineral profiles (Figure 8.1) demonstrated larger

TABLE 8.1   Different Calcium Orthophosphate Phases Used in Resin-Based Materials concerning Ca/P Ratios

Calcium Phosphate	Chemical Formula	Ca/P Ratio	log (K_{sp}) at 25°	log (K_{sp}) at 37°
Dicalcium phosphate dihydrate (DCPD)	$CaHPO_4H_2O$	1.0	6.59	6.63
Dicalcium phosphate anhydrous (DCPA)	$CaHPO_4$	1.0	6.90	7.02
Amorphous calcium phosphate (ACP)	$Ca_xH_y(PO_4)_{zn}H_2O$	1.2–2.2	*	*
Tetracalcium phosphate (TTCP)	$Ca_4(PO_4)_2O$	2	38-44	42.4
Hydroxyapatite (HA)	$Ca_{10}(PO_4)_6(OH)_2$	1.67	58.4	58.6
ß-Tricalcium phosphate	$ß-Ca_3(PO_4)_2$	1.5	28.9	29.5

Source: Adapted from Balhaddad et al. (2019b), with permission from © 2019 Elsevier.
    ACP, amorphous calcium phosphate; DCPA, dicalcium phosphate anhydrous; DCPD, dicalcium phosphate dihydrate; HA, hydroxyapatite; TTCP, tetracalcium phosphate.
    *ACP solubility cannot be measured accurately.

demineralized surface and higher mineral loss in enamel-contacting conventional composite compared to enamel-contacting NACP composite (Melo et al. 2013) (Figure 8.2).

The main concern about NACP resin composites is related to the robust initial ion release, which may impact the sustained release over time, and may also reduce the mechanical properties of the restoration. This issue was solved by constructing a resin composite formulation that can be recharged using recharging solutions used as a mouthwash (Al-Dulaijan et al. 2018a,b). The rechargeable NACP resin composite consisted of ethoxylated bisphenol A dimethacrylate (EBPADMA) and pyromellitic glycerol dimethacrylate (PMGDM) to allow the frequent recharging ability. The amount of calcium and phosphate ion release was maintained at the same level (Figure 8.3) with each recharging cycle (Al-Dulaijan et al. 2018a).

Combining the NACP fillers with dimethylaminohexadecyl methacrylate (DMAHDM), as an antibacterial monomer, was attempted in several studies (Balhaddad et al. 2019a; Al-Dulaijan et al. 2018a; Cheng et al. 2016). DMAHDM-NACP resin composite demonstrates the ability to preserve the mechanical properties and antibacterial functions after one year of water aging. Metabolic activities, lactic acid production, biofilm viability, and colony-forming units were reduced after one year in the same pattern compared to those samples tested at the baseline time point, and

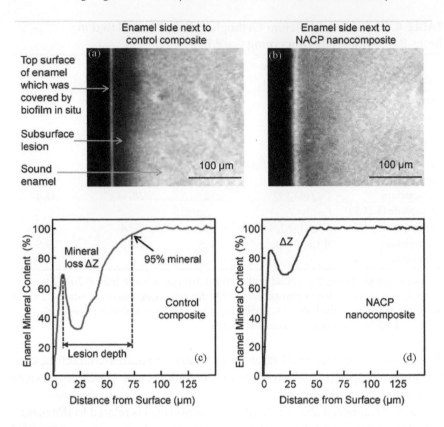

Figure 8.1   A representative of subsurface enamel lesion contacting conventional resin composite (a) and resin composite containing NACP (b) via transverse microradiography analysis. (c and d) The lesion depth profile can be observed in both conventional and NACP composites. Greater lesion is seen concerning the conventional resin composite (c) compared to the NACP resin composite that showed a less pronounced demineralized lesion (d). (Adapted from Melo et al. (2013), with permission from © 2015 Elsevier.)

indicating the long-term effect of this bioactive resin composite (Cheng et al. 2016).

DMAHDM antibacterial monomer and NACP fillers were incorporated in a resin composite formulation that is able to recharge the calcium and phosphate ions through specific solutions used as mouthwashes. The rechargeability is an important feature for NACP-containing resin composite to assure the replacement of calcium and phosphate ions (Al-Dulaijan et al. 2018a). This approach can assure preserving the structural stability of the resin composite and also the ability to release the ions several times to promote remineralization for a long term. The rationale of combining

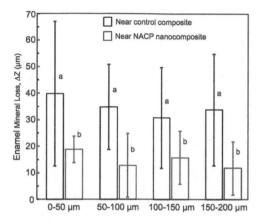

Figure 8.2 Enamel mineral loss observed in situ in both conventional and NACP resin composites concerning the distance from the restoration-enamel interface. NACP resin composite significantly demonstrated a less amount of mineral loss at each distance. (Adapted from Melo et al. (2013), with permission from © 2015 Elsevier.)

DMAHDM and NACP fillers in one formulation is to have dual benefits of the contact-killing mechanism of DMAHDM and the remineralization ability of NACP ion release (Ibrahim et al. 2019). More investigations are needed to understand how far NACP ion release may contribute to the advancement of secondary caries prevention. Table 8.2 summarizes all the calcium phosphate compounds used in the dental literature and their remineralizing and neutralizing activities.

8.3 Metallic and Metallic/Oxide Nanoparticles in Restorative Dentistry

The use of metallic nanoparticle fillers has been suggested as an approach to target cariogenic species. Several metallic nanoparticle platforms such as bioactive glass, silver, zinc oxide, copper oxide, and diamond nanoparticles were found effective in the perspective of bacterial growth inhibition (Balhaddad et al. 2019b). Multiple studies have demonstrated the ability of bioactive glass to reduce the growth and activity of *S. mutans* (Khvostenko et al. 2016; Chatzistavrou et al. 2015; Tezvergil-Mutluay et al. 2017).

In one study, the amount of bacterial penetration in resin composite with bioactive glass was reduced by 40% compared to resin composite with no bioactive glass (Khvostenko et al. 2016). These results could be

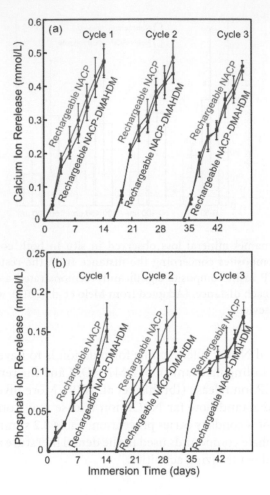

Figure 8.3 Three cycles of calcium (a) and phosphate (b) ion recharge and re-release by the NACP resin composite. (Adapted from Al-Dulaijan et al. (2018a), with permission from © 2015 Elsevier.)

elaborated to reduce the risk of secondary caries around resin composite restorations. The suggested mechanism of bioactive glass is that the release of calcium and phosphate ions could be bactericidal to the *S. mutans* biofilm, also helping in reducing the acidity and enhancing the remineralization of the surrounding tooth structure (Khvostenko et al. 2016). The combining effect of silver and bioactive glass can reduce *S. mutans* biofilm and increase the formation of the appetite layer (Chatzistavrou et al. 2015). The synergetic effect of fluoride ions and calcium phosphate ions released by bioactive glass demonstrates greater remineralization capability and

TABLE 8.2 Outlines of Studies Investigating the Bioactivity of Calcium Phosphate Compounds Incorporated into Resin Composites and Their Effects on Dental Biofilms and Surrounding Tissues

Agent	References	Concentration	Mechanical Properties	Remarks
ACP ZrOCl$_2$-ACP TEOS-ACP	Skrtic et al. (1996)	40%		Sustained release of Ca and PO$_4$ ions that is able to induce remineralization
ACP reinforced with silica or zirconia	Skrtic et al. (2000)	40%	Biaxial flexure strength values were significantly lower compared to control samples	
Nano DCPA	Xu et al. (2006)	60%	Mixed with nano silica fused whisker, flexural strength values were comparable to control samples and higher than previous CaP compounds	Comparable or higher amount of Ca and PO$_4$ ion release compared to previous CaP compounds
Nano DCPA	Xu et al. (2007)	Varied from 0% to 75%	Compared to control, nano DCPA demonstrated higher elastic modulus and hardness, but comparable flexural strength values	
TTCP	Xu et al. (2009)	Varied from 0% to 75%	TTCP with whisker reinforcement demonstrated flexural strength values that were not significantly different compared to control hybrid resin composites. TTCP with whisker reinforcement demonstrated significantly high flexural strength compared to TTCP alone	Ca and PO$_4$ ion release increased by about 6-fold when the pH changed from 6 to 4. TTCP resin composites demonstrated higher amount of released ions compared to TTCP with whisker reinforcement
TTCP	Cheng et al. (2012b)	40%	No significant differences were found in flexural strength and elastic modulus between TTCP-QADM and control samples	TTCP-QADM resin composites demonstrated higher antibacterial action against S. mutans compared to control. CFU, metabolic activity, and lactic acid production were 50% lower in TTCP-QADM samples compared to control

(Continued)

TABLE 8.2 (Continued) Outlines of Studies Investigating the Bioactivity of Calcium Phosphate Compounds Incorporated into Resin Composites and Their Effects on Dental Biofilms and Surrounding Tissues

Agent	References	Concentration	Mechanical Properties	Remarks
NACP	Xu et al. (2011)	10%, 15%, and 20%	No significant differences were found in flexural strength and elastic modulus between all NACP samples and control	Increasing NACP amount was associated with higher ion release
NACP	Moreau et al. (2011)	10%–40%	10%–30% NACP resin composite demonstrated comparable flexural strength and elastic modulus to hybrid resin composite control. 40% NACP resin composite demonstrated significantly low flexural strength and elastic modulus compared to control, but was similar to microfill resin composite control	NACP resin composites raised the pH and neutralized the acid, higher capability to raise the pH and neutralize the acid was observed and the NACP concentration increased. NACP resin composite demonstrated a significant ability to resist the adherence of S. mutans compared to control samples
NACP	Moreau et al. (2012)	10%, 15% and 20%	Flexural strength and elastic modulus were higher or matching that of control samples before and after thermal cycling. With water aging, the flexural strength of NACP samples decreased significantly, but they were higher than their control counterparts Increasing the NACP mass fraction significantly increased the amount of wear compared to control, but the values were lower than that of RMGI	—

(Continued)

TABLE 8.2 (*Continued*) Outlines of Studies Investigating the Bioactivity of Calcium Phosphate Compounds Incorporated into Resin Composites and Their Effects on Dental Biofilms and Surrounding Tissues

Agent	References	Concentration	Mechanical Properties	Remarks
NACP	Melo et al. (2013)	40%	—	This in situ study demonstrated that biofilms collected from NACP restored samples had a higher amount of Ca and PO$_4$ ions compared to control. Biofilm CFU values of *S. mutans*, *Lactobacillus* and total *Streptococcus* were lower, but not significant, in NACP samples. Also, NACP samples demonstrated fewer subsurface enamel lesions compared to control
DCPD	Chiari et al. (2015)	Varied from 0% to 20%	Adding DCPD filler did not affect the degree of conversion of resin composites. Increasing the mass fraction of filler negatively compromised the material strength. However, the optimum mass friction of DCPD that demonstrated proper mechanical properties after water aging was 10%	10% Mass fraction of DCPD demonstrated a constant ion release for 28 days
NACP	Zhang et al. (2016)	20%	No significant differences were found in flexural strength and elastic modulus between PE-NACP and control samples	A novel rechargeable NACP resin composite was invented with sustainable and long-term ion release
NACP+TTCP	Weir et al. (2017)	40% NACP, 20% TTCP	—	NACP-TTCP resin composite was able to remineralize dentin and neutralizes pH. However, no significant differences were found in ion release and remineralization capability between NACP and NACP-TTCP

(Continued)

TABLE 8.2 (Continued)   Outlines of Studies Investigating the Bioactivity of Calcium Phosphate Compounds Incorporated into Resin Composites and Their Effects on Dental Biofilms and Surrounding Tissues

Agent	References	Concentration	Mechanical Properties	Remarks
NACP	Al-Dulaijan et al. (2018a)	20%	Flexural strength and elastic modulus were similar to control	No effect on the recharging capability and ion release after adding 3% of DMAHDM into the NACP mixture. The ion release was maintained as the number of recharging cycles increased. NACP-DMAHDM resin composite reduced the lactic acid, metabolic activities, and colony-forming units of S. *mutans*, total *Streptococcus*, and total microorganisms by around 3 log
NACP	Al-Dulaijan et al. (2018b)	20%	Flexural strength and elastic modulus were similar to control	NACP mixed with 3% of MPC demonstrated excellent rechargeability and ion release. The ion release was maintained as the number of recharging cycles increased. NACP-MPC resin composites reduced the lactic acid, metabolic activities, and colony-forming units of S. *mutans*, total *Streptococcus*, and total microorganisms by 2 log. NACP-MPC resin composites

Source: Adapted from Balhaddad et al. (2019b), with permission from © 2019 Elsevier.

Ag, silver; DCPA, dicalcium phosphate anhydrate; DCPD, dicalcium phosphate dehydrate; DMAHDM, dimethylaminohexadecyl methacrylate; MPC, 2-methacryloyloxyethyl phosphorylcholine; NACP, nano amorphous calcium phosphate; PE-NACP, NACP mixed with pyromellitic glycerol dimethacrylate (PMGDM) and ethoxylated bisphenol A dimethacrylate (EBPADMA) at 1:1 ratio; QADM, quaternary ammonium dimethacrylate; TEOS-ACP, tetraethoxysilane-modified ACP; TTCP, tetracalcium phosphate; $ZrOCl_2$-ACP, zirconyl chloride-modified ACP.

degradation resistance compared to bioactive glass alone (Tezvergil-Mutluay et al. 2017). These results may indicate combining bioactive glass with another antibacterial or remineralizing particle to enhance the performance of such restoration.

Silver nanoparticles have been used in medicine for centuries due to its unique antibacterial effect and biocompatibility. Silver ions can interact with the cell membrane and DNA confirmation of many bacterial species (Balhaddad et al. 2019b). In restorative dentistry, silver-containing resin composite has demonstrated the ability to reduce the pathogenicity of caries-related pathogens. The incorporation of 0.028% of silver into resin composite was found effective to reduce the *S. mutans* biofilm by 75%, and decreasing the metabolic activities and lactic acid production of multispecies pathogens isolated from saliva by 50% and 60%, respectively. Increasing the silver weight in different fractions from 0.028% to 0.175% was associated with more bacterial inhibition, but less mechanical properties. The maximum bacterial inhibition with acceptable mechanical properties compared to the control was found with 0.088% of silver in resin composite (Cheng et al. 2012b). Silver ions released from resin composite are also effective in reducing the biofilm of *Lactobacillus* species, one of the main microorganisms of root caries (Kasraei et al. 2014).

Zinc oxide nanoparticles are effective in killing many oral species. The antibacterial activities of zinc oxide in resin composite were investigated first time in 2010. Compared to zinc oxide weights of 3% and 10% added to resin composites, 5% of zinc oxide demonstrates good antibacterial properties without compromising the mechanical properties. However, the antibacterial efficiency is reduced with aging (Niu et al. 2010). It is suggested that zinc oxide nanoparticles have the ability to produce reactive oxygen species, which then reduce the growth of bacterial species. In another study, the zinc oxide nanoparticles were incorporated in different weights: 1%, 5%, and 10%. While zinc oxide resin composites demonstrated higher antibacterial activities compared to unmodified resin composites, resin composites with incorporated silver nanoparticles demonstrated the highest antibacterial properties, which may indicate the superiority of silver over zinc oxide nanoparticles (Aydin Sevinç and Hanley 2010).

Zinc oxide nanoparticles demonstrate the ability to reduce *Lactobacillus* growth, but the antibacterial activities were found less compared to silver-containing resin composites (Kasraei et al. 2014). The limitations associated with zinc oxide-containing resin composites are the reduced antibacterial efficiency with aging and against multispecies biofilm, and also the reduced depth of cure compared with resin composites without zinc oxide nanoparticles (Aydin Sevinç and Hanley 2010; Tavassoli Hojati et al. 2013).

The use of copper oxide nanoparticles has limited uses to target caries-related pathogens. The important use of copper oxide nanoparticles in restorative dentistry is to reduce the polymerization shrinkage of resin composites (Song et al. 2016). The construction of copper oxide-containing resin composite showed 1–2 log reduction of *S. mutans* biofilm and reduced luciferase activity (Zajdowicz et al. 2018). The suggested mechanism of antibacterial action referred to the ability of copper oxide nanoparticles to generate reactive hydroxyl radicals, thereby inhibiting the growth of many microorganisms (Balhaddad et al. 2019b).

In nanotechnology, the use of nanodiamonds in polymer engineering has improved the mechanical and antibacterial properties of several materials in the industrial and medical fields. Nanodiamonds are suggested to have the ability to manipulate the permeability of the bacterial cell walls causing bacterial death. Besides the abroad antibacterial properties, nanodiamonds present suitable biocompatibility and structural stability (Turcheniuk and Mochalin 2017). Adding nanodiamonds with silver nanoparticles into resin composite was achieved with different mass fractions between 0.1% and 1.5%. A significant increase in the microhardness and flexural strength was observed with decreased viability of *S. mutans* biofilm. Unfortunately, only nanodiamonds' mass fractions of less than 1% revealed acceptable biocompatibility as concentrations of higher than 1% was associated with cytotoxicity (Cao et al. 2018). Table 8.3 outlines bioactive metallic nanoparticles used as reinforcing fillers in the resin composite system to target dental biofilms.

8.4 Bioactive Materials in Vital Pulp Therapy

The use of bioactive materials in vital dental pulp therapy is a hot-spot area in dental research. In case of reversible pulpitis due to caries progression toward the pulp, it is recommended to use specific liners as pulp-capping materials before the placement of the final restoration to enhance the formation of reparative dentin and remineralizing the surrounding dentin (Zhang and Yelick 2010).

Odontoblasts and undifferentiated mesenchymal cells can be recruited to induce reparative dentin formation by the use of pulp-capping materials to protect the dental pulp from further insults and prevent the onset of pulpitis (Goldberg and Smith 2004). Zinc oxide eugenol was found ineffective in healing the pulp (Glass and Zander 1949). Most probably, the release of eugenol is highly toxic and interferes with diminishing the pulpal inflammation (Hume 1984).

TABLE 8.3 Outlines of Studies Investigating the Bioactivity of Metal/Metal Oxide Nanoparticles Incorporated into Resin Composites and Their Biological and Antimicrobial Effects

Agent	Bioactive Function	References	Concentration	Mechanical Properties	Remarks
Silver nanoparticles	Silver ion release with bacterial damage and cell death	Cheng et al. (2012b)	0.028%	Flexural strength and elastic modulus were comparable to commercial control	Significant reduction of S. mutans metabolic activity, lactic acid, and colony-forming units by around 50%, 60%, and 90%, respectively
Silver nanoparticles		das Neves et al. (2014)	0.35%	Roughness and the compressive strength were comparable to the control samples	Inhibition of S. mutans and Lactobacillus acidophilus by around 90%
Silver nanoparticles		Kasraei et al. (2014)	1%	–	Proximally 95% and 80% significant colonies reduction of S. mutans and Lactobacillus, respectively
Ag bromide-cationic polymer (AgBr/BHPVP)	Silver ion release with bacterial damage and cell death	Cao et al. (2017)	<0.1%	Flexural strength and elastic modulus were not affected with higher Vicker's hardness compared to control	Greater antibacterial activities against S. mutans compared to control
Tetrapod-like ZnO whisker	A specific reaction that releases H_2O_2	Niu et al. (2010)	5%	Higher flexural, compressive, and diametral tensile strength compared to control	Enhanced antibacterial activity against S. mutans
ZnO	and reactive oxygen species forming	Aydin Sevinç and Hanley (2010)	1%–10%	–	80% Bacterial count reduction against S. mutans, but low antibacterial activities against multispecies biofilm
ZnO nanoparticles	hydroxyl radicals that limit the bacterial growth	Kasraei et al. (2014)	1%	–	Approximately >99% and 70% significant colonies reduction of S. mutans and Lactobacillus, respectively

(Continued)

TABLE 8.3 (Continued)   Outlines of Studies Investigating the Bioactivity of Metal/Metal Oxide Nanoparticles Incorporated into Resin Composites and Their Biological and Antimicrobial Effects

Agent	Bioactive Function	References	Concentration	Mechanical Properties	Remarks
CuO	Generation of reactive hydroxyl radicals which are toxic to the bacterial cells	Zajdowicz et al. (2018)	0.5%–4%	–	Around 90%–95% reduction of S. *mutans*
BG	Ca and PO$_4$ ion release and increasing the pH	Chatzistavrou et al. (2015)	5 and 15 wt.%	Bonding strength was comparable to the control samples	>99% Reduction against S. *mutans* was associated with 15 wt.% BG
BG	are the suggested two antibacterial mechanisms. BG	Khvostenko et al. (2016)	15 wt.%	–	Around 40% less bacterial penetration compared to free-BG resin composite
Fluoride-containing phosphate-rich BG	also induces remineralization with and without fluoride	Tezvergil-Mutluay et al. (2017)	50 wt.%	–	Significantly higher capability to remineralize dentin and higher protection of dentin-matrix interface from degradation compared to control samples
Nanodiamonds	Negatively or positively charged particles change the membrane permeability which might cause bacterial death	Cao et al. (2018)	0.1 wt.%–1.5 wt.%	Higher Vicker's hardness, flexural strength, modulus of elasticity. Higher toxicity was reported as the concentration of nanodiamonds increased	The number of viable S. *mutans* decreased by about 80%–90% compared to unmodified samples

Source: Adapted from Balhaddad et al. (2019b), with permission from © 2019 Elsevier.

The use of glass ionomer and RMGI as direct pulp-capping materials was also associated with chronic inflammation and no bridge formation (do Nascimento et al. 2000). Instead, calcium hydroxide is successful and has been used as a gold standard for direct pulp capping for centuries. Calcium hydroxide is effective in reducing the number of microorganisms after 1 h contact (Stuart et al. 1991). In addition to its high pH, it is suggested that calcium hydroxide may solubilize bone morphogenic protein (BMP) and transforming growth factor-beta one (TBF-β1) in order to induce the pulpal repair via dentinogenesis (Hilton 2009). The data retrieved from several human studies illustrated that MTA has a higher success rate than calcium hydroxide in reducing dental pulp inflammation and enhancing dentin bridge formation (Asgary et al. 2008; Mohammadi and Dummer 2011).

Mineral trioxide aggregate (MTA) has been introduced to overcome the drawbacks of calcium hydroxide. Human studies in primary teeth did not reveal any significant difference between calcium hydroxide and MTA (Schwendicke et al. 2016). Higher success rate than calcium hydroxide in reducing dental pulp inflammation and enhancing dentin bridge formation (Li et al. 2015; Zhu et al. 2015). The mechanism of action of MTA is believed to be similar to that found with calcium hydroxide with a greater sealing ability observed with the use of MTA (Fridland and Rosado 2003, 2005). However, using a layer of glass ionomer or RMGI is suggested after applying calcium hydroxide or MTA to enhance the sealing and protect the capping materials during the restoration placement (Hilton 2009).

Several drawbacks were reported with the use of MTA, such as the delayed setting time and the poor handling properties (Asgary et al. 2008). The use of other strategies such as the incorporation of antibiotics was suggested, but the clinical benefits were less compared to MTA AlShwaimi et al. 2016). Therefore, more efforts have been directed to modify MTA to improve the setting time and the handling properties. As a result, materials such as Angelus MTA, BioAggregate, EndoSequence BC RRM, and Biodentine were designed (Komabayashi et al. 2016).

Growing attention has been directed toward Biodentine because of its ability to deposit hydroxyapatite and increasing the sealing ability of the material (Malkondu et al. 2014).

The use of Biodentine was found effective in proliferating odontoblasts by the induction of TGFβ-1, which demonstrated promising results in vital pulp therapy even in challenging cases (Laurent et al. 2012). To overcome the problem related to the setting time, a light-cured resin-modified calcium silicate (TheraCal) was designed. However, the clinical outcomes of Biodentine concerning bridge formation, inflammatory response, and pulpal regeneration were better than TheraCal (Giraud et al. 2017; Bakhtiar et al. 2017).

8.5 Conclusion

While the use of metallic nanoparticles platforms and antibacterial monomers has shown promising results related to their remineralization and antibacterial actions, we are still far away to consider these platforms as alternatives for conventional resin composites. Many questions should be answered related to the long-term mechanical properties and performance of these materials. Materials with high mechanical properties may reveal a significant decay after physical or water aging, especially for those materials with ion release behavior. It is unknown if the release of ions may compromise the mechanical properties, and then accelerate the degradation and failure of such material. Also, most of the studies did not evaluate all the required parameters related to mechanical properties. While most of the studies reported the values of flexural strength and elastic modulus, other parameters such as hardness, fatigue behavior, wear resistance, solubility, and sorption were not measured in most of the studies.

Another concern is related to the polymerization behavior of these materials. Most of the studies did not investigate important parameters such as degree of conversion, depth of cure, and polymerization shrinkage, which can highlight a better understanding of the polymerization behavior of such materials. Incomplete polymerization is associated with a considerable amount of unreacted monomers. Unreacted monomers have the ability to enhance plaque accumulation and increase the attachment of dental microorganisms. Besides, unreacted monomers may induce a cytotoxic effect on the surrounding dental tissues (Beriat et al. 2010; Mayanagi et al. 2017; Al-Hiyasat et al. 2005). Other concerns are related to biocompatibility and degradation behavior, and very small numbers of the previously discussed bioactive resin composites were subjected to cytotoxicity and degradation tests. Materials with a high amount of cytotoxicity may affect the surrounding tissues inside the oral cavity causing serious complications, and materials with high susceptibility for degradation may detach causing microleakage and restoration failure. To conclude, with a long-term assessment, bioactive resin composites should have a strong antibacterial action, excellent mechanical properties, acceptable polymerization behavior, and low cytotoxicity with no degradation over time.

References

Al-Dulaijan, Y. A., L. Cheng, M. D. Weir, M. A. S. Melo, H. Liu, T. W. Oates, L. Wang, and H. H. K. Xu. 2018a. "Novel Rechargeable Calcium Phosphate

Nanocomposite with Antibacterial Activity to Suppress Biofilm Acids and Dental Caries." *Journal of Dentistry* 72: 44–52. https://doi.org/10.1016/j.jdent .2018.03.003.

Al-Dulaijan, Y. A., M. D. Weir, M. A. S. Melo, J. Sun, T. W. Oates, K. Zhang, and H. H. K. Xu. 2018b. "Protein-Repellent Nanocomposite with Rechargeable Calcium and Phosphate for Long-Term Ion Release." *Dental Materials* 34 (12): 1735–47. https://doi.org/10.1016/j.dental.2018.09.005.

Al-Hiyasat, A. S., H. Darmani, and M. M. Milhem. 2005. "Cytotoxicity Evaluation of Dental Resin Composites and Their Flowable Derivatives." *Clinical Oral Investigations* 9 (1): 21–5. https://doi.org/10.1007/s00784-004-0293-0.

AlShaafi, M. M. 2017. "Factors Affecting Polymerization of Resin-Based Composites: A Literature Review." *The Saudi Dental Journal* 29 (2): 48–58. https://doi.org/10.1016/j.sdentj.2017.01.002.

AlShwaimi, E., A. Majeed, and A. A. Ali. 2016. "Pulpal Responses to Direct Capping with Betamethasone/Gentamicin Cream and Mineral Trioxide Aggregate: Histologic and Micro-Computed Tomography Assessments." *Journal of Endodontics* 42 (1): 30–5. https://doi.org/10.1016/j.joen.2015.09.016.

Asgary, S., M. J. Eghbal, M. Parirokh, F. Ghanavati, and H. Rahimi. 2008. "A Comparative Study of Histologic Response to Different Pulp Capping Materials and a Novel Endodontic Cement." *Oral Surgery, Oral Medicine, Oral Pathology, Oral Radiology, and Endodontics* 106 (4): 609–14. https://doi .org/10.1016/j.tripleo.2008.06.006.

Aydin Sevinç, B., and L. Hanley. 2010. "Antibacterial Activity of Dental Composites Containing Zinc Oxide Nanoparticles." *Journal of Biomedical Materials Research: Part B, Applied Biomaterials* 94 (1): 22–31. https://doi.org/10.1002 /jbm.b.31620.

Bakhtiar, H., M. H. Nekoofar, P. Aminishakib, F. Abedi, F. N. Moosavi, E. Esnaashari, A. Azizi, et al. 2017. "Human Pulp Responses to Partial Pulpotomy Treatment with TheraCal as Compared with Biodentine and ProRoot MTA: A Clinical Trial." *Journal of Endodontics* 43 (11): 1786–91. https://doi.org/10.1016/j.joen .2017.06.025.

Balhaddad, A. A., A. A. Kansara, D. Hidan, M. D. Weir, H. H. K. Xu, and M. A. S. Melo. 2019b. "Toward Dental Caries: Exploring Nanoparticle-Based Platforms and Calcium Phosphate Compounds for Dental Restorative Materials." *Bioactive Materials* 4 (1): 43–55. https://doi.org/10.1016/j.bioactmat.2018. 12.002.

Balhaddad, A. A., M. A. S. Melo, and R. L. Gregory. 2019c. "Inhibition of Nicotine-Induced Streptococcus Mutans Biofilm Formation by Salts Solutions Intended for Mouthrinses." *Restorative Dentistry & Endodontics* 44 (1): e4. https://doi.org/10.5395/rde.2019.44.e4.

Balhaddad, A. A., M. Ibrahim, M. D. Weir, H. H. K. Xu, and M. A. S. Melo. 2019a. "Anti-Biofilm and Mechanically Stable Bioactive Composite for Root Caries Restorations." *Dental Materials*, Abstracts of the Academy of Dental Materials Annual Meeting, 02–05 October 2019—Jackson Hole, USA, 35 (January): e4–5. https://doi.org/10.1016/j.dental.2019.08.008.

Baras, B. H., M. A. S. Melo, V. Thumbigere-Math, F. R. Tay, A. F. Fouad, T. W. Oates, M. D. Weir, L. Cheng, and H. H. K. Xu. 2020. "Novel Bioactive and Therapeutic Root Canal Sealers with Antibacterial and Remineralization Properties." *Materials* 13 (5). https://doi.org/10.3390/ma13051096.

Beriat, N. C., A. A. Ertan, S. Canay, A. Gurpinar, and M. A. Onur. 2010. "Effect of Different Polymerization Methods on the Cytotoxicity of Dental Composites." *European Journal of Dentistry* 4 (3): 287–92.

Cabral, M. F. C., R. L. de Menezes Martinho, M. V. Guedes-Neto, M. A. B. Rebelo, D. G. Pontes, and F. Cohen-Carneiro. 2015. "Do Conventional Glass Ionomer Cements Release More Fluoride than Resin-Modified Glass Ionomer Cements?" *Restorative Dentistry & Endodontics* 40 (3): 209–15. https://doi.org/10.5395/rde.2015.40.3.209.

Cao, W., X. Wang, Q. Li, Z. Ye, and X. Xing. 2018. "Mechanical Property and Antibacterial Activity of Silver-Loaded Polycation Functionalized Nanodiamonds for Use in Resin-Based Dental Material Formulations." *Materials Letters* 220 (June): 104–7. https://doi.org/10.1016/j.matlet.2018.03.027.

Cao, W., Y. Zhang, X. Wang, Y. Chen, Q. Li, X. Xing, Y. Xiao, X. Peng, and Z. Ye. 2017. "Development of a Novel Resin-Based Dental Material with Dual Biocidal Modes and Sustained Release of Ag$^+$ Ions Based on Photocurable Core-Shell AgBr/Cationic Polymer Nanocomposites." *Journal of Materials Science: Materials in Medicine* 28 (7): 103. https://doi.org/10.1007/s10856-017-5918-3.

Chatzistavrou, X., S. Velamakanni, K. DiRenzo, A. Lefkelidou, J. C. Fenno, T. Kasuga, A. R. Boccaccini, and P. Papagerakis. 2015. "Designing Dental Composites with Bioactive and Bactericidal Properties." *Materials Science & Engineering: C, Materials for Biological Applications* 52: 267–72. https://doi.org/10.1016/j.msec.2015.03.062.

Cheng, L., K. Zhang, C.-C. Zhou, M. D. Weir, X.-D. Zhou, and H. H. K. Xu. 2016. "One-Year Water-Ageing of Calcium Phosphate Composite Containing Nano-Silver and Quaternary Ammonium to Inhibit Biofilms." *International Journal of Oral Science* 8 (3): 172–81. https://doi.org/10.1038/ijos.2016.13.

Cheng, L., K. Zhang, M. D. Weir, M. A. S. Melo, X. Zhou, and H. H. K. Xu. 2015. "Nanotechnology Strategies for Antibacterial and Remineralizing Composites and Adhesives to Tackle Dental Caries." *Nanomedicine (London, England)* 10 (4): 627–41. https://doi.org/10.2217/nnm.14.191.

Cheng, L., M. D. Weir, H. H. K. Xu, J. M. Antonucci, N. J. Lin, S. Lin-Gibson, S. M. Xu, and X. Zhou. 2012b. "Effect of Amorphous Calcium Phosphate and Silver Nanocomposites on Dental Plaque Microcosm Biofilms." *Journal of Biomedical Materials Research: Part B, Applied Biomaterials* 100 (5): 1378–86. https://doi.org/10.1002/jbm.b.32709.

Cheng, L., M. D. Weir, P. Limkangwalmongkol, G. D. Hack, H. H. K. Xu, Q. Chen, and X. Zhou. 2012a. "Tetracalcium Phosphate Composite Containing Quaternary Ammonium Dimethacrylate with Antibacterial Properties."

Journal of Biomedical Materials Research: Part B, Applied Biomaterials 100 (3): 726–34. https://doi.org/10.1002/jbm.b.32505.

Chiari, M. D. S., M. C. Rodrigues, T. A. Xavier, E. M. N. de Souza, V. E. Arana-Chavez, and R. R. Braga. 2015. "Mechanical Properties and Ion Release from Bioactive Restorative Composites Containing Glass Fillers and Calcium Phosphate Nano-Structured Particles." *Dental Materials* 31 (6): 726–33. https://doi.org/10.1016/j.dental.2015.03.015.

das Neves, P. B. A., J. A. M. Agnelli, C. Kurachi, C. W. O. de Souza, P. B. A. das Neves, J. A. M. Agnelli, C. Kurachi, and C. W. O. de Souza. 2014. "Addition of Silver Nanoparticles to Composite Resin: Effect on Physical and Bactericidal Properties In Vitro." *Brazilian Dental Journal* 25 (2): 141–5. https://doi.org /10.1590/0103–6440201302398.

do Nascimento, A. B., U. F. Fontana, H. M. Teixeira, and C. A. Costa. 2000. "Biocompatibility of a Resin-Modified Glass-Ionomer Cement Applied as Pulp Capping in Human Teeth." *American Journal of Dentistry* 13 (1): 28–34.

Fridland, M., and R. Rosado. 2003. "Mineral Trioxide Aggregate (MTA) Solubility and Porosity with Different Water-to-Powder Ratios." *Journal of Endodontics* 29 (12): 814–7. https://doi.org/10.1097/00004770–200312000–00007.

Fridland, M., and R. Rosado. 2005. "MTA Solubility: A Long Term Study." *Journal of Endodontics* 31 (5): 376–9. https://doi.org/10.1097/01.don.0000140566 .97319.3e.

Giraud, T., P. Rufas, F. Chmilewsky, C. Rombouts, J. Dejou, C. Jeanneau, and I. About. 2017. "Complement Activation by Pulp Capping Materials Plays a Significant Role in Both Inflammatory and Pulp Stem Cells' Recruitment." *Journal of Endodontics* 43 (7): 1104–10. https://doi.org/10.1016/j.joen.2017.02.016.

Glass, R. L., and H. A. Zander. 1949. "Pulp Healing." *Journal of Dental Research* 28 (2): 97–107. https://doi.org/10.1177/00220345490280021101.

Goldberg, M., and A. J. Smith. 2004. "Cells and Extracellular Matrices of Dentin and Pulp: A Biological Basis for Repair and Tissue Engineering." *Critical Reviews in Oral Biology and Medicine* 15 (1): 13–27. https://doi.org/10.1177 /154411130401500103.

Hamba, H., T. Nikaido, G. Inoue, A. Sadr, and J. Tagami. 2011. "Effects of CPP-ACP with Sodium Fluoride on Inhibition of Bovine Enamel Demineralization: A Quantitative Assessment Using Micro-Computed Tomography." *Journal of Dentistry* 39 (6): 405–13. https://doi.org/10.1016/j.jdent.2011.03.005.

Hasan, A. M. H. R., S. K. Sidhu, and J. W. Nicholson. 2019. "Fluoride Release and Uptake in Enhanced Bioactivity Glass Ionomer Cement ('Glass Carbomer™') Compared with Conventional and Resin-Modified Glass Ionomer Cements." *Journal of Applied Oral Science* 27 (February). https://doi.org/10.1590/1678–7757–2018–0230.

Hilton, T. J. 2009. "Keys to Clinical Success with Pulp Capping: A Review of the Literature." *Operative Dentistry* 34 (5): 615–25. https://doi.org/10.2341/ 09–132–0.

Hume, W. R. 1984. "Effect of Eugenol on Respiration and Division in Human Pulp, Mouse Fibroblasts, and Liver Cells In Vitro." *Journal of Dental Research* 63 (11): 1262–5. https://doi.org/10.1177/00220345840630110101.

Ibrahim, M. S., A. S. Ibrahim, A. A. Balhaddad, M. D. Weir, N. J. Lin, F. R. Tay, T. W. Oates, H. H. K. Xu, and M. A. S. Melo. 2019. "A Novel Dental Sealant Containing Dimethylaminohexadecyl Methacrylate Suppresses the Cariogenic Pathogenicity of Streptococcus Mutans Biofilms." *International Journal of Molecular Sciences* 20 (14). https://doi.org/10.3390/ijms20143491.

Kaisarly, D., and M. El Gezawi. 2016. "Polymerization Shrinkage Assessment of Dental Resin Composites: A Literature Review." *Odontology* 104 (3): 257–70. https://doi.org/10.1007/s10266-016-0264-3.

Kasraei, S., L. Sami, S. Hendi, M.-Y. Alikhani, L. Rezaei-Soufi, and Z. Khamverdi. 2014. "Antibacterial Properties of Composite Resins Incorporating Silver and Zinc Oxide Nanoparticles on Streptococcus Mutans and Lactobacillus." *Restorative Dentistry & Endodontics* 39 (2): 109–14. https://doi.org/10.5395/rde.2014.39.2.109.

Kermanshahi, S., J. P. Santerre, D. G. Cvitkovitch, and Y. Finer. 2010. "Biodegradation of Resin-Dentin Interfaces Increases Bacterial Microleakage." *Journal of Dental Research* 89 (9): 996–1001. https://doi.org/10.1177/0022034510372885.

Khvostenko, D., T. J. Hilton, J. L. Ferracane, J. C. Mitchell, and J. J. Kruzic. 2016. "Bioactive Glass Fillers Reduce Bacterial Penetration into Marginal Gaps for Composite Restorations." *Dental Materials* 32 (1): 73–81. https://doi.org/10.1016/j.dental.2015.10.007.

Kitasako, Y., A. Sadr, H. Hamba, M. Ikeda, and J. Tagami. 2012. "Gum Containing Calcium Fluoride Reinforces Enamel Subsurface Lesions in Situ." *Journal of Dental Research* 91 (4): 370–5. https://doi.org/10.1177/0022034512439716.

Komabayashi, T., Q. Zhu, R. Eberhart, and Y. Imai. 2016. "Current Status of Direct Pulp-Capping Materials for Permanent Teeth." *Dental Materials Journal* 35 (1): 1–12. https://doi.org/10.4012/dmj.2015-013.

Laurent, P., J. Camps, and I. About. 2012. "Biodentine(TM) Induces TGF-B1 Release from Human Pulp Cells and Early Dental Pulp Mineralization." *International Endodontic Journal* 45 (5): 439–48. https://doi.org/10.1111/j.1365-2591.2011.01995.x.

Li, Z., L. Cao, M. Fan, and Q. Xu. 2015. "Direct Pulp Capping with Calcium Hydroxide or Mineral Trioxide Aggregate: A Meta-Analysis." *Journal of Endodontics* 41 (9): 1412–7. https://doi.org/10.1016/j.joen.2015.04.012.

Maktabi, H., A. A. Balhaddad, Q. Alkhubaizi, H. Strassler, and M. A. S. Melo. 2018. "Factors Influencing Success of Radiant Exposure in Light-Curing Posterior Dental Composite in the Clinical Setting." *American Journal of Dentistry* 31 (6): 320–8.

Malkondu, Ö., M. K. Kazandağ, and E. Kazazoğlu. 2014. "A Review on Biodentine, a Contemporary Dentine Replacement and Repair Material." *BioMed Research International* 2014: 160951. https://doi.org/10.1155/2014/160951.

Mayanagi, G., K. Igarashi, J. Washio, and N. Takahashi. 2017. "pH Response and Tooth Surface Solubility at the Tooth/Bacteria Interface." *Caries Research* 51 (2): 160–6. https://doi.org/10.1159/000454781.

Melo, M. A. S., M. D. Weir, L. K. A. Rodrigues, and H. H. K. Xu. 2013. "Novel Calcium Phosphate Nanocomposite with Caries-Inhibition in a Human in Situ Model." *Dental Materials* 29 (2): 231–40. https://doi.org/10.1016/j.dental .2012.10.010.

Mohammadi, Z., and P. M. H. Dummer. 2011. "Properties and Applications of Calcium Hydroxide in Endodontics and Dental Traumatology." *International Endodontic Journal* 44 (8): 697–730. https://doi.org/10.1111/j.1365-2591.2011 .01886.x.

Moreau, J. L., L. Sun, L. C. Chow, and H. H. K. Xu. 2011. "Mechanical and Acid Neutralizing Properties and Bacteria Inhibition of Amorphous Calcium Phosphate Dental Nanocomposite." *Journal of Biomedical Materials Research: Part B, Applied Biomaterials* 98 (1): 80–8. https://doi.org/10.1002/jbm.b.31834.

Moreau, J. L., M. D. Weir, A. A. Giuseppetti, L. C. Chow, J. M. Antonucci, and H. H. K. Xu. 2012. "Long-Term Mechanical Durability of Dental Nanocomposites Containing Amorphous Calcium Phosphate Nanoparticles." *Journal of Biomedical Materials Research: Part B, Applied Biomaterials* 100 (5): 1264–73. https://doi.org/10.1002/jbm.b.32691.

Niu, L. N., M. Fang, K. Jiao, L. H. Tang, Y. H. Xiao, L. J. Shen, and J. H. Chen. 2010. "Tetrapod-Like Zinc Oxide Whisker Enhancement of Resin Composite." *Journal of Dental Research* 89 (7): 746–50. https://doi.org/10 .1177/0022034510366682.

Philip, N. 2019. "State of the Art Enamel Remineralization Systems: The Next Frontier in Caries Management." *Caries Research* 53 (3): 284–95. https://doi .org/10.1159/000493031.

Pitts, N. B., D. T. Zero, P. D. Marsh, K. Ekstrand, J. A. Weintraub, F. Ramos-Gomez, J. Tagami, S. Twetman, G. Tsakos, and A. Ismail. 2017. "Dental Caries." *Nature Reviews Disease Primers* 3 (May): 17030. https://doi.org/10.1038/nrdp. 2017.30.

Price, R. B., A. C. Shortall, and W. M. Palin. 2014. "Contemporary Issues in Light Curing." *Operative Dentistry* 39 (1): 4–14. https://doi.org/10.2341/13-067-LIT.

Price, R. B., J. L. Ferracane, and A. C. Shortall. 2015. "Light-Curing Units: A Review of What We Need to Know." *Journal of Dental Research* 94 (9): 1179– 86. https://doi.org/10.1177/0022034515594786.

Reynolds, E. C., F. Cai, P. Shen, and G. D. Walker. 2003. "Retention in Plaque and Remineralization of Enamel Lesions by Various Forms of Calcium in a Mouthrinse or Sugar-Free Chewing Gum." *Journal of Dental Research* 82 (3): 206–11. https://doi.org/10.1177/154405910308200311.

Schwendicke, F., F. Brouwer, A. Schwendicke, and S. Paris. 2016. "Different Materials for Direct Pulp Capping: Systematic Review and Meta-Analysis and Trial Sequential Analysis." *Clinical Oral Investigations* 20 (6): 1121–32. https://doi.org/10.1007/s00784-016-1802-7.

Skrtic, D., J. M. Antonucci, and E. D. Eanes. 1996. "Improved Properties of Amorphous Calcium Phosphate Fillers in Remineralizing Resin Composites." *Dental Materials* 12 (5): 295–301. https://doi.org/10.1016/s0109-5641 (96)80037-6.

Skrtic, D., J. M. Antonucci, E. D. Eanes, F. C. Eichmiller, and G. E. Schumacher. 2000. "Physicochemical Evaluation of Bioactive Polymeric Composites Based on Hybrid Amorphous Calcium Phosphates." *Journal of Biomedical Materials Research* 53 (4): 381–91. https://doi.org/10.1002/1097-4636 (2000)53:4<381::aid-jbm12>3.0.co;2-h.

Song, H. B., N. Sowan, P. K. Shah, A. Baranek, A. Flores, J. W. Stansbury, and C. N. Bowman. 2016. "Reduced Shrinkage Stress via Photo-Initiated Copper(I)-Catalyzed Cycloaddition Polymerizations of Azide-Alkyne Resins." *Dental Materials* 32 (11): 1332–42. https://doi.org/10.1016/j.dental.2016.07.014.

Stuart, K. G., C. H. Miller, C. E. Brown, and C. W. Newton. 1991. "The Comparative Antimicrobial Effect of Calcium Hydroxide." *Oral Surgery, Oral Medicine, and Oral Pathology* 72 (1): 101–4. https://doi.org/10.1016/0030-4220(91)90198-l.

Tavassoli Hojati, S., H. Alaghemand, F. Hamze, F. A. Babaki, R. Rajab-Nia, M. B. Rezvani, M. Kaviani, and M. Atai. 2013. "Antibacterial, Physical and Mechanical Properties of Flowable Resin Composites Containing Zinc Oxide Nanoparticles." *Dental Materials* 29 (5): 495–505. https://doi.org/10.1016/j .dental.2013.03.011.

Tezvergil-Mutluay, A., R. Seseogullari-Dirihan, V. P. Feitosa, G. Cama, D. S. Brauer, and S. Sauro. 2017. "Effects of Composites Containing Bioactive Glasses on Demineralized Dentin." *Journal of Dental Research* 96 (9): 999–1005. https:// doi.org/10.1177/0022034517709464.

Turcheniuk, K., and V. N. Mochalin. 2017. "Biomedical Applications of Nanodiamond (Review)." *Nanotechnology* 28 (25): 252001. https://doi.org/10 .1088/1361-6528/aa6ae4.

Weir, M. D., J. Ruan, N. Zhang, L. C. Chow, K. Zhang, X. Chang, Y. Bai, and H. H. K. Xu. 2017. "Effect of Calcium Phosphate Nanocomposite on In Vitro Remineralization of Human Dentin Lesions." *Dental Materials* 33 (9): 1033–44. https://doi.org/10.1016/j.dental.2017.06.015.

Xu, H. H. K., J. L. Moreau, L. Sun, and L. C. Chow. 2011. "Nanocomposite Containing Amorphous Calcium Phosphate Nanoparticles for Caries Inhibition." *Dental Materials* 27 (8): 762–9. https://doi.org/10.1016/j.dental.2011.03.016.

Xu, H. H. K., L. Sun, M. D. Weir, J. M. Antonucci, S. Takagi, L. C. Chow, and M. Peltz. 2006. "Nano DCPA-Whisker Composites with High Strength and Ca and PO_4 Release." *Journal of Dental Research* 85 (8): 722–7.

Xu, H. H. K., M. D. Weir, and L. Sun. 2009. "Calcium and Phosphate Ion Releasing Composite: Effect of pH on Release and Mechanical Properties." *Dental Materials* 25 (4): 535–42. https://doi.org/10.1016/j.dental.2008.10.009.

Xu, H. H. K., M. D. Weir, L. Sun, S. Takagi, and L. C. Chow. 2007. "Effects of Calcium Phosphate Nanoparticles on Ca-$_{PO4}$ Composite." *Journal of Dental Research* 86 (4): 378–83.

Zajdowicz, S., H. B. Song, A. Baranek, and C. N. Bowman. 2018. "Evaluation of Biofilm Formation on Novel Copper-Catalyzed Azide-Alkyne Cycloaddition (CuAAC)-Based Resins for Dental Restoratives." *Dental Materials* 34 (4): 657–66. https://doi.org/10.1016/j.dental.2018.01.011.

Zhang, K., B. Baras, C. D. Lynch, M. D. Weir, M. A. S. Melo, Y. Li, M. A. Reynolds, et al. 2018. "Developing a New Generation of Therapeutic Dental Polymers to Inhibit Oral Biofilms and Protect Teeth." *Materials* 11 (9). https://doi.org /10.3390/ma11091747.

Zhang, L., M. D. Weir, L. C. Chow, J. M. Antonucci, J. Chen, and H. H. K. Xu. 2016. "Novel Rechargeable Calcium Phosphate Dental Nanocomposite." *Dental Materials* 32 (2): 285–93. https://doi.org/10.1016/j.dental.2015.11.015.

Zhang, N., Y. Ma, M. D. Weir, H. H. K. Xu, Y. Bai, and M. A. S. Melo. 2017. "Current Insights into the Modulation of Oral Bacterial Degradation of Dental Polymeric Restorative Materials." *Materials (Basel, Switzerland)* 10 (5). https://doi.org/10.3390/ma10050507.

Zhang, W., and P. C. Yelick. 2010. "Vital Pulp Therapy-Current Progress of Dental Pulp Regeneration and Revascularization." *International Journal of Dentistry* 2010: 856087. https://doi.org/10.1155/2010/856087.

Zhu, C., B. Ju, and R. Ni. 2015. "Clinical Outcome of Direct Pulp Capping with MTA or Calcium Hydroxide: A Systematic Review and Meta-Analysis." *International Journal of Clinical and Experimental Medicine* 8 (10): 17055–60.

9

Methods for Characterization of Bioactivity Using Confocal Microscopy[*]

Jirun Sun, Joy P. Dunkers, Sheng Lin-Gibson, and Nancy J. Lin

National Institute of Standards and Technology

Contents

9.1 Introduction

One common tissue engineering (TE) approach for regenerating or replacing damaged tissues involves a porous polymeric scaffold. The scaffolds serve as the mechanical framework for cell attachment and growth, and generate an environment with features that span multiple-length scales to guide cell differentiation and tissue regeneration (Langer and Vacanti 1993,

---

[*] Jirun Sun and Nancy J. Lin have contributed equally to this work.

Seliktar 2012, Wheeldon et al. 2011, Sun et al. 2011, McCullen et al. 2011, Hasirci and Kenar 2006, Stevens and George 2005, Gonzalez-Bonet et al. 2015, Yang et al. 2016). Robust cell attachment and vigorous cell growth are the first and essential steps for successful tissue restorations (Roach et al. 2007, Simon and Lin-Gibson 2011). Effective methods to evaluate cell density in three-dimensional (3D) scaffolds are vital for the development of TE (Cancedda et al. 2007, Jones et al. 2007).

Laser scanning confocal microscopy (LSCM) is a useful technique to evaluate cell adhesion and spatial distribution within a scaffold since it is designed to collect image slices through the sample thickness (Allan et al. 2009, Hutmacher et al. 2001). However, common synthetic polymers used for preparing scaffolds, including polycaprolactone, poly(lactic acid), and their copolymers, are highly scattering, which limits the imaging depth to less than 1 mm (Rai et al. 2004, Yang et al. 2008). The reason for this depth limitation is twofold: the light scattering that occurs within semi-crystalline thermoplastics and the scattering due to refractive index mis-match between the polymer scaffold and the material occupying the pores (e.g., cells or medium) (Landis et al. 2006, Lin-Gibson et al. 2007, Lin-Gibson et al. 2006).

We previously developed TE scaffolds based on photo-polymerizable amorphous polymers for deep optical imaging (Landis et al. 2006, Lin-Gibson et al. 2007). These scaffolds are well suited for visible and near-infrared microscopy since they have no crystallinity and, therefore, minimal scattering. Besides, they exhibit essentially no autofluorescence and do not adsorb common fluorescent cell stains.

Other advantages of the photo-polymerized salt-leaching process include a relatively facile fabrication, absence of toxic solvent, and the ability to tailor mechanical properties, scaffold architecture, and chemical composition [for example, encapsulating bone morphogenetic protein (BMP) (Giri et al. 2011)] to meet specific applications. They have also shown good cell adhesion and growth, and are hydrolytically stable over several weeks in cell growth media. The latter property is important for long-term in vitro studies of cell penetration and proliferation. Furthermore, they have been used to produce micro- and nano-environments to guide cell alignment and morphology (Sun et al. 2010, Ding et al. 2011).

This study developed and evaluated three methods to characterize cell-material interactions by quantifying the 3D spatial distribution of cells in scaffolds using LSCM and assessing the kinetics of cell distribution as a function of time in static culture systems. These methods utilized the technical capabilities of LSCM and the optical and mechanical proper-ties of the amorphous polymeric scaffolds. One method was selected to characterize cell number and distribution within 3D scaffolds of optimized porosity and porogen size using two seeding densities at multiple time points. The progression of cell growth and cell distribution as a function of culture time obtained using these methods agreed well with computational prediction and experimental results (Sengers et al. 2007, Galban and Locke 1999, Dunn et al. 2006, Chung et al. 2006).

9.2 Methods[*]

9.2.1 Reagents

Ethoxylated bisphenol-A dimethacrylate (EDMA, degree of ethoxylation ≈ 6), was obtained from Esstech, Inc. Camphorquinone (CQ) and ethyl 4-N,N-dimethylaminobenzoate (4E) were purchased from Aldrich Corp. All reagents were used as received. The resin monomer was activated with a redox photoinitiator system consisting of 0.2% CQ and 0.8% 4E (by mass), and stored in the dark until use. Sodium chloride crystals were ground into small particles using a mortar and pestle and then separated into defined size ranges using brass sieves.

9.2.2 Fabrication of EDMA Tissue Engineering Scaffolds

Scaffolds were prepared using procedures described in literature (Landis et al. 2006). Briefly, activated EDMA was blended with sieved NaCl crystals. The mass fraction of NaCl was set at 84% to achieve optimal scaffold porosity and strength according to our previous publication (Lin-Gibsonet al. 2006). First, a scaffold bar (L × W × H = 30 mm × 5 mm × 3.5 mm) was prepared to optimize porogen size. The bar was composed of six equal volume sections (L × W × H = 5 mm × 5 mm × 3.5 mm) with different porogen sizes (Table 9.1). The EDMA-salt mixtures were packed into a Teflon mold with each section confined by Mylar films. After packing, Mylar films were removed, and bars were cured for 5 min per side using a tungsten halogen light (250 W, 120 V) and post-cured at 100°C for 1 h. The composite samples were soaked in deionized water for five days with multiple changes of water to dissolve the salt porogen and

---

[*] Certain equipment, instruments, or materials are identified in this chapter in order to adequately specify the experimental details. Such identification does not imply recommendation by the National Institute of Standards and Technology nor does it imply the materials are necessarily the best available for the purpose.

air-dried. Scaffolds were sterilized and seeded as described below. Based on cell density results from these scaffolds, an optimal porogen size was selected for cylindrical scaffold samples. To prepare cylindrical scaffolds, activated EDMA-salt mixture (with optimal salt size) was packed into a Teflon mold (L × W × H = 100 mm × 100 mm × 3.5 mm), pressed together between two glass plates, and processed as described above. Cylindrical scaffolds were punched out of the resultant sheet of porous material using an 8 mm punch. Final scaffold dimensions were 8 mm in diameter and 3.5 mm thick.

9.2.3 Cell Seeding and Staining

The MC3T3-E1 subclone 4 murine pre-osteoblast cell line was purchased from the American Type Culture Collection and maintained in alpha Minimum Essential Medium Eagle (α-MEM) supplemented with 10% (volume fraction) fetal bovine serum, 2 mmol/L L-glutamine, and 1% (volume fraction) penicillin/streptomycin at 37°C, 5% (by volume) CO_2. Cells of passages 3–6 were used in this study. Scaffolds were sterilized using ethylene oxide, degassed for at least three days, and hydrated through an ethanol series with moderate vacuum to facilitate wetting throughout the scaffold pores. Scaffolds were then transferred to a 48-well plate and prewetted with growth medium for 1 h prior to seeding. For scaffold bars, 1.4×10^6 cells were evenly distributed along the bar. Cylindrical scaffolds were each seeded with 1×10^5 or 5×10^5 cells. (The seeding density for the scaffold bars is equivalent to 2.5×10^5 cells on the cylindrical scaffolds.) The drop-wise seeding protocol for the cylindrical scaffolds was optimized in preliminary studies. Briefly, after removing the medium used for prewetting, half of the cells were suspended in 250 μL and added to the scaffold by pipetting up and down. After 1 h incubation at 37°C, the scaffolds were turned bottom-up and seeded dropwise (without pipetting) with the remaining cells suspended in 125 μL medium. After 1 h incubation, scaffolds were placed top-up in new 12-well plates, covered with 3 mL medium, and returned to the incubator. The growth medium was changed every three days.

At the designated times, scaffolds were fixed using 3.7% (by volume) formaldehyde in phosphate-buffered saline (PBS) for 20 min. The cells were permeabilized with 0.5% (by volume) Triton X-100 for 15 min, blocked with 10 mg/mL bovine serum albumin in PBS for 30 min, and rinsed with PBS. Cell nuclei were stained with Sytox Green (Invitrogen) at a 1:5,000 dilution in PBS for 30 min, and the actin cytoskeleton was stained for

1 h with Alexa Fluor 546-Phalloidin (Invitrogen) diluted 40-fold in PBS. Samples were rinsed three times with PBS and imaged in PBS.

9.2.4 Laser Scanning Confocal Microscopy (LSCM)

LSCM was carried out using an upright Zeiss LSCM 510 with 1 Airy-disk-unit pinhole in reflectance mode. A 5× objective [numerical aperture (NA): 0.15 and working distance (WD): 13.7 mm] and 10×W objective (W stands for water immersion, NA: 0.30 and WD: 3.1 mm) were used to image a field of view approximately 3.2 and 0.8 mm², respectively. A water immersion 40×W (NA: 0.80 and WD: 3.6 mm) objective was used to evaluate cell morphology.

A three-channel configuration was applied to monitor scaffold structure, cell nuclei, and cytoskeletal actin. One channel (reflectance of a 488 nm light source, pseudo-colored white) was assigned to the scaffold material. The second channel (pseudo-colored green) monitored cell nuclei labeled with Sytox Green using 488 nm excitation and a band-pass emission filter (505–550 nm). The third channel (pseudo-colored red) gathered signals from Alexa Fluor 546-phalloidin labeled actin excited using a 532 nm laser and collected through a 560 nm long-pass filter.

The imaging depth of the green channel was determined using fluorescently labeled polystyrene microspheres with an average diameter of 10 μm (FluoSpheres® polystyrene microspheres, Invitrogen #F8836) adsorbed throughout the scaffolds. The absorbance/emission wavelengths of the fluorescent dye covalently attached to the microspheres were (505/515) nm. To load the microspheres inside the scaffolds, a microsphere/water blend (3.6 × 10⁵ microspheres/mL) was gently rocked with the scaffolds overnight.

The acquisition settings of the LSCM, including laser power, filter selection, pinhole size, and other optical parameters, were optimized for image quality and resolution. A custom-built sample holder was used, along with a vibration isolation table, to eliminate scaffold movement during imaging and enable high-quality images to be captured. The holder consisted of a piece of foam secured to the bottom of a polystyrene petri dish, with a hole in the center of the foam slightly smaller than the scaffolds. Scaffolds were gently pressed into the hole to physically stabilize the scaffolds and prevent movement.

Images were collected as single x-y images, tiles of x-y images (via a motorized stage), and stacks of x-y images taken as a function of the depth (z). Image size was 512 pixels × 512 pixels. Image stacks were reconstructed to form 3D projection images using the manufacturer's software.

9.2.5 Quantification of Cell Density

Custom macros were written in ImagePro Plus 6.0 (Media Cybernetics, Bethesda, MD, USA) to quantify the number of nuclei per image. Cell nuclei (green) images were imported and converted to 8-bit grayscale images, and intensity was best-fit equalized. The number of nuclei per image was counted using an automatic threshold to detect nuclei and a minimum area filter ($\approx 16\ \mu m^2$) to remove noise. Actin staining (red) was used to visualize cell bodies. Cell number (number of nuclei per image) and cell area were exported for data analysis. Standard uncertainty associated with these measurements is 5%.

Each LSCM image represents a three-dimensional volume within the scaffold, enabling cell number to be converted to cell density per volume (cells/mm^3). The optical section height in the z-direction, which depended upon the NA of the objective and the pinhole setup, was calculated by the microscope software to be 21.2 μm and 7.0 μm for 5× and 10×W objectives, respectively, based on the full-width at half-maximum axial resolution.

9.3 Results

9.3.1 Maximum Depth of Imaging

The maximum depth of imaging for the 10×W objective was determined using scaffolds containing fluorescently labeled polystyrene microspheres. The average diameter of 30 microspheres imaged with the 10×W objective was 10.5±1 μm, similar to the diameter of the nuclei ($\approx 20\ \mu$m). The top of the scaffold where the green signal was first visible was defined as depth zero. Depth was measured as the travel distance of the objective and was used as a reference for evaluating cell distribution. A drop in microsphere fluorescence was observed at depths of $\approx 1,200\ \mu$m (Figure 9.1). Based on these results, all subsequent imaging was performed to a maximum depth of 1,000 μm.

9.3.2 Optimization of Scaffold Porogen Size

A scaffold bar with six sections each containing different porogen sizes (Table 9.1) was prepared to optimize porogen size based on cell density. Porogen size increased from sections 2 to 6, while section 1 had a 50:50

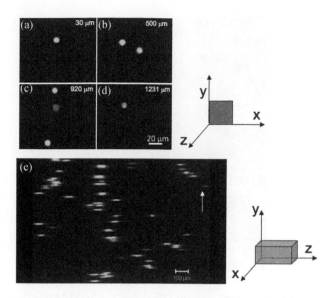

Figure 9.1 Determination of maximum imaging depth using the 10×W objective and fluorescently labeled polystyrene microspheres adsorbed to the scaffold. Images (a)–(d) are x-y slices at depths noted in the images. Image (e) is an x-axis projection of a stack of 2D images. The arrow indicates the drop in fluorescence intensity at a depth of ~1,300 µm. The x-z-y coordinates indicate the orientation of the images.

TABLE 9.1   Mesh and Porogen Sizes for Each Section of the Scaffold Bar

Section	Mesh Size	Porogen Size (µm)
1	100–200, 40–45	Equal mass mixture of 2 and 6
2	100–200	75–150
3	60–100	150–250
4	50–60	250–300
5	45–50	300–355
6	40–45	355–425

(by mass) mixture of salt crystals used in sections 2 and 6 to provide a complex pore size distribution. Figure 9.2 shows representative 3D projection images of cells within the six sections of the scaffold bar after 24 h culture. From sections 2 to 4, the density of nuclei increased, whereas nuclei density was similar throughout sections 4–6. Based on these results, the middle of these three sections (section 5, porogen size of 300–350 µm) was used for the remainder of the study.

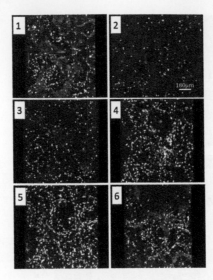

Figure 9.2   Effect of porogen size on cell density. LSCM projection images of cells in sections 1–6 of a representative scaffold bar. Porogen sizes were 75–150, 150–250, 250–300, 300–355, and 355–425 µm for sections 2, 3, 4, 5, and 6, respectively. Section 1 contained a 50:50 mixture (by mass) of 75–150 and 355–425 µm porogens.

9.3.3 Imaging Methods

Three methods were developed to evaluate cell distribution in the scaffolds using LSCM (Figure 9.3). Method I quantifies cell distribution in an x-y plane of the scaffold at multiple depths to obtain cell density as a function of x-y location and z-depth for a limited portion of the scaffold (Figure 9.3a). To image the entire x-y cross-sectional area of the 8 mm diameter scaffold, a 6 × 6 tile of x-y images was collected using the 5× objective, with each image covering an area of 1.8 × 1.8 mm (Figure 9.3b). Nuclei within each tile image (Figure 9.3c) were counted using ImagePro. To determine cell density as a function of depth, tile images were collected at intervals of 100 µm to ~1 mm below the top surface of the scaffold. The scaffold was then inverted and imaged from the bottom surface to obtain the cell distribution within the lower 1 mm portion of the scaffold.

Method II evaluates cell distribution throughout the entire scaffold by physically sectioning the scaffold through the center into two semicylindrical halves and positioning these halves so the cut surface is up for imaging (Figure 9.3a). These images provide information to calculate relative cell distribution from top to bottom of the scaffold. The 10×W

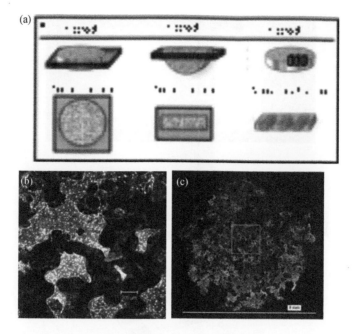

Figure 9.3 Methods to evaluate the spatial distribution of cells in 3D scaffolds (a). Method I combines adjacent x-y images collected using the low-magnification objective (5×) to create a tile image and determine cell distribution in a number of x-y planes. Method II involves sectioning the scaffold into two halves and collecting x-z tile images of the full depth of the scaffold through the newly exposed cross-sectional surfaces. Method III determines cell density and morphology by collecting and analyzing a series of precisely positioned stacks of 2D x-y images with a higher resolution (40×W) objective. An example single image (b) and 6 × 6 tile image of the entire scaffold surface (c) are shown for Method I.

objective was used, and tile images (10 × 5 images) were collected at depths of 200, 300, and 400 μm from each cut surface.

Method III determines cell number and morphology at specific locations using a series of precisely positioned stacks of 2D images collected with the 40×W objective (Figure 9.3a). The higher magnification objective provides spatially rich information particularly with regard to cell morphology. Figure 9.4 provides a representative z-axis projection view of a stack of 2D images (207 images at a 0.76 μm z-interval) from a scaffold seeded with 500,000 cells and cultured for 24h. Images are shown for actin (Figure 9.4a), nuclei (Figure 9.4b), and reflected light, which visualizes both the cells and the scaffold (white in Figure 9.4c), along with an overlay image. The reflection image is useful in visualizing scaffold structure to correlate it with cell location. For instance, the empty space in Figure 9.4a

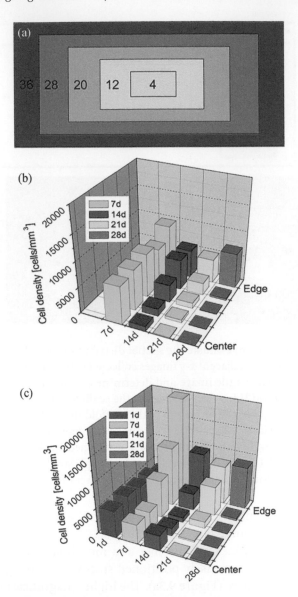

Figure 9.4   Cell distribution in 3D as a function of culture time for two seeding densities using Method II. Tile images were collected and divided into 100 small identical units that were then organized into five regions from the edge to the center of the scaffolds (a). The first (center) region contains four units and is surrounded by the second region which includes 12 units. The third, fourth, and fifth regions have 20, 28, and 36 units, respectively. Cell distribution at different culture times was determined for seeding densities of 100,000 (b) and 500,000 (c) cells/scaffold, respectively.

is a scaffold pore, as outlined in Figure 9.4c; thus, the lack of cells in this space is explained.

9.3.4 Comparison of Methods I and II

Methods I and II were selected to quantify cell density as a function of depth (travel distance of the objective) in scaffolds seeded with 500,000 cells and cultured for 24 h. Figure 9.4 shows tile images of the scaffold at a depth of 100 μm using Method I and 200 μm into the fresh-cut cross-sectional surface from Method II showing the full-depth profile. For both methods, the top surface of the scaffold was defined as depth zero, and the bottom surface (the surface in contact with the culture dish) was depth 3.5 mm. The results from Method I revealed a reproducible trend in cell distribution for the three scaffolds, with the highest cell density at depth zero, a significant decrease in cell density near the center to almost zero, and a slight recovery of cell density at the bottom. Method II has a similar trend, with the highest cell density at the top surface, and further demonstrated that cell density as a function of depth agreed between the two corresponding scaffold halves. Thus, the two methods were in agreement in sections near the top and bottom surfaces of the scaffolds that could be accurately measured by both methods.

9.3.5 Tracking Cell Distribution over Time

Based on the comparison study, we selected Method II to quantify cell distribution as a function of culture time (1, 7, 14, 21, and 28 days) and seeding density (Figure 9.4). During image analysis, the area of the fresh-cut surface was defined manually to avoid empty space (broken scaffold) within the tile image. The selected area was divided into 100 identical units ($\approx 0.8 \times 0.35$ mm each) organized into five regions. The center region contained four units and was surrounded by the second region (12 units). The third, fourth, and fifth regions had 20, 28, and 36 units, respectively. In developing the region layout, we also considered rectangular regions stacked from the top to bottom of the scaffold, but these were ruled out due to variations in cell density from the edge (whether top/bottom or side) to the center of the scaffold. Thus, a concentric-like approach was taken.

Cell distribution was determined after seeding either 100,000 or 500,000 cells/scaffold. Cell density depended on location within the scaffold, seeding density, and time point. The higher seeding density initially resulted in increased cell numbers, particularly in seven days near the scaffold edges. However, differences in cell number due to seeding density disappeared, such that cell number and distribution were similar on both scaffolds for 28 days. For both seeding densities, cell distribution increased in heterogeneity throughout the scaffold as time progressed, with cell density much greater at the surface than in the center of the scaffolds. The transition to this nonuniform cell distribution with a near-zero density at the center was more rapid (<7 days) for the higher seeding density.

9.4 Discussion

Cell distribution in 3D scaffolds was characterized using new methods developed for the LSCM. Further, amorphous, optically clear scaffolds were utilized to enhance light penetration into the scaffolds without sacrificing intensity, providing a 1 mm workable depth for imaging. The combination of these scaffolds and the imaging LSCM methods enabled a full characterization of cell distribution throughout the scaffold depth as a function of time.

Cell density was determined by the number of nuclei per unit volume, so commercially available microspheres were used to determine the maximum imaging depth within the scaffolds using the green channel. The measured microsphere diameter matched with the expected diameter of 10 μm and agreed well with the resolution (0.8 μm) of the 10×W objective used.

Scaffold porosity and pore size are important factors for cell proliferation and distribution in 3D. Porosity affects diffusion and is vital for nutrient distribution and waste removal (Sun et al. 2008, Leddy et al. 2004, Schwartz et al. 1993). In general, higher porosity is preferable for increased nutrient and waste exchange. In our polymeric scaffolds, there exists a maximum porosity above which the scaffolds collapse during cell culture and imaging (Lin-Gibsonet al. 2006, Landis et al. 2006). The maximum acceptable porosity is ≈77% [with 84% (by mass) NaCl] as previously determined by microcomputed tomography. Using this porosity, porogens of 300–350 μm in diameter resulted in optimal cell attachment and growth, based on cell data from scaffold bars with multiple porogen sizes. These scaffold bars enabled simultaneous evaluation of multiple porogen sizes to screen the effect of porogen size on initial cell density.

The 5×W and 10×W objectives were chosen for Methods I and II, respectively, rather than the 40×W objective to obtain larger viewing areas and reduce the time needed to map the cell distribution throughout the scaffold. Using the 5× or 10×W objective, the diameter of a 20 µm nucleus covered approximately 5–6 pixels or 11–12 pixels in a 512 pixel × 512 pixel image, respectively, which was sufficient to distinguish nuclei from background noise. Method III utilized a 40×W objective to enable higher magnification imaging.

Each of the three imaging methods developed in this study has advantages and drawbacks. All methods utilized the imaging capabilities of the LSCM while also taking advantage of the low-scattering nature of the amorphous polymers, and Methods I and II can run automatically with very little user input once the scaffold is prepared and positioned.

For the 3.5 mm thick and 8 mm diameter scaffolds used in this study, Method I provided a rapid and nondestructive way to quantify cell distribution but only evaluated approximately half of the scaffold volume. Analyzing the entire cross-sectional area provided a more thorough characterization of the cell density at accessible depths and is useful in evaluating cell uniformity at a given depth, but cells within the central depths of the scaffold could not be imaged due to limitations in maximum depth of imaging. A thinner scaffold could be used, but the relevance of the study would decrease, as thinner scaffolds may not be of sufficient size to meet regenerative needs. The 5× objective was used for proof of concept due to the efficiency of imaging and image quality. Method I should be easily adaptable to a 10×W objective, if desired, but it would require a fourfold increase in the number of images (12 × 12 images) to image the entire x-y area of the scaffold.

Method II enabled a full-depth analysis of the cell distribution for cylindrical scaffolds, with the assumption that cell distribution depends on depth and radial location, but not angular location. The data is based on a small sampling area and may, therefore, be easily skewed by nonuniform densities. To overcome this limitation and increase the area considered for each depth, several images were taken (200, 300, and 400 µm into the scaffold section), each of which contains data for all scaffold depths. Data from these multiple images can be combined to increase the sample size for each scaffold depth. While this method works well for the cylinders, it may not work well for other scaffold shapes (e.g., cubes, rectangular prisms, and irregular shapes).

The strength of Method III is the imaging of cell morphology at higher resolution. While this method could provide spatial distribution of cells over an entire scaffold for a thin or sectioned scaffold, it would require a tremendous amount of time compared with the other two methods and is therefore not practical if one or both of the other methods provide reasonable results.

When considering all of these three methods, Method III is best for collecting detailed information of cell morphology and cell-scaffold interactions in 3D. Actin filaments are clearly shown and can be used to evaluate cell spreading (Figure 9.4). Method I is preferred for determining cell distribution in thinner scaffolds where sample thickness allows for imaging through the entire scaffold depth. It would also work well for nonuniform, noncylindrical shapes. Method II, the sectioned-scaffold approach, provides a full-depth analysis of cell distribution in symmetric scaffolds and only requires one cut of the scaffold, versus other sectioning and imaging techniques that require multiple slices through the scaffold. Further, Method II may be acceptable for other materials with reduced imaging depths.

Methods I and II were compared in their ability to determine cell distribution throughout a set of three representative scaffolds. Method III was not used in this comparison, as it is not recommended for a more complete scaffold characterization. Method I covered a large volume and a large scaffold area per depth but only approximately half of the scaffold height, whereas Method II measured a smaller volume with much less area per depth but the full scaffold height range. Method II also offers an internal control via evaluation of both scaffold halves. Trends in cell density were comparable for the two methods, with one exception—Method I suggests a near-zero cell density approaching the center of the scaffold (i.e., very few cells imaged at depths of 1 and 2.5 mm). These positions are 1 mm from the scaffold top/bottom and within the imaging range determined using the fluorescent microspheres. However, data from Method II reveals that cells are present in the central portion of the scaffold, suggesting that the maximum imaging depth may be reduced when cells are adherent, likely due to increased scattering on the interfaces present between cells, extracellular matrix, medium, and scaffold. Absolute cell densities from Method I were higher than those from Method II. Edge effects contribute to these differences. In an x-y plane of the scaffold, cell density on the edge is higher than in the scaffold interior due to increased nutrients and oxygen. Tile images from Method I contain more cell-rich scaffold edge relative to scaffold interior as compared to Method II, increasing the average cell density per depth. Future optimization of the imaging protocol via a combination of Methods I and II, along with the evaluation of cell density as a function of depth and radius, is expected to further increase data accuracy (due to large sampling volumes of Method I) while at the same time providing full-depth imaging (from Method II).

For our thick scaffolds, imaging the entire depth was critical, so Method II was selected to evaluate the effect of culture time and seeding density on 3D cell distribution. Other applications with thinner scaffolds would likely benefit from using Method I, due to the higher amount of data collected per depth. Further, Method III could be used in conjunction with either Method I or II to provide complementary information on cell morphology within the scaffold. For instance, after scaffolds were sectioned and imaged via Method II, Method III could then be used to evaluate cell morphology at any scaffold depth.

Cell distribution changed greatly as culture time progressed, transitioning from a nearly uniform distribution throughout the scaffold to a surface-only cell distribution. These changes are likely due to variations in the supply of nutrients and partial pressure of oxygen throughout the scaffold (Leddy et al. 2004, Kellner et al. 2002, Brunelle and Chandel 2002). At the time of seeding, scaffolds are thoroughly wetted with growth medium and should have sufficient nutrients and oxygen throughout the scaffold to support initial cell attachment and growth, even in the center of the scaffold. As local nutrients are expended, cells must rely on diffusion from the bulk medium into the scaffold. Previous studies suggest that nutrients may diffuse as fast in medium-wetted scaffolds as in pure water (Sun et al. 2008). However, the consumption of nutrients and oxygen by cells near the scaffold surface will be substantial. As surface cell density increases due to longer culture times and/or higher seeding densities, the available supply of nutrients and oxygen for cells deeper within the scaffolds will drop significantly, decreasing the internal cell density over time. This study was performed with a static culture system and highlights the need for medium flow and/or perfusion to sustain the cells within larger scaffolds such as the ones used here.

9.5 Conclusions

Using an amorphous, biocompatible dimethacrylate scaffold, three methods were developed for deep optical microscopy to image cells in 3D, and one method was selected to study the anisotropy of cell distribution in 3D scaffolds. Amorphous polymeric scaffolds were selected to enable deep light penetration with reduced scattering, enabling images to be collected as deep as 1,200 μm into the scaffolds. These scaffolds also allow for controlled pore size, which was optimized using a scaffold bar with multiple porogen sizes. One imaging method (Method III), which uses 3D image stacks and a higher magnification objective, is effective in characterizing cell morphology in 3D but is not useful for evaluating the full cell distribution within a scaffold. The other two methods (Methods I and II) utilize 2D tile images of the scaffold. Although both methods provide cell density data, halving and imaging the scaffolds near the freshly cut surface (Method II) enabled a more complete imaging of cells at all depths. Method II was thus applied to evaluate changes in cell density and distribution as a function of culture time and seeding density. Cells may initially be dispersed throughout the scaffold, but cell distribution quickly becomes nonhomogeneous, likely due to increased numbers of cells near the surface that consume nutrients and oxygen, reducing their availability further into the scaffold. Overall, these LSCM methods and amorphous polymeric scaffolds are a useful tool and model system to obtain visual and quantitative information on cell-material interactions in 3D.

Acknowledgments

Official contribution of the National Institute of Standards and Technology; not subject to copyright in the United States. Dr. Sun would like to thank for financial support provided through National Institute of Dental and Craniofacial Research (U01DE023752) and the ADA Foundation. The authors would like to thank American Dental Association for their supports. The EDMA resins were kindly donated by Esstech, Inc. The authors would like to thank Drs. Marcus Cicerone, Forrest A. Landis, and Yuexin Liu for their advice and technical recommendations.

References

Allan, I. U., R. V. Shevchenko, B. Rowshanravan, B. Kara, C. A. Jahoda, and S. E. James. 2009. "The use of confocal laser scanning microscopy to assess the potential suitability of 3D scaffolds for tissue regeneration, by monitoring extra-cellular matrix deposition and by quantifying cellular infiltration and proliferation." *Soft Materials* 7 (4):319–341. doi: 10.1080/15394450903372679.

Brunelle, J. K., and N. S. Chandel. 2002. "Oxygen deprivation induced cell death: An update." *Apoptosis* 7 (6):475–482. doi: 10.1023/a:1020668923852.

Cancedda, R., A. Cedola, A. Giuliani, V. Komlev, S. Lagomarsino, M. Mastrogiacomo, F. Peyrin, and F. Rustichelli. 2007. "Bulk and interface investigations of scaffolds and tissue-engineered bones by X-ray microtomography and X-ray microdiffraction." *Biomaterials* 28 (15):2505–2524. doi: 10.1016/j.biomaterials.2007.01.022.

Chung, C. A., C. W. Yang, and C. W. Chen. 2006. "Analysis of cell growth and diffusion in a scaffold for cartilage tissue engineering." *Biotechnology and Bioengineering* 94 (6):1138–1146. doi: 10.1002/bit.20944.

Ding, Y. F., J. R. Sun, H. W. Ro, Z. Wang, J. Zhou, N. J. Lin, M. T. Cicerone, C. L. Soles, and S. Lin-Gibson. 2011. Thermodynamic underpinnings of cell alignment on controlled topographies. *Advanced Materials* 23 (3):421–5.

Dunn, J. C. Y., W. Y. Chan, V. Cristini, J. S. Kim, J. Lowengrub, S. Singh, and B. M. Wu. 2006. "Analysis of cell growth in three-dimensional scaffolds." *Tissue Engineering* 12 (4):705–716. doi: 10.1089/ten.2006.12.705.

Galban, C. J., and B. R. Locke. 1999. "Analysis of cell growth kinetics and substrate diffusion in a polymer scaffold." *Biotechnology and Bioengineering* 65 (2):121–132. doi: 10.1002/(sici)1097–0290(19991020)65:2<121::aid-bit1>3.0 .co;2–6.

Giri, J., W.-J. Li, R. S. Tuan, and M. T. Cicerone. 2011. "Stabilization of proteins by nanoencapsulation in sugar–glass for tissue engineering and drug delivery applications." *Advanced Materials* 23 (42):4861–4867. doi: 10.1002/adma.201102267.

Gonzalez-Bonet, A., G. Kaufman, Y. Yang, C. Wong, A. Jackson, G. Huyang, R. Bowen, and J. Sun. 2015. "Preparation of dental resins resistant to enzymatic and hydrolytic degradation in oral environments." *Biomacromolecules* 16:-3381–3388. doi: 10.1021/acs.biomac.5b01069.

Hasirci, V., and H. Kenar. 2006. "Novel surface patterning approaches for tissue engineering and their effect on cell behavior." *Nanomedicine* 1 (1):73–89. doi: 10.2217/17435889.1.1.73.

Hutmacher, D. W., T. Schantz, I. Zein, K. W. Ng, S. H. Teoh, and K. C. Tan. 2001. "Mechanical properties and cell cultural response of polycaprolactone scaffolds designed and fabricated via fused deposition modeling." *Journal of Biomedical Materials Research* 55 (2):203–216.

Jones, J. R., G. Poologasundarampillai, R. C. Atwood, D. Bernard, and P. D. Lee. 2007. "Non-destructive quantitative 3D analysis for the optimisation of tissue scaffolds." *Biomaterials* 28 (7):1404–1413. doi: 10.1016/j. biomaterials.2006.11.014.

Kellner, K., G. Liebsch, I. Klimant, O. S. Wolfbeis, T. Blunk, M. B. Schulz, and A. Gopferich. 2002. "Determination of oxygen gradients in engineered tissue using a fluorescent sensor." *Biotechnology and Bioengineering* 80 (1):73–83. doi: 10.1002/bit.10352.

Landis, F. A., J. S. Stephens, J. A. Cooper, M. T. Cicerone, and S. Lin-Gibson. 2006. "Tissue engineering scaffolds based on photocured dimethacrylate polymers for in vitro optical imaging." *Biomacromolecules* 7 (6): 1751–1757.

Langer, R., and J. P. Vacanti. 1993. "Tissue engineering." *Science* 260 (5110):920–926.

Leddy, H. A., H. A. Awad, and F. Guilak. 2004. "Molecular diffusion in tissue-engineered cartilage constructs: Effects of scaffold material, time, and culture conditions." *Journal of Biomedical Materials Research Part B—Applied Biomaterials* 70B (2):397–406. doi: 10.1002/jbm.b.30053.

Lin-Gibson, S., F. A. Landis, and P. L. Drzal. 2006. "Combinatorial investigation of the structure-properties characterization of photopolymerized dimethacrylate networks." *Biomaterials* 27 (9):1711–1717. doi: 10.1016/j.biomaterials.2005.10.040.

Lin-Gibson, S., J. A. Cooper, F. A. Landis, and M. T. Cicerone. 2007. "Systematic investigation of porogen size and content on scaffold morphometric parameters and properties." *Biomacromolecules* 8 (5):1511–1518. doi: 10.1021/bm061139q.

McCullen, S. D., A. G. Y. Chow, and M. M. Stevens. 2011. "In vivo tissue engineering of musculoskeletal tissues." *Current Opinion in Biotechnology* 22 (5):715–720. doi: 10.1016/j.copbio.2011.05.001.

Rai, B., S. H. Teoh, K. H. Ho, D. W. Hutmacher, T. Cao, F. Chen, and K. Yacob. 2004. "The effect of rhBMP-2 on canine osteoblasts seeded onto 3D bioactive polycaprolactone scaffolds." *Biomaterials* 25 (24):5499–5506. doi: 10.1016/j.biomaterials.2004.01.007.

Roach, P., D. Eglin, K. Rohde, and C. C. Perry. 2007. "Modern biomaterials: A review-bulk properties and implications of surface modifications." *Journal of Materials Science-Materials in Medicine* 18 (7):1263–1277.

Schwartz, L. M., N. Martys, D. P. Bentz, E. J. Garboczi, and S. Torquato. 1993. "Cross-property relations and permeability estimation in model porous-media." *Physical Review E* 48 (6):4584–4591. doi: 10.1103/PhysRevE.48.4584.

Seliktar, D. 2012. "Designing cell-compatible hydrogels for biomedical applications." *Science* 336 (6085):1124–1128. doi: 10.1126/science.1214804.

Sengers, B. G., M. Taylor, C. P. Please, and R. O. C. Oreffo. 2007. "Computational modelling of cell spreading and tissue regeneration in porous scaffolds." *Biomaterials* 28 (10):1926–1940. doi: 10.1016/j.biomaterials.2006.12.008.

Simon, C. G., and S. Lin-Gibson. 2011. "Combinatorial and high-throughput screening of biomaterials." *Advanced Materials* 23 (3):369–387. doi: 10.1002/adma.201001763.

Stevens, M. M., and J. H. George. 2005. "Exploring and engineering the cell surface interface." *Science* 310 (5751):1135–1138.

Sun, H. L., F. H. Meng, A. A. Dias, M. Hendriks, J. Feijen, and Z. Y. Zhong. 2011. "Alpha-amino acid containing degradable polymers as functional biomaterials: Rational design, synthetic pathway, and biomedical applications." *Biomacromolecules* 12 (6):1937–1955. doi: 10.1021/bm200043u.

Sun, J., B. F. Lyles, K. H. Yu, J. Weddell, J. Pople, M. Hetzer, D. De Kee, and P. S. Russo. 2008. "Diffusion of dextran probes in a self-assembled fibrous gel composed of two-dimensional arborols." *Journal of Physical Chemistry B* 112 (1):29–35.

Sun, J. R., Y. F. Ding, N. J. Lin, J. Zhou, H. Ro, C. L. Soles, M. T. Cicerone, and S. Lin-Gibson. 2010. "Exploring cellular contact guidance using gradient nanogratings." *Biomacromolecules* 11 (11):3067–3072. doi: 10.1021/bm100883m.

Wheeldon, I., A. Farhadi, A. G. Bick, E. Jabbari, and A. Khademhosseini. 2011. "Nanoscale tissue engineering: Spatial control over cell-materials interactions." *Nanotechnology* 22 (21). doi: 10.1088/0957-4484/22/21/212001.

Yang, Y., A. Urbas, A. Gonzalez-Bonet, R. J. Sheridan, J. E. Seppala, K. L. Beers, and J. R. Sun. 2016. "A composition-controlled cross-linking resin network through rapid visible-light photo-copolymerization." *Polymer Chemistry* 7 (31):5023–5030. doi: 10.1039/c6py00606j.

Yang, Y., D. Bolikal, M. L. Becker, J. Kohn, D. N. Zeiger, and C. G. Simon. 2008. "Combinatorial polymer scaffold libraries for screening cell-biomaterial interactions in 3D." *Advanced Materials* 20 (11):2037–2043. doi: 10.1002/adma.200702088.

10

Quantum Dots as Biointeractive and Non-Agglomerated Nanoscale Fillers for Dental Resins

Isadora Martini Garcia and Fabrício Mezzomo Collares
Federal University of Rio Grande do Sul

Contents

10.1 Inorganic Particles in Adhesive Resins

Dental caries is a chronic disease with major prevalence worldwide, with almost 100% of adults and approximately 60%–90% of children being affected (WHO 2012). To replace the lost hard dental tissues, restorative procedures with resins are the most common treatment due to their conservative and esthetic approach. However, the survival of this treatment decreases over time, mainly after seven years from the restorative technique, due to the recurrence of caries (Opdam et al. 2014). Restorations placed with composite resins show a lifespan of around 4.5 years (Burke et al. 2001; Rho et al. 2013). In general, dentistry, the replacement of restorations is the most common practice, and it constitutes 50%–70% of dentists' operative time (Deligeorgi et al. 2001; Sunnegardh-Gronberg et al. 2009).

The replacement of restorations involves patients in a restorative spiral circle (Sheiham 2002), with a gradual increase of cavities size, leading to the loss of dental structures over time (Schwendicke et al. 2016; Deligeorgi et al. 2001). A reliable dental-resin interface is not simple to be created, mostly when the restoration involves the hybridization of dentin. Dentin is a more heterogeneous tissue and has more water content in comparison to enamel (Nakabayashi 1998). In this context, the long-lasting performance of composite resins restorations is affected by the bonding performance and by the maintenance of dentin-adhesive interface stability over time. Unfortunately, this site is the most susceptible area of failure (Spencer et al. 2010).

To overcome this problem and to improve the predictability of the treatments, researches have been developed to modify the adhesive systems, especially the adhesive resins. Adhesive systems have been innovated to have antibacterial activity (Collares et al. 2017; Makvandi et al. 2018; Andreet al. 2018; Melo et al. 2016), less hydrolytic degradation (Salz et al. 2005; Rodrigues et al. 2018) and to provide less collagen degradation by collagenolytic enzymes (Frassetto et al. 2016; Tezvergil-Mutluay et al. 2015), and greater dentin remineralization (Tay and Pashley 2009; Schwendicke et al. 2019).

One way to provide some of these characteristics to adhesive systems is by incorporating inorganic fillers into them. Silicon dioxide (Van Landuyt et al. 2007), barium borosilicate glass particles (Martins et al. 2014), and fluoraluminosilicate glass (Van Landuyt et al. 2007) are the widest fillers incorporated into adhesive resins. Others have been tested to support the development of biointeractive adhesives, such as zirconium oxide (Lohbauer et al. 2010; Provenzi et al. 2018), niobium pentoxide (Leitune, Collares, Takimi et al. 2013; Marins et al. 2017), tantalum oxide (Garcia, Leitune, Ferreira et al. 2018; Schulz et al. 2008), titanium oxide (Jowkar et al. 2018; Sun et al. 2011, 2016), calcium phosphates (Leitune, Collares, Trommer et al. 2013; Garcia et al. 2017; Schwendicke et al. 2019), zinc oxide (Osorio, Cabello et al. 2014; Mahshid Saffarpour 2016; Gutierrez et al. 2019), copper (Gutierrez et al. 2019; Gutierrez et al. 2017), silver (Jowkar et al. 2018), gold, and platinum nanoparticles (Hashimoto et al. 2016). Inorganic materials such as nanotubes have also been added to adhesive resins to carry antibacterial agents (Feitosa et al. 2014, 2019) or to improve their physicochemical properties (Degrazia et al. 2017).

The addition of inorganic fillers in adhesive resins helps to reinforce the polymer via a crack deflection and plastic deformation in the sites around the particles (Bartczak et al. 1999). Moreover, the particles may increase the elastic modulus of the resin via simply decreased of organic/inorganic rate. Besides the fact that inorganic particles could reinforce the material, their use in the nanoscale range has called attention in the research field because of the exciting properties that they can assume.

In the nanometric scale, materials have different properties in comparison to their bulk state, leading to wide-ranging applications (Roduner 2006). Roduner (2006) made an interesting analogy to introduce this theme in his previous review: we have already accepted that some materials can present different allotropic forms and, consequently, show entirely different chemical and physical properties, as occurs with carbon. Similarly, materials' properties depend on their size.

Some of the most differentiated properties involve nanoparticle's photoelectric behavior, especially in semiconductor materials (Efros and Nesbitt 2016). Another feature is the higher antimicrobial activity presented with decreased size (Raghupathi et al. 2011). For instance, titanium dioxide (TiO_2) has been widely investigated in nanoscale size not only due to its photocatalytic activity (Hashimoto et al. 2005) but also because of its antimicrobial effect via generation of reactive oxygen species (ROS) (Sun et al. 2017).

For dentistry, another compelling reason to use fillers with this dimension is that they could permeate through the entire length of the hybrid layer, reaching dentin interfibrillar spaces. Interfibrillar spaces are around 20 nm after acid demineralization process in the restorative procedures (Tay et al. 1999) and the intermolecular collagen spaces in the fibers are around 1.26–1.33 nm (Bertassoni et al. 2012). Therefore, in addition to reinforcing the adhesive blend and hybrid layer with dentin, nanoparticles could be used to provide bioactive property for interface and support the remineralization process of caries affected dentin.

10.2 The Agglomeration Concern

Despite the remarkable properties that nanoparticles can provide when added to biopolymers, there are problems related to their stability in the blend. Researchers face concern about the high-frequent nanoparticle agglomeration, which probably occurs due to the high surface area available for electrostatic interactions (Jordan et al. 2005; Cai et al. 2012; Sun et al. 2017; Garcia, Leitune, Ferreira et al. 2018). As seen in Figures 10.1–10.3, the nanoparticles agglomerate in the polymer in larger inorganic contents. Instead of reinforcing the polymers, agglomerates may impair polymers' properties.

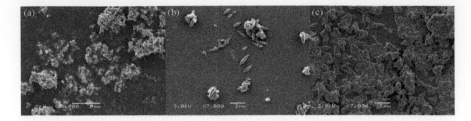

Figure 10.1 Scanning electron microscopy (SEM) images of tantalum dioxide (Ta_2O_5) powder (a) and Ta_2O_5 in adhesive resin at 1 wt.% (b) and 10 wt.% (c). Images (b) and (c) show the particles on the surface of the polymerized adhesive after mixture of an experimental uncured resin and powder of Ta_2O_5. The powder of nanoparticles is clearly arranged in larger agglomerates. (Chapter authors.)

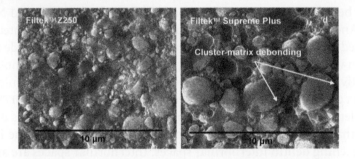

Figure 10.2 SEM images of two commercial composite resins: a microhybrid composite (Filtek™ Z250) and a nanofill composite (Filtek™ Supreme Plus). The presence of protruding fillers with arrangement in larger agglomerates can be observed on the surface of the nanofill composite resin. The agglomerates of nanoparticles debond from resin matrix on the nanofill composite resin, and this resin showed a decreased fatigue threshold in comparison to the microhybrid composite. (Adapted from Shah et al. (2009).)

The agglomerates have lower adhesion to resin matrix in comparison to well-dispersed particles, and they can detach from the polymer, as previously observed with composite resins for filling (Shah et al. 2009). Furthermore, the agglomerates can perform as sites with high-stress concentration, jeopardizing the tensile dissipation along with the material (Jordan et al. 2005). These features might turn the filled resin more susceptible to failures over time (Palaniappan et al. 2011). Besides the issues mentioned above, when added to adhesive resins, nanoparticles' agglomerates do not permeate through all the hybrid layer, and they are kept at the top of it. In this chapter, we are going to present two approaches recently used to overcome this issue in polymers with applicability for dentistry.

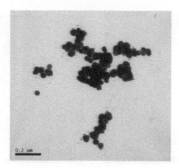

Figure 10.3   Transmission electron microscopy (TEM) image of silver nanoparticles with 25–100 nm arranged in agglomerates (Degrazia et al. 2016).

10.3 Quantum Dots: Background and Their Use to Overcome Nanoparticles Agglomeration Concern

Nanoparticles with a mean size of 1–100 nm dispersed in liquids constitute colloidal systems, and they suffer attraction and repulsion electrostatically during the Brownian movement (Chebbi 2015). When there is an equilibrium between the attraction and repulsion potentials, the colloidal kinetic stability can be achieved. One way to formulate composites filled with non-agglomerated nanoparticles was suggested via the development of a dental adhesive with quantum dots (Garcia et al. 2016).

Quantum dots are inorganic particles of about 1–10 nm obtained via semiconductor materials (Singh and Kumar 2006). These nanocrystals, also known as "artificial atoms," have been studied for having various applications in materials engineering (Buatong et al. 2015; Jahantigh et al. 2020) and bioengineering (Pleskova et al. 2018; Samadikhah et al. 2017), mainly due to the fluorescence that semiconductors exhibit when they present this dimension. Interestingly, these nanoparticles showed reliable equilibrium without agglomeration even after six months of storage in liquid (Garcia et al. 2016). As seen in Figure 10.4, quantum dots could be promising nanoparticles to be incorporated into polymers.

Quantum dots have broad applicability in vitro and in vivo. As shown in Figure 10.5, the properties of quantum dots, such as their fluorescence, may be a promising strategy for many purposes. In health sciences, quantum dots have been used as biomarkers due to their feature of intermittent luminescence. These nanoparticles are so small that their radius is smaller than the gap between the valence band and electron position in the conduction band when a bulk semiconductor material is excited. When this gap, also called as "exciton Bohr radius," is higher than the particle radius,

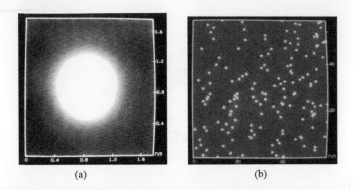

Figure 10.4 Scanning tunneling microscopy (STM) images of quantum dots. Image (a) shows a single quantum dot of iron-doped zinc sulfide. Each quantum dots showed about 1 nm of diameter. Image (b) shows the set of quantum dots of iron-doped zinc sulfide. All the particles showed the spherical shape and nano-size compatible with particles in the tridimensional quantum confinement effect. (Adapted from Khani et al. (2011).)

electrons and holes (in the vacancy band) undergo quantum confinement and are not free to move (Bimberg and Pohl 2011), making the particle stable if controlled from the external environment.

Photoemission can occur from the quantum dots when the electron-hole pair is recombined after incident energy higher than the band-gap (a gap between vacancy and conduction band) is applied on these nanoparticles. Thus, the confinement changes the density of energy states (Bimberg and Pohl 2011) and can observe this phenomenon via intermittency of light or "blinking" (Efros and Nesbitt 2016). Therefore, a way to verify if nanoparticles are in quantum confinement and, consequently, incompatible nanometric dimension (1–10 nm) (Bimberg and Pohl 2011) is via high-resolution fluorescence microscopy by analyzing the intermittence of light emitted by quantum dots even in the polymerized material (Garcia et al. 2016, 2019).

10.4 ZnO Quantum Dots in an Experimental Dental Adhesive: The First Step

The first step proposed to incorporate quantum dots in dental adhesive was via the synthesis of these nanoparticles by self-organization of the particles or the so-called bottom-up process based on a previous study (Meulenkamp 1998). The authors decided to synthesize ZnO quantum

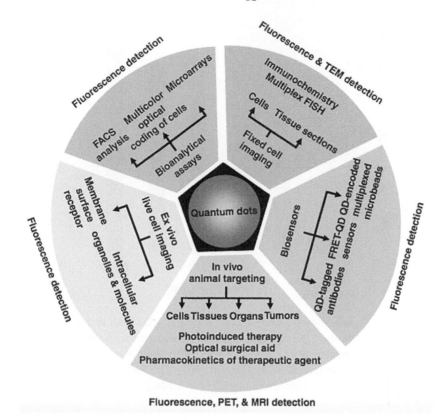

Figure 10.5 Scheme of possible applications of quantum dots that use their fluorescence (Michalet et al. 2005).

dots because this oxide has desired properties to be used in dentistry, and it could be an interesting filler to provide biointeractivity for the polymer.

ZnO is a very versatile semiconductor with applications not only in engineering, such as diodes and electroluminescent devices but also in biosensors, bioelectrodes, and in daily life in the form of cosmetics and drugs (Mirzaei and Darroudi 2017). Moreover, ZnO shows biocompatibility (Mutoh and Tani-Ishii 2011), bioactivity via the precipitation and maturation of calcium phosphates on its surface (Osorio, Cabello et al. 2014), antimicrobial activity (Mahshid Saffarpour 2016; Tavassoli Hojati et al. 2013; Dananjaya et al. 2018), and ability to affect metalloproteinases (Osorio, Osorio et al. 2014) negatively. Noteworthily, the smaller the ZnO particles, the higher the antibacterial activity provided by this oxide due to the enlargement of the total surface area available to interact with the microorganisms (Raghupathi et al. 2011). This effect can be clearly

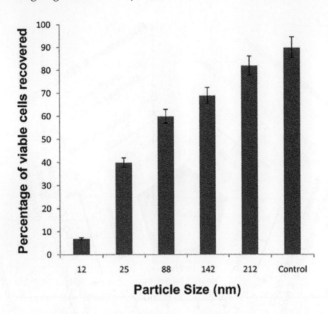

Figure 10.6   Graph showing the effect of ZnO particles with different sizes on the viability of *S. aureus*. The bacterial cultures were grown with 6 mm of ZnO for 6 h. Note that the bacterial viability decreased with the reduction of nanoparticles of ZnO.(Raghupathi et al. 2011). (Reprinted with permission from (*Langmuir* 2011, 27, 7, 4020–4028, https://doi.org/10.1021/la104825u). © 2011 American Chemical Society.)

observed in Figure 10.6, in which the graph shows the percentage of viable bacteria after the exposition of ZnO at different sizes.

ZnO has antibacterial activity through the injury of phospholipids' molecular structure, leading to the disruption of the bacterial membrane. Subsequently, internalization of particles in the cytoplasmic matrix can occur (Huang et al. 2008) as observed in Figure 10.7, with the development of ROS such as superoxide radical ($O_2^-\bullet$), hydroxyl radical (OH•), and singlet oxygen ($1O_2$) (Leung et al. 2016) on the surface of ZnO (Mirzaei and Darroudi 2017). Therefore, studies started to highly explore the effects of ZnO nanoparticles in adhesive resins in order to assist in the best mechanical and biological performance of adhesive resins (Dananjaya et al. 2018).

Zinc oxide quantum dots (ZnO_{QDs}) are easily synthesized via particle self-organization processes using common solvents such as ethanol and isopropanol (Garcia et al. 2016; Meulenkamp 1998; Hsueh et al. 2015; Hsu et al. 2016). To develop a dental resin with quantum dots, the authors decided to synthesize ZnO_{QDs} via this route and incorporate these

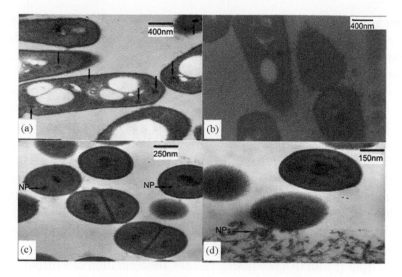

Figure 10.7 TEM images of *Streptococcus agalactiae* (a and b) and *Staphylococcus aureus* (c and d) after contact with ZnO nanoparticles. The antibacterial activity of ZnO nanoparticles can occur via the formation of ROS and penetration of the nanoparticles into the bacterial cell. In these images, the internalization of the ZnO nanoparticles is indicated by the arrows (Huang et al. 2008). (Reprinted with permission from (*Langmuir* 2008, 24, 8, 4140–4144, https://doi.org/10.1021/la7035949). © 2008 American Chemical Society.)

nanoparticles into an experimental dental adhesive from a conventional etch-and-rinse adhesive system (Garcia et al. 2016).

10.5 Synthesis and Characterization of ZnO$_{QDs}$

The synthesis of ZnO$_{QDs}$ was performed via the self-organization of the particles or the so-called bottom-up process based on a previous study (Meulenkamp 1998). For this purpose, firstly, 125 mL of isopropyl alcohol was cooled up to 4°C. Zinc acetate dihydrate (Zn(CH$_3$COO)$_2$·2H$_2$O, 0.25 mmol: 0.0548 g) was added to 42 mL of isopropyl alcohol in a glass vial, and the solution was sonicated until complete dissolution of the zinc acetate dihydrate. Parallelly, lithium hydroxide anhydrous (LiOH·H$_2$O, 0.7 mmol: 0.0167 g) was added to 8 mL of ethanol in another glass vial, which was also sonicated until the complete dissolution of the solute. Then, both solutions were cooled to 4°C.

The solution containing zinc acetate dihydrate in isopropyl alcohol, followed by that of lithium hydroxide anhydrous in ethanol, was added, under vigorous manual stirring, to the 125 mL of isopropyl alcohol previously cooled to 4°C. The final solution containing zinc acetate dihydrate, lithium hydroxide anhydrous, ethanol and isopropanol was heated in a water bath up to 40°C.

To evaluate if the nanoparticles of ZnO were in the size range of quantum dots, the solution was analyzed via ultraviolet-visible spectroscopy (UV-Vis) and stored at −20°C. The solution was analyzed immediately after the synthesis, and 24 h, 2 months, and 6 months later (Garcia et al. 2016). The results showed that the mean particle size was at 1.20 ± 0.01 nm, and it kept stable after 24 h from the synthesis. ZnO_{QDs} were stable after two months and six months from the synthesis with size at 1.19 ± 0.01 nm.

Although the methodology used for the synthesis is simple, several factors determine the reproducibility of the technique. During attempts to reproduce the synthesis, the waiting time for solutes to dissolve in alcohol ranged from 15 min to a few hours. Besides, the formation of a turbid liquid with a white precipitate was observed in the vials with $LiOH \cdot H_2O$ with ethanol in some of the times when the dilution attempt time was greater than 1 h. This precipitate is probably due to the formation of lithium carbonate (Li_2CO_3) after $LiOH \cdot H_2O$ contacts with CO_2. While LiOH is partially soluble in alcohol, carbonated salts are difficult to dissolve and therefore tend to precipitate in the aqueous or alcoholic medium. The reagents must always be weighed in a controlled environment with a dehumidifier. Then, the dilution time became short and standardized, and there was no formation of Li_2CO_3.

The formulated ZnO_{QDs} tend to increase their average diameter with the increase of temperature up to 4°C (Meulenkamp 1998). The reaction yields may not reach 100%, and reagent remains may react or become new nuclei of growth with increasing temperature. The high temperature increases the kinetic energy of the particles, boosting the chances of a particle collision in the alcohol medium, and increases the solubility of the reagents.

To evaluate if the quantum dots synthesized were of ZnO, the authors washed the product via changing liquid media and centrifugation. After a sequence of centrifugation, a powder was isolated. This powder was analyzed via Fourier Transform Infrared (FTIR) Spectroscopy. As observed in Figure 10.8, FTIR analysis revealed the characteristic peak related to Zn-O bonding, suggesting the formation of ZnO_{QDs}.

Even though the washing step seems feasible to isolate the product and obtain a powder, this process brings disadvantages for the stability of the particles, making them agglomerate. This process hampers the redispersion of the particles in another medium due to their agglomeration. Thus, the washing steps should be used only if it is desired to analyze the product, such as via FTIR chemically.

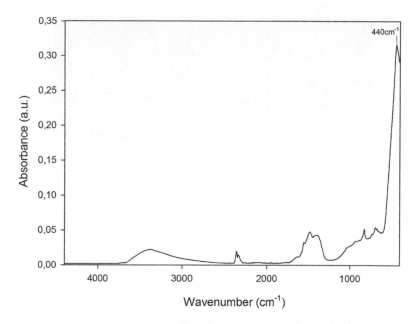

Figure 10.8 The chemical characterization of the synthesized ZnO$_{QDs}$ was performed via FTIR-ATR. The spectrum indicates the peak in the region of 440 cm^{-1} related to Zn-O bond in the powder of ZnO$_{QDs}$ (Garcia et al. 2016).

The authors used a system with low pressure to boil the alcohol at low temperature, not exceeding 4°C, in order to exchange the liquid media of the synthesis (ethanol and isopropanol) for a dental monomer without the necessity to have the ZnO$_{QDs}$ in powder and agglomerated. When there was not too much alcohol remained in the flask, the classical dental monomer hydroxyethyl methacrylate (HEMA) was added. The remaining alcohol was evaporated, and the HEMA containing the particles was evaluated via UV-Vis immediately and after two months of storage. With this sequence of methods, it was possible to keep ZnO$_{QDs}$ stabilized since their synthesis up to two months in HEMA with 1.24 nm of mean diameter. The HEMA containing ZnO$_{QDs}$ was further used for dental adhesive formulation.

10.6 Dental Adhesive with ZnO$_{QDs}$

A dental resin was formulated using the HEMA containing ZnO$_{QDs}$, bisphenol A glycerolate dimethacrylate (BisGMA), and photoinitiators (Garcia et al. 2016; Garcia, Leitune, Visioli et al. 2018).

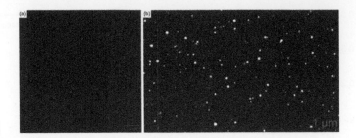

Figure 10.9   Images of high-resolution fluorescence microscopy used to analyze the light intermittency by quantum dots incorporated into the adhesive resin. The images were performed with the polymerized samples of adhesive without prior treatment(a). Both images were captured with the objective of 100×. Digital zoom at 1.4× was performed in image (b). The light emissions of the ZnO_{QDs} differ among the particles within the polymerized sample (Garcia et al. 2016).

Via SEM-EDS, the authors quantified the Zn present in the group containing ZnO_{QDs}, suggesting 1.54 ($\pm$0.46)% of it in the polymerized adhesive. Polymerized samples with ZnO_{QDs} were analyzed via super-resolution confocal microscopy to evaluate if the ZnO_{QDs} kept the quantum dots size after the preparation of the adhesive resin. Figure 10.9 shows the quantum dots in the polymerized resin. The high fluorescence of ZnO_{QDs} in the polymerized samples prevented the measurement of each particle in the polymer. However, due to the blinking of the ZnO_{QDs} via intermittent fluorescence, the author could confirm that the quantum dot confinement was present for the nanoparticles, suggesting the maintenance of stability and non-agglomeration. In this way, the UV-Vis spectroscopy showed no agglomeration of the ZnO_{QDs} in the alcohol and HEMA, and the findings of confocal microscopy corroborated these outcomes.

The use of super-resolution confocal microscopy to evaluate the blinking of the nanoparticles and, consequently, their quantum confinement effect and nano size, is very attractive for many reasons. First, via this technique, there is no need for sample preparation. The samples were made using a silicone mold with a 4 mm diameter hole and 1 mm thickness. The polymerized sample of dental adhesive containing ZnO_{QDs} was simply positioned in the microscope, surrounded by oil, and the fluorescence of the ZnO_{QDs} was observed after the wavelength hit the sample. Second, it is very difficult to find a methodology able to analyze nanoparticles with such a small size, asof 1 nm, which makes them contain only a small number of atoms. This is even harder if the nanoparticles are incorporated in another medium, such as a polymer. Techniques such as scanning tunneling microscopy may be possible to use. The authors used confocal microscopy not only to take images but mainly to obtain movies of the fluorescence profile. Therefore, as the third advantage, this is a microscopy technique that can be used not only to observe if there is confinement effect of the nanoparticles but also to evaluate the fluorescence profile of them (analysis of time on and off of fluorescence during the blinking). Other areas of knowledge use the quantum dots' fluorescence, and it is crucial for them to analyze the profile of this phenomenon.

The dental adhesive with ZnO_{QDs} was compared to the same adhesive without ZnO_{QDs}. Regarding the degree of conversion, it was observed that both adhesive resins reached values above 50%, which corresponds to the values of commercial adhesives according to the literature (Gaglianone et al. 2012). Interestingly, the adhesive with ZnO_{QDs} reached higher value than the control group, but the initial Knoop hardness value of the group with ZnO_{QDs} was lower than the control. The rationale for this outcome may be that the control group achieved more cross-linking density with a lower degree of conversion in comparison to ZnO_{QDs} group. While the ZnO_{QDs} group had a favorable conversion of monomers based on a more linear resulting polymer. However, the measurement of softening after solvent and the evaluation of the ultimate tensile strength of the adhesives showed no differences between them.

Moreover, the incorporation of ZnO_{QDs} did not affect the microtensile bond strength between dentin and adhesive interface after 24 h from the restoration procedure. Interestingly, after six months of storage in distilled water, there was no difference between both groups, but that one with ZnO_{QDs} showed a lower difference for itself between the immediate and the long-term analyses. In other words, it seems that the addition of ZnO_{QDs} could assist in preserving the bonding interface from degradation.

Attempts have been made to develop materials with therapeutic activity, such as antibacterial property and bioactivity. On the one hand, ZnO_{QDs} could show interesting antibacterial activity because of their small size (Raghupathi et al. 2011). On the other hand, with the decreasing size of the particles, the toxicity against cells may increase (Sahu et al. 2014). Thus, the second step after the formulation of the dental adhesive with ZnO_{QDs} and its evaluation regarding physicochemical properties was the analysis of antibacterial activity and cytotoxicity effect.

In this study, the dental adhesive formulated with ZnO_{QDs} was exposed to a 24 h biofilm model with a single-species of *Streptococcus mutans*. The chosen for this bacterium was due to its positive correlation with caries (Kirstila et al. 1998). The samples were exposed to form biofilm on their surface; the biofilm was mechanically removed from them and analyzed via counting of colonies number in an agar Petri-dish. This method provides us a reliable result about the viability of the bacteria on biofilm. The group with ZnO_{QDs} presented less biofilm formation on the samples' surface in comparison to the neat adhesive. This outcome may be justified due to the antibacterial activity of both components: ZnO and acetate from zinc acetate dihydrate used for ZnO_{QDs} synthesis (Lee et al. 2002).

For the cytotoxicity evaluation, the polymerized samples were stored for 24 h in a culture medium. Then, this medium with possible leaching (eluate) from the samples was placed on human pulp cells. Cells and eluates were kept in contact for 72 h. The viability of cells after this period was analyzed via sulforhodamine B (SRB) colorimetric assay, which determines the cell density by staining proteins of viable cells. The viability of cells, according to ISO 10993-5 standardization, must be at least 70% to infer that the material has no cytotoxicity. The adhesives with and without ZnO_{QDs} showed values higher than 70%, without difference between them. The method used in this study is an exciting alternative to the typical assay using tetrazolium salt (MTT). SRB method has the advantage not to be related to metabolic activity, but to enable cell enumeration based on protein content. Fewer compounds (intracellular and extracellular) interfere in the SRB outcome in comparison to MTT assay, and SRB shows a better predictive power than MTT (van Tonder et al. 2015).

The outcomes observed in these studies presented a method to develop nanocomposites for dentistry without agglomerated nanoparticles. Also, the use of ZnO_{QDs} in the polymer provided antibacterial property to the dental adhesive without inducing toxicity to pulp cells.

10.7 From Sol-Gel Routes to Chemical Ionic-Liquid Routes

Despite the promising results found for ZnO_{QDs}, traditional syntheses via sol-gel process and self-organization of the nanoparticles with common solvents (such as alcohol, acetone, and methanol) present low yield, making it challenging to develop and to study materials with different amounts of quantum dots. Moreover, as previously stated, the quantum dots must remain in the liquid medium at low temperatures (Meulenkamp 1998) to not agglomerate.

Currently, other routes to synthesize quantum dots have been proposed through ionic liquids (ILs) (Dupont and Scholten 2010). Most liquids are made up of neutral molecules because charged species generally lead to strong ionic interactions that drive the material to the solid arrangement. On the other side, "molten salts at room temperature" or "ionic liquids" are organic salts with low melting points (below 100°C), and they are often liquid at room temperature (Dupont and Scholten 2010). ILs have low vapor pressure, high thermal and chemical stability, and different density and viscosity depending on their cations and anions (Luczak et al. 2016). These salts comprise a cationic nucleus, usually an organic nitrogen group (such as those from imidazole and pyridine), attached to an alkyl chain (Modaressi et al. 2007). This cationic part of the IL interacts with an anion, that can be as simple as halides, or more complex such as negatively charged sugars and amino acids. Due to the fact that the charge is displaced in bulky cyclic nuclei, there is a lack of salt symmetry (Earle and Seddon 2002), leading to poor coordination and ionic packaging, preventing the formation of a stable crystal lattice, resulting in low melting point and liquid physical state (Pendleton and Gilmore 2015).

ILs have molecular properties such as geometry and dipolar moment and a highly organized structure in comparison to traditional liquids, with a network of cations and anions interacting through electrostatic forces and hydrogen bonds (Dupont and Scholten 2010). The ability to form preorganized structures, mainly by means of hydrogen bonds, inducing structural directionality, is a property that distinguishes ILs from simple salts or classic quaternary ammonium compounds (Dupont and Scholten 2010).

Initially employed in studies related to electrochemistry, in recent years ILs have proven their versatility in synthetic and catalytic applications, provoking great interest in academic and industrial research (Pendleton and Gilmore 2015). With their unique and adjustable properties, ILs have become increasingly used in micro- and nanometer-scale particle synthesis by changing the length of the alkyl chain, incorporating cationic groups, or varying the anion (Dupont and Scholten 2010). In some chemical reactions, ILs act as solvents and particle stabilizers. In others, the ionic liquid itself carries the reducing agent (such as imidazole cation), participating directly in the synthesis (Prechtl et al. 2010). Due to the structural organization of ILs, as well as their affinity with other molecules (due to their ability to donate/receive electrons and create hydrogen bonds), ILs have become an interesting key tool to prepare new nanostructures (Dupont and Scholten 2010).

The morphology of nano- and microstructures, such as particle shape and size, the porosity and the density of crystalline defects, can be controlled by using appropriate ILs and different conditions (temperature, pressure, and reaction duration) (Dupont and Scholten 2010). Nanostructures of stable size are usually obtained by the synthesis in the presence of protective or stabilizing agents such as amphiphilic compounds, polymers, dendrimers, or micelle dispersion systems (Luczak et al. 2016). The composition of ILs and their physicochemical properties influence not only particle synthesis (Souza et al. 2016) but also their stability. ILs are able to act as stabilizing agents via the creation of a protective layer around the nanoparticles (Luczak et al. 2016).

After washing the product of a quantum dots synthesis that used ILs as a reagent, the quantum dots can be reintroduced in another medium without the loss of their stability. Contrary to what happened with sol-gel synthesis using alcohol as a surfactant, ILs still remain around the quantum dots even after the washing steps, and the layers of ILs around these nanoparticles ensure their non-agglomeration. It is possible to identify this IL after washing the quantum dots via usual technical methods, such as thermogravimetric analysis (Souza et al. 2016). Although there are several theories about how ILs act as structuring agents, it is known that the principal means for this area is the formation of protective layers, steric stabilization, electrostatic stabilization, higher viscosity of the medium, as well as a mold that limits the growth of nanoparticles in their chains (or "IL tunnels") during the synthesis (Souza et al. 2016). Therefore, nanoparticles can be maintained in ILs in two ways: the product of the synthesis can be washed, and powder of quantum dots surrounded by nanolayers of ILs can be obtained; the product of the synthesis can be maintained in the liquid media where they were synthesized; in other words, the quantum dots can be maintained in the IL.

Previous researchers decided to synthesize quantum dots using IL using a route of synthesis (Garcia et al. 2019), knowing that it is possible to obtain a powder of quantum dots by using ILs, that is, a much more profitable synthetic route in comparison to self-organization synthesis (such as that used for ZnO_{QDs} synthesis). This was performed using a previously reported synthesis of titanium dioxide (TiO_2) quantum dots with the IL 1-butyl-3-methylimidazolium tetrafluoroborate ($BMI·BF_4$) ($TiO_{2QDs/BMI·BF4}$).

10.8 $TiO_{2QDs/BMI·BF4}$ in an Experimental Adhesive Resin: The Second Step

TiO_2 nanoparticles are widely studied because of their photocatalytic activity (Hashimoto et al. 2016) and antimicrobial effect via generation of ROS (Sun et al. 2017). ROS are formed when this semiconductor material is irradiated with photons (Sun et al. 2017) with higher energy (or shorter waves) than their band-gap (Hashimoto et al. 2016). Electrons move from the valence band to the conduction band, creating a vacancy (hole) in the valence band, making it positive (h+) (charge equal to the electron charge, but with opposite signal), and giving rise to the electron-hole pair (exciton) on the catalyst surface (Garvey et al. 2016; Zhang et al. 2014). Oxidation reactions occur in the valence band and reduction in the conduction band, leading to a photocatalytic process (Souza et al. 2016) and generation of ROS (Garvey et al. 2016). ROS can damage the molecular structure of phospholipids, disrupting the bacterial membrane (Garvey et al. 2016).

For these properties, TiO_2 has been used on self-cleaning surfaces (Isaifan et al. 2017), in the development of antimicrobial materials (Garvey et al. 2016; Kim et al. 2017), as coinitiators in photo-activated reactions (Sun et al. 2011, 2016), as photovoltaic cells in solar panels, for hydrogen production by water splitting (Hashimoto et al. 2016), and as filler to mechanically reinforce polymers (Pinto et al. 2015), such as those for dental use (Sun et al. 2011).

In addition to the benefits mentioned for TiO_2 and ILs, ILs can provide antimicrobial properties. Significant advances in the understanding of ILs' physicochemical and biological properties have been boosting their broad application in health sciences. Some authors suggest that the set of properties, versatility, and potential for multiple functionalities of ILs could present innovative antimicrobial strategies to combat, for instance, bacteria resistant to antibiotics (Pendleton and Gilmore 2015).

ILs have been shown to disrupt biofilms, and their antimicrobial effects are attributed to the cationic group, alkyl chain, or anion. ILs share structural and functional analogies with quaternary ammonium compounds due to their similar structure composed by positively charged organic groups with one or more alkyl chains. Besides their ability to disrupt the structure and integrity of cytoplasmic membranes, ILs may coagulate matrix constituents, causing enzyme denaturation, as well as may occur with quaternary ammonium compounds (Pernak and Chwala 2003).

The antimicrobial characteristics of ILs have been documented since the 1990s, showing that these organic salts can exhibit broad-spectrum antimicrobial activity, affecting Gram-positive and Gram-negative bacteria, mycobacteria, and fungi (Pendleton and Gilmore 2015). In general, the antimicrobial activity of ILs increases with increased lipophilicity, usually manipulated by alkyl chain extension. However, as previously mentioned, the cationic group of the IL may also present antimicrobial action via its interaction with negative charges on the prokaryotic cell membrane (Pernak et al. 2007). Among the most commonly used cations in the formation of the cationic group of ILs, the imidazoles have gained prominence because of its high positive charge and previously reported antimicrobial activity (Ferraz et al. 2011). The possibility of multiple antimicrobial activities may also occur due to the anions of the ILs, which generally play a secondary role (Łuczak et al. 2010). In the constitution of ILs, chlorine ions are the most used for bio purposes because of their more accepted biocompatibility (Pendleton and Gilmore 2015).

ILs have been used in drug delivery systems (Halayqa et al. 2019), in the synthesis of antimicrobial coatings (Ran et al. 2018). Moreover, these salts have been investigated as active pharmaceutical compounds to surpass the polymorphism issue of salts used in drug formulation (Ferraz et al. 2011). Imidazolium-based ILs were tested to coat titanium implants and provide them antimicrobial and anticorrosion properties (Gindri, Palmer et al. 2016; Gindri et al. 2015; Gindri, Siddiqui et al. 2016). Imidazolium-based ILs were also suggested to synthesize silver nanoparticles to be used for endodontic disinfection solutions (Abbaszadegan et al. 2015). More recently, another imidazolium-based IL was incorporated into an orthodontic adhesive resin to provide its antibacterial activity against the biofilm formation of *S. mutans* (Martini Garcia et al. 2019).

In this context, ILs showed attractive properties to be used as a stabilizer of nanoparticles that could be used as a filler for dental resins. With this approach, it would be possible to use quantum dots synthesis routes with higher yield and versatility for the formulation and study of dental resins.

10.9 Synthesis and Characterization of $TiO_{2QDs/BMI\cdot BF4}$

For filler synthesis, $TiCl_4$ (0.5 mL) was mixed with $BMI\cdot BF_4$ (5 mL) (Souza et al. 2016). The mixture was stirred at room temperature, 1 mL of deionized water was added, and the mixture was stirred at 80°C for 12 h. The product was washed with acetonitrile, distilled water, and acetone by centrifugation and dried under vacuum for 24 h. This process generated a powder of $TiO_{2QDs/BMI\cdot BF4}$.

To characterize the $TiO_{2QDs/BMI\cdot BF4}$, it was chemically evaluated via μ-Raman spectroscopy, which indicated characteristic peaks of anatase and rutile of TiO_2. Thermogravimetry was used to quantify the $BMI\cdot BF_4$ remained probably around the $TiO_{2QDs/BMI\cdot BF4}$ after washing it. This method showed around 26 wt.% of $BMI\cdot BF_4$. Lastly, $TiO_{2QDs/BMI\cdot BF4}$ presented a minimum size of 1.19 nm, a maximum size of 7.11 nm, and a mean size of 3.54±1.08 nm via transmission electron microscopy (TEM). The good dispersal of $TiO_{2QDs/BMI\cdot BF4}$ encouraged the researchers to continue and to evaluate the effect of these particles in a dental adhesive.

10.10 $TiO_{2QDs/BMI\cdot BF4}$ in Dental Adhesive

A dental adhesive was formulated with HEMA, BisGMA, and photoinitiators (Garcia et al. 2016, 2019; Garcia, Leitune, Visioli et al. 2018). $TiO_{2QDs/BMI\cdot BF4}$

was incorporated at 2.5, 5, and 0 wt.%. TEM of the polymerized adhesive indicated that $TiO_{2QDs/BMI\cdot BF4}$ were well dispersed. High-resolution fluorescence microscopy showed that $TiO_{2QDs/BMI\cdot BF4}$ had fluorescence intermittency, singular behavior of particles in quantum confinement effect, which was also previously noted when ZnO_{QDs} were added to a dental adhesive. As observed in Figure 10.10, quantum dots present fluorescence in the same area of the polymer at different moments, indicating that they blink in the polymerized material.

The dental adhesives were physicochemically evaluated first via FTIR to investigate the conversion of monomers. The adhesives showed different polymerization kinetics, but all groups maintained a reliable degree of conversion, with values higher than 50%. The addition of 2.5 wt.% did not affect the softening in the solvent of the polymer, and it did not influence

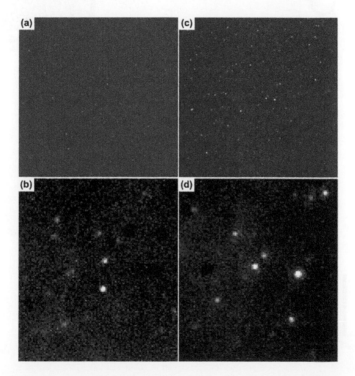

Figure 10.10 Images of high-resolution fluorescence microscopy used to analyze the light intermittency by $TiO_{2QDs/BMI\cdot BF4}$ incorporated into the adhesive resin. Image (a) is the high magnification, and (b) is the lower magnification to the polymerized adhesive with 2.5 wt.% of $TiO_{2QDs/BMI\cdot BF4}$; image (c) is the high magnification, and image (d) is the lower magnification of the polymerized adhesive with 5 wt.% of $TiO_{2QDs/BMI\cdot BF4}$. (Adapted from Garcia et al. (2019).)

the bonding strength to dentin either immediately or after six months of storage in water.

The adhesives were further evaluated for its antibacterial properties and cytotoxic effects against pulp cells. As shown in Figure 10.11, the adhesives with $TiO_{2QDs/BMI·BF4}$ presented antibacterial activity against biofilm formation after 24 h and after three months of storage of samples in water. The SRB assay indicated that these particles did not induce cytotoxicity against pulp cells. In this way, there were no adverse effects observed on

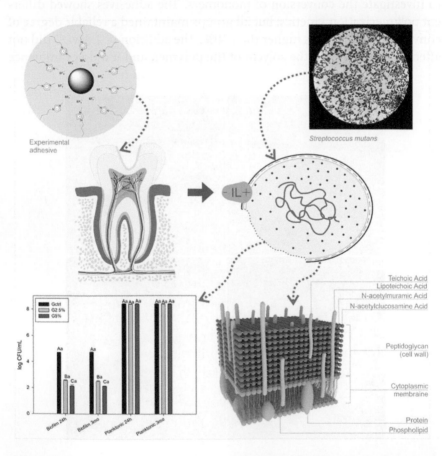

Figure 10.11   Scheme to illustrate the antibacterial mechanism of IL from $TiO_{2QDs/BMI·BF4}$ that was incorporated into the adhesive resin. Data from immediate and long-term antibacterial analyses are indicated in the graph. The most critical negative charged elements in the *S. mutans*' membrane is illustrated in orange and green, and they may have interacted with the positive charge of the IL (Garcia et al. 2019).

physical, chemical, or biological properties when it was added 2.5 wt.% of $TiO2_{QDs/BMI\cdot BF4}$ into the dental adhesive.

For the first time, quantum dots synthesized with an IL as stabilizer were used to formulate a dental adhesive. The outcomes of this study support that it is possible to achieve biopolymers with non-agglomerated nanoparticles using ionic liquid as a stabilizer, which may also be an interesting alternative to provide antibacterial activity against *S. mutans* without cytotoxicity for pulp cells.

10.11 Future Perspectives

The studies performed so far showed the reliability to formulate dental resins with quantum dots. The process of synthesis was refined over the years from the auto-organization of particles to chemical reactions involving ILs to stabilize the particles. This progress will provide further investigation on resins with quantum dots, mainly in the biological field.

In addition to the properties already evaluated, TiO_2 and ZnO are bioactive materials. TiO_2 incorporated into polymers formulation induced mineral deposition on resins' surfaces when they were immersed in simulated body fluid solution (Saito et al. 2011; Shimizu et al. 2016), as well as ZnO (Osorio, Cabello et al. 2014). The dental adhesives formulated with quantum dots of ZnO or TiO_2 should be investigated regarding this property, mainly to be proposed for the biomimetic remineralization approach. Noteworthily, with the advent of restorative techniques involving the selective removal of carious tissue, materials capable of improving the dentin remineralization process, and the properties of dentine affected by caries are desired in dentistry (Tay and Pashley 2009; Schwendicke et al. 2019). The particles evaluated so far for biomimetic remineralization do not have a size compatible with the dentin intrafibrillar spaces (Bertassoni et al. 2012). They often do not penetrate the entire length of the hybrid layer (Tay et al. 1999), which may improve the therapeutic effect of newly developed restorative materials.

Quantum dots such as those proposed currently may serve as ion nucleation sites in places where larger particles do not access (Bertassoni et al. 2012). Even surrounded by IL, previous works show that when surrounded by a relatively hydrophilic material (such as triethylene glycol dimethacrylates, TEGDMA), the particles continue to present important characteristics for bioactivity, such as the release of ions in the case of phosphates (Alania et al. 2016). Therefore, the bioactivity of the adhesives with quantum dots and their possible remineralizing effect on dentin should be evaluated.

In addition to the use of conventional adhesive as proposed in this study, quantum dots with ionic liquids could be added and evaluated in other materials; for instance, in self-etching adhesive systems. Self-etching adhesive systems show advantages over conventional systems, and it is possible to plan the synthesis of acidic ionic liquids to be used in these systems. Another component of adhesive systems that could be modified is the primer. Primers could better carry quantum dots to the inter- and intrafibrillar spaces.

Furthermore, the quantum dots could be tested in composite resins, also in an attempt to reduce the problem of nanoparticle agglomeration (Shahet al. 2009). Endodontic sealers and solutions for endodontic disinfection could also be formulated. In this way, quantum dots could deliver therapeutic agents in areas of difficult access to dental anatomies, such as inside the tubular dentin. The so-called artificial atoms will continue to be extensively tested for biomaterials application.

References

Abbaszadegan, A., M. Nabavizadeh, A. Gholami, Z. S. Aleyasin, S. Dorostkar, M. Saliminasab, Y. Ghasemi, B. Hemmateenejad, and H. Sharghi. 2015. "Positively charged imidazolium-based ionic liquid-protected silver nanoparticles: a promising disinfectant in root canal treatment." *Int Endod J* 48 (8):790–800. doi: 10.1111/iej.12377.

Alania, Y., M. D. S. Chiari, M. C. Rodrigues, V. E. Arana-Chavez, A. H. A. Bressiani, F. M. Vichi, and R. R. Braga. 2016. "Bioactive composites containing TEGDMA-functionalized calcium phosphate particles: degree of conversion, fracture strength and ion release evaluation." *Dent Mater* 32 (12):e374–e381. doi: https://doi.org/10.1016/j.dental.2016.09.021.

Andre, C. B., D. C. Chan, and M. Giannini. 2018. "Antibacterial-containing dental adhesives' effects on oral pathogens and on *Streptococcus mutans* biofilm: current perspectives." *Am J Dent* 31 (Sp Is B):37b–41b.

Bartczak, Z., A. S. Argon, R. E. Cohen, and M. Weinberg. 1999. "Toughness mechanism in semi-crystalline polymer blends: II. High-density polyethylene toughened with calcium carbonate filler particles." *Polymer* 40 (9):2347–65. https://doi.org/10.1016/S0032-3861(98)00444-3.

Bertassoni, L. E., J. P. Orgel, O. Antipova, and M. V. Swain. 2012. "The dentin organic matrix—limitations of restorative dentistry hidden on the nanometer scale." *Acta Biomater* 8 (7):2419–33. doi: 10.1016/j.actbio.2012.02.022.

Bimberg, D., and U. W. Pohl. 2011. "Quantum dots: promises and accomplishments." *Mater Today* 14 (9):388–97. https://doi.org/10.1016/S1369-7021(11)70183-3.

Buatong, N., I.-M. Tang, and W. Pon-On. 2015. "Quantum dot-sensitized solar cells having 3D-TiO$_2$ flower-like structures on the surface of titania nanorods with CuS counter electrode." *Nanoscale Res Lett* 10:146.

Burke, F. J., N. H. Wilson, S. W. Cheung, and I. A. Mjor. 2001. "Influence of patient factors on age of restorations at failure and reasons for their placement and replacement." *J Dent* 29 (5):317–24. doi: 10.1016/s0300-5712(01)00022-7.

Cai, X., B. Li, Y. Pan, and G. Wu. 2012. "Morphology evolution of immiscible polymer blends as directed by nanoparticle self-agglomeration." *Polymer* 53 (1):259–66. https://doi.org/10.1016/j.polymer.2011.11.032.

Chebbi, R. 2015. "Thermal conductivity of nanofluids: effect of Brownian motion of nanoparticles." *AIChE J* 61 (7):2368–9. doi: 10.1002/aic.14847.

Collares, F. M., V. C. B. Leitune, P. Franken, C. F. Parollo, F. A. Ogliari, and S. M. W. Samuel. 2017. "Influence of addition of [2-(methacryloyloxy)ethyl]trimethylammonium chloride to an experimental adhesive." *Braz Oral Res* 31:e31. doi: 10.1590/1807-3107BOR-2017.vol31.0031.

Dananjaya, S. H. S., R. S. Kumar, M. Yang, C. Nikapitiya, J. Lee, and M. De Zoysa. 2018. "Synthesis, characterization of ZnO-chitosan nanocomposites and evaluation of its antifungal activity against pathogenic *Candida albicans*." *Int J Biol Macromol* 108:1281–8 doi: 10.1016/j.ijbiomac.2017.11.046.

Degrazia, F. W., V. C. B. Leitune, I. M. Garcia, R. A. Arthur, S. M. Samuel, and F. M. Collares. 2016. "Effect of silver nanoparticles on the physicochemical and antimicrobial properties of an orthodontic adhesive." *J Appl Oral Sci* 24 (4):404–10. doi: 10.1590/1678-775720160154.

Degrazia, F. W., V. C. B. Leitune, S. M. W. Samuel, and F. M. Collares. 2017. "Boron nitride nanotubes as novel fillers for improving the properties of dental adhesives." *J Dent* 62:85–90 doi: 10.1016/j.jdent.2017.05.013.

Deligeorgi, V., I. A. Mjor, and N. H. Wilson. 2001. "An overview of reasons for the placement and replacement of restorations." *Prim Dent Care* 8 (1):5–11. doi: 10.1308/135576101771799335.

Dupont, J., and J. D. Scholten. 2010. "On the structural and surface properties of transition-metal nanoparticles in ionic liquids." *Chem Soc Rev* 39 (5):1780–804. doi: 10.1039/B822551F.

Earle, M. J., and K. R. Seddon 2002. "Ionic liquids: green solvents for the future." Clean solvents. Alternative media for chemical reactions and processing. 819 (2):10–25. American Chemical Society (Distributed by Oxford University Press): Washington, DC.

Efros, A. L., and D. J. Nesbitt. 2016. "Origin and control of blinking in quantum dots." *Nat Nanotechnol* 11 (8):661–71. doi: 10.1038/nnano.2016.140.

Feitosa, S. A., J. Palasuk, K. Kamocki, S. Geraldeli, R. L. Gregory, J. A. Platt, L. J. Windsor, and M. C. Bottino. 2014. "Doxycycline-encapsulated nanotube-modified dentin adhesives." *J Dent Res* 93 (12):1270–6. doi: 10.1177/0022034514549997.

Feitosa, S. A., J. Palasuk, S. Geraldeli, L. J. Windsor, and M. C. Bottino. 2019. "Physicochemical and biological properties of novel chlorhexidine-loaded nanotube-modified dentin adhesive." *J Biomed Mater Res B Appl Biomater* 107 (3):868–75. doi: 10.1002/jbm.b.34183.

Ferraz, R., L. C. Branco, C. Prudencio, J. P. Noronha, and Z. Petrovski. 2011. "Ionic liquids as active pharmaceutical ingredients." *ChemMedChem* 6 (6):975–85. doi: 10.1002/cmdc.201100082.

Frassetto, A., L. Breschi, G. Turco, G. Marchesi, R. Di Lenarda, F. R. Tay, D. H. Pashley, and M. Cadenaro. 2016. "Mechanisms of degradation of the hybrid layer in adhesive dentistry and therapeutic agents to improve bond durability—a literature review." *Dent Mater* 32 (2):e41–53. doi: 10.1016/j. dental.2015.11.007.

Gaglianone, L. A., A. F. Lima, L. S. Goncalves, A. N. Cavalcanti, F. H. Aguiar, and G. M. Marchi. 2012. "Mechanical properties and degree of conversion of etch-and-rinse and self-etch adhesive systems cured by a quartz tungsten halogen lamp and a light-emitting diode." *J Mech Behav Biomed Mater* 12:- 139–43. doi: 10.1016/j.jmbbm.2012.01.018.

Garcia, I. M., V. C. B. Leitune, C. J. Ferreira, and F. M. Collares. 2018. "Tantalum oxide as filler for dental adhesive resin." *Dent Mater J* 37 (6):897–903. doi: 10.4012/dmj.2017–308.

Garcia, I. M., V. C. B. Leitune, F. Visioli, S. M. W. Samuel, and F. M. Collares. 2018. "Influence of zinc oxide quantum dots in the antibacterial activity and cyto- toxicity of an experimental adhesive resin." *J Dent* 73:57–60. doi: 10.1016/j. jdent.2018.04.003.

Garcia, I. M., V. C. B. Leitune, S. M. W. Samuel, and F. M. Collares. 2017. "Influence of different calcium phosphates on an experimental adhesive resin." *J Adhes Dent* 19 (5):379–84. doi: 10.3290/j.jad.a38997.

Garcia, I. M., V. C. B. Leitune, T. L. Kist, A. Takimi, S. M. Samuel, and F. M. Collares. 2016. "Quantum dots as nonagglomerated nanofillers for adhesive resins." *J Dent Res* 95 (12):1401–7. doi: 10.1177/0022034516656838.

Garcia, I. M., V. S. Souza, C. Hellriegel, J. D. Scholten, and F. M. Collares. 2019. "Ionic liquid-stabilized titania quantum dots applied in adhesive resin." *J Dent Res* 98 (6):682–8. doi: 10.1177/0022034519835203.

Garvey, M., E. Panaitescu, L. Menon, C. Byrne, S. Dervin, S. J. Hinder, and S. C. Pillai. 2016. "Titania nanotube photocatalysts for effectively treating water- borne microbial pathogens." *J Catal* 344:631–9. https://doi.org/10.1016/j.jcat .2016.11.004.

Gindri, I. M., D. A. Siddiqui, C. P. Frizzo, M. A. P. Martins, and D. C. Rodrigues. 2015. "Ionic liquid coatings for titanium surfaces: effect of IL structure on coat- ing profile." *ACS Appl Mater Interfaces* 7 (49):27421–31. doi: 10.1021/acsami. 5b09309.

Gindri, I. M., D. A. Siddiqui, C. P. Frizzo, M. A. P. Martins, and D. C. Rodrigues. 2016. "Improvement of tribological and anti-corrosive performance of tita- nium surfaces coated with dicationic imidazolium-based ionic liquids." *RSC Adv* 6 (82):78795–802. doi: 10.1039/C6RA13961B.

Gindri, I. M., K. L. Palmer, D. A. Siddiqui, S. Aghyarian, C. P. Frizzo, M. A. P. Martins, and D. C. Rodrigues. 2016. "Evaluation of mammalian and bacterial cell activity on titanium surface coated with dicationic imidazolium-based ionic liquids." *RSC Adv* 6 (43):36475–83. doi: 10.1039/C6RA01003B.

Gutierrez, M. F., L. F. Alegria-Acevedo, L. Mendez-Bauer, J. Bermudez, A. Davila- Sanchez, S. Buvinic, N. Hernandez-Moya, A. Reis, A. D. Loguercio, P. V. Farago, J. Martin, and E. Fernandez. 2019. "Biological, mechanical and adhesive properties of universal adhesives containing zinc and copper nanoparticles." *J Dent* 82:45–55. doi: 10.1016/j.jdent.2019.01.012.

Gutierrez, M. F., P. Malaquias, T. P. Matos, A. Szesz, S. Souza, J. Bermudez, A. Reis, A. D. Loguercio, and P. V. Farago. 2017. "Mechanical and microbiological properties and drug release modeling of an etch-and-rinse adhesive containing copper nanoparticles." *Dent Mater* 33 (3):309–20. doi: 10.1016/j.dental.2016.12.011.

Halayqa, M., M. Zawadzki, U. Domańska, and A. Plichta. 2019. "Polymer – ionic liquid – pharmaceutical conjugates as drug delivery systems." *J Mol Struct* 1180:573–84. https://doi.org/10.1016/j.molstruc.2018.12.023.

Hashimoto, K., H. Irie, A. Fujishima. 2005. "TiO_2 photocatalysis: a historical overview and future prospects." *Jpn J Appl Phys* 44 (12):8269–85.

Hashimoto, M., K. Kawai, H. Kawakami, and S. Imazato. 2016. "Matrix metalloproteases inhibition and biocompatibility of gold and platinum nanoparticles." *J Biomed Mater Res A* 104 (1):209–17. doi: 10.1002/jbm.a.35557.

Hsu, C. C., Y. X. Chen, H. W. Li, and J. S. Hsu. 2016. "Low switching voltage ZnO quantum dots doped polymer-dispersed liquid crystal film." *Opt Express* 24 (7):7063–8. doi: 10.1364/oe.24.007063.

Hsueh, Y. H., W. J. Ke, C. T. Hsieh, K. S. Lin, D. Y. Tzou, and C. L. Chiang. 2015. "ZnO nanoparticles affect bacillus subtilis cell growth and biofilm formation." *PLoS One* 10 (6):e0128457. doi: 10.1371/journal.pone.0128457.

Huang, Z., X. Zheng, D. Yan, G. Yin, X. Liao, Y. Kang, Y. Yao, D. Huang, and B. Hao. 2008. "Toxicological effect of ZnO nanoparticles based on bacteria." *Langmuir* 24 (8):4140–4. doi: 10.1021/la7035949.

Isaifan, R. J., A. Samara, W. Suwaileh, D. Johnson, W. Yiming, A. A. Abdallah, and B. Aïssa. 2017. "Improved self-cleaning properties of an efficient and easy to scale up TiO_2 thin films prepared by adsorptive self-assembly." *Sci Rep* 7 (1):9466. doi: 10.1038/s41598-017-07826-0.

Jahantigh, F., S. M. B. Ghorashi, and A. Bayat. 2020. "Hybrid dye sensitized solar cell based on single layer graphene quantum dots." *Dyes Pigments* 175: 108118. doi: 10.1016/j.dyepig.2019.108118.

Jordan, J., K. I. Jacob, R. Tannenbaum, M. A. Sharaf, and I. Jasiuk. 2005. "Experimental trends in polymer nanocomposites—a review." *Mater Sci Eng A* 393 (1):1–11. https://doi.org/10.1016/j.msea.2004.09.044.

Jowkar, Z., N. Farpour, F. Koohpeima, M. J. Mokhtari, and F. Shafiei. 2018. "Effect of silver nanoparticles, zinc oxide nanoparticles and titanium dioxide nanoparticles on microshear bond strength to enamel and dentin." *J Contemp Dent Pract* 19 (11):1404–11.

Khani, O., H. R. Rajabi, M. H. Yousefi, A. A. Khosravi, M. Jannesari, and M. Shamsipur. 2011. "Synthesis and characterizations of ultra-small ZnS and Zn(1-x)Fe(x)S quantum dots in aqueous media and spectroscopic study of their interactions with bovine serum albumin." *Spectrochim Acta A Mol Biomol Spectrosc* 79 (2):361–9. doi: 10.1016/j.saa.2011.03.025.

Kim, C. H., E. S. Lee, S. M. Kang, E. de Josselin de Jong, and B. I. Kim. 2017. "Bactericidal effect of the photocatalystic reaction of titanium dioxide using visible wavelengths on *Streptococcus mutans* biofilm." *Photodiagnosis Photodyn Ther* 18:279–83. doi: 10.1016/j.pdpdt.2017.03.015.

Kirstila, V., P. Hakkinen, H. Jentsch, P. Vilja, and J. Tenovuo. 1998. "Longitudinal analysis of the association of human salivary antimicrobial agents with caries increment and cariogenic microorganisms: a two-year cohort study." *J Dent Res* 77 (1):73–80. doi: 10.1177/00220345980770011101.

Lee, Y. L., T. Cesario, J. Owens, E. Shanbrom, and L. D. Thrupp. 2002. "Antibacterial activity of citrate and acetate." *Nutrition* 18 (7–8):665–6. doi: 10.1016/s0899-9007(02)00782-7.

Leitune, V. C., F. M. Collares, A. Takimi, G. B. de Lima, C. L. Petzhold, C. P. Bergmann, and S. M. Samuel. 2013. "Niobium pentoxide as a novel filler for dental adhesive resin." *J Dent* 41 (2):106–13. doi: 10.1016/j.jdent.2012.04.022.

Leitune, V. C., F. M. Collares, R. M. Trommer, D. G. Andrioli, C. P. Bergmann, and S. M. Samuel. 2013. "The addition of nanostructured hydroxyapatite to an experimental adhesive resin." *J Dent* 41 (4):321–7. doi: 10.1016/j.jdent.2013.01.001.

Leung, Y. H., X. Xu, A. P. Ma, F. Liu, A. M. Ng, Z. Shen, L. A. Gethings, M. Y. Guo, A. B. Djurisic, P. K. Lee, H. K. Lee, W. K. Chan, and F. C. Leung. 2016. "Toxicity of ZnO and TiO_2 to *Escherichia coli* cells." *Sci Rep* 6:35243. doi: 10.1038/srep35243.

Lohbauer, U., A. Wagner, R. Belli, C. Stoetzel, A. Hilpert, H. D. Kurland, J. Grabow, and F. A. Muller. 2010. "Zirconia nanoparticles prepared by laser vaporization as fillers for dental adhesives." *Acta Biomater* 6 (12):4539–46. doi: 10.1016/j.actbio.2010.07.002.

Łuczak, J., C. Jungnickel, I. Łącka, S. Stolte, and J. Hupka. 2010. "Antimicrobial and surface activity of 1-alkyl-3-methylimidazolium derivatives." *Green Chem* 12 (4):593–601. doi: 10.1039/B921805J.

Luczak, J., M. Paszkiewicz, A. Krukowska, A. Malankowska, and A. Zaleska-Medynska. 2016. "Ionic liquids for nano- and microstructures preparation. Part 1: Properties and multifunctional role." *Adv Colloid Interface Sci* 230:-13–28. doi: 10.1016/j.cis.2015.08.006.

Mahshid Saffarpour, M. R., M. Tahriri, A. Peymani. 2016. "Antimicrobial and bond strength properties of a dental adhesive containing zinc oxide nanoparticles." *Braz J Oral Sci* 15 (1):66–9.

Makvandi, P., R. Jamaledin, M. Jabbari, N. Nikfarjam, and A. Borzacchiello. 2018. "Antibacterial quaternary ammonium compounds in dental materials: a systematic review." *Dent Mater* 34 (6):851–67. doi: 10.1016/j.dental.2018.03.014.

Marins, N. H., C. T. W. Meereis, R. M. Silva, C. P. Ruas, A. S. Takimi, N. L. V. Carreno, F. A. Ogliari. 2017. "Radiopaque dental adhesive with addition of niobium pentoxide nanoparticles." *Polym Bull* 6:2301–14.

Martini Garcia, I., C. Jung Ferreira, V. S. de Souza, V. C. Branco Leitune, S. M. W. Samuel, G. de Souza Balbinot, A. de Souza da Motta, F. Visioli, J. Damiani Scholten, and F. Mezzomo Collares. 2019. "Ionic liquid as antibacterial agent for an experimental orthodontic adhesive." *Dent Mater* 35 (8):1155–65. doi: 10.1016/j.dental.2019.05.010.

Martins, G. C., M. M. Meier, A. D. Loguercio, A. Reis, J. C. Gomes, and O. M. Gomes. 2014. "Effects of adding barium-borosilicate glass to a simplified etch-and-rinse adhesive on radiopacity and selected properties." *J Adhes Dent* 16 (2):107–14. doi: 10.3290/j.jad.a30687.

Melo, M. A., S. Orrego, M. D. Weir, H. H. Xu, and D. D. Arola. 2016. "Designing multiagent dental materials for enhanced resistance to biofilm damage at the bonded interface." *ACS Appl Mater Interfaces* 8 (18):11779–87. doi: 10.1021/acsami.6b01923.

Meulenkamp, E. A. 1998. "Synthesis and growth of ZnO nanoparticles." *J Phys Chem B* 102:5566–72.

Michalet, X., F. F. Pinaud, L. A. Bentolila, J. M. Tsay, S. Doose, J. J. Li, G. Sundaresan, A. M. Wu, S. S. Gambhir, and S. Weiss. 2005. "Quantum dots for live cells, in vivo imaging, and diagnostics." *Science* 307 (5709):538–44. doi: 10.1126/science.1104274.

Mirzaei, H., and M. Darroudi. 2017. "Zinc oxide nanoparticles: biological synthesis and biomedical applications." *Ceram Int* 43 (1, Part B):907–14. https://doi .org/10.1016/j.ceramint.2016.10.051.

Modaressi, A., H. Sifaoui, M. Mielcarz, U. Domańska, and M. Rogalski. 2007. "Influence of the molecular structure on the aggregation of imidazolium ionic liquids in aqueous solutions." *Colloid Surf A Physicochem Eng Asp* 302 (1):181–5. https://doi.org/10.1016/j.colsurfa.2007.02.020.

Mutoh, N., and N. Tani-Ishii. 2011. "A biocompatible model for evaluation of the responses of rat periapical tissue to a new zinc oxide-eugenol sealer." *Dent Mater J* 30 (2):176–82. doi: 10.4012/dmj.2010–095.

Nakabayashi, N., and D. Pashley. 1998. *Hybridization of dental hard tissues.* Chicago: Quintessence Publishing.

Opdam, N. J., F. H. van de Sande, E. Bronkhorst, M. S. Cenci, P. Bottenberg, U. Pallesen, P. Gaengler, A. Lindberg, M. C. Huysmans, and J. W. van Dijken. 2014. "Longevity of posterior composite restorations: a systematic review and meta-analysis." *J Dent Res* 93 (10):943–9. doi: 10.1177/0022034514544217.

Osorio, R., E. Osorio, A. L. Medina-Castillo, and M. Toledano. 2014. "Polymer nanocarriers for dentin adhesion." *J Dent Res* 93 (12):1258–63. doi: 10.1177/ 0022034514551608.

Osorio, R., I. Cabello, and M. Toledano. 2014. "Bioactivity of zinc-doped dental adhesives." *J Dent* 42 (4):403–12. doi: 10.1016/j.jdent.2013.12.006.

Palaniappan, S., D. Bharadwaj, D. L. Mattar, M. Peumans, B. Van Meerbeek, and P. Lambrechts. 2011. "Nanofilled and microhybrid composite restorations: five-year clinical wear performances." *Dent Mater* 27 (7):692–700. doi: 10.1016/j. dental.2011.03.012.

Pendleton, J. N., and B. F. Gilmore. 2015. "The antimicrobial potential of ionic liquids: a source of chemical diversity for infection and biofilm control." *Int J Antimicrob Agents* 46 (2):131–9. doi: 10.1016/j.ijantimicag.2015.02.016.

Pernak, J., A. Syguda, I. Mirska, A. Pernak, J. Nawrot, A. Pradzynska, S. T. Griffin, and R. D. Rogers. 2007. "Choline-derivative-based ionic liquids." *Chemistry* 13 (24):6817–27. doi: 10.1002/chem.200700285.

Pernak, J., and P. Chwala. 2003. "Synthesis and antimicrobial activities of choline-like quaternary ammonium chlorides." *Eur J Med Chem* 38 (11–12):1035–42. doi: 10.1016/j.ejmech.2003.09.004.

Pinto, D., L. Bernardo, A. Amaro, and S. Lopes. 2015. "Mechanical properties of epoxy nanocomposites using titanium dioxide as reinforcement – a review." *Constr Build Mater* 95:506–24. https://doi.org/10.1016/j.conbuildmat.2015 .07.124.

Pleskova, S., E. Mikheeva, and E. Gornostaeva. 2018. "Using of quantum dots in biology and medicine." *Adv Exp Med Biol* 1048:323–34. doi: 10.1007/978-3-319 -72041-8_19.

Prechtl, M. H., P. S. Campbell, J. D. Scholten, G. B. Fraser, G. Machado, C. C. Santini, J. Dupont, and Y. Chauvin. 2010. "Imidazolium ionic liquids as promoters and stabilising agents for the preparation of metal(0) nanoparticles by reduction and decomposition of organometallic complexes." *Nanoscale* 2 (12):2601–6. doi: 10.1039/c0nr00574f.

Provenzi, C., F. M. Collares, M. Cuppini, S. M. W. Samuel, A. K. Alves, C. P. Bergmann, and V. C. B. Leitune. 2018. "Effect of nanostructured zirconium dioxide incorporation in an experimental adhesive resin." *Clin Oral Investig* 22 (6):2209–18. doi: 10.1007/s00784-017-2311-z.

Raghupathi, K. R., R. T. Koodali, and A. C. Manna. 2011. "Size-dependent bacterial growth inhibition and mechanism of antibacterial activity of zinc oxide nanoparticles." *Langmuir* 27 (7):4020–8. doi: 10.1021/la104825u.

Ran, B., Z. Zhang, L. Yin, T. Hu, Z. Jiang, Q. Wang, et al. 2018. "A facile antibacterial coating based on UV-curable acrylated imidazoliums." *J Coat Technol Res* 15:345–9.

Rho, Y. J., C. Namgung, B. H. Jin, B. S. Lim, and B. H. Cho. 2013. "Longevity of direct restorations in stress-bearing posterior cavities: a retrospective study." *Oper Dent* 38 (6):572–82. doi: 10.2341/12-432-C.

Rodrigues, S. B., C. L. Petzhold, D. Gamba, V. C. B. Leitune, and F. M. Collares. 2018. "Acrylamides and methacrylamides as alternative monomers for dental adhesives." *Dent Mater* 34 (11):1634–44. doi: 10.1016/j.dental.2018.08.296.

Roduner, E. 2006. "Size matters: why nanomaterials are different." *Chem Soc Rev* 35 (7):583–92. doi: 10.1039/b502142c.

Sahu, D., G. M. Kannan, and R. Vijayaraghavan. 2014. "Size-dependent effect of zinc oxide on toxicity and inflammatory potential of human monocytes." *J Toxicol Environ Health A* 77 (4):177–91. doi: 10.1080/15287394.2013.853224.

Saito, T., M. Takemoto, A. Fukuda, Y. Kuroda, S. Fujibayashi, M. Neo, D. Honjoh, T. Hiraide, T. Kizuki, T. Kokubo, and T. Nakamura. 2011. "Effect of titania-based surface modification of polyethylene terephthalate on bone-implant bonding and peri-implant tissue reaction." *Acta Biomater* 7 (4):1558–69. doi: 10.1016/j.actbio.2010.11.018.

Salz, U., J. Zimmermann, F. Zeuner, and N. Moszner. 2005. "Hydrolytic stability of self-etching adhesive systems." *J Adhes Dent* 7 (2):107–16.

Samadikhah, H. R., M. Nikkhah, and S. Hosseinkhani. 2017. "Enhancement of cell internalization and photostability of red and green emitter quantum dots upon entrapment in novel cationic nanoliposomes." *Luminescence* 32 (4):-517–28. doi: 10.1002/bio.3207.

Schulz, H., B. Schimmoeller, S. E. Pratsinis, U. Salz, and T. Bock. 2008. "Radiopaque dental adhesives: dispersion of flame-made Ta_2O_5/SiO_2 nanoparticles in methacrylic matrices." *J Dent* 36 (8):579–87. doi: 10.1016/j.jdent.2008. 04.010.

Schwendicke, F., A. Al-Abdi, A. Pascual Moscardo, A. Ferrando Cascales, and S. Sauro. 2019. "Remineralization effects of conventional and experimental ion-releasing materials in chemically or bacterially-induced dentin caries lesions." *Dent Mater* 35 (5):772–9. doi: 10.1016/j.dental.2019.02.021.

Schwendicke, F., J. E. Frencken, L. Bjorndal, M. Maltz, D. J. Manton, D. Ricketts, K. Van Landuyt, A. Banerjee, G. Campus, S. Domejean, M. Fontana, S. Leal, E. Lo, V. Machiulskiene, A. Schulte, C. Splieth, A. F. Zandona, and N. P. Innes. 2016. "Managing carious lesions: consensus recommendations on carious tissue removal." *Adv Dent Res* 28 (2):58–67. doi: 10.1177/0022034516639271.

Shah, M. B., J. L. Ferracane, and J. J. Kruzic. 2009. "Mechanistic aspects of fatigue crack growth behavior in resin based dental restorative composites." *Dent Mater* 25 (7):909–16. doi: 10.1016/j.dental.2009.01.097.

Sheiham, A. 2002. "Minimal intervention in dental care." *Med Princ Pract* 11 (Suppl 1):2–6.

Shimizu, T., S. Fujibayashi, S. Yamaguchi, K. Yamamoto, B. Otsuki, M. Takemoto, M. Tsukanaka, T. Kizuki, T. Matsushita, T. Kokubo, and S. Matsuda. 2016. "Bioactivity of sol-gel-derived TiO_2 coating on polyetheretherketone: in vitro and in vivo studies." *Acta Biomater* 35:305–17. doi: 10.1016/j. actbio.2016.02.007.

Singh, V. A., and Kumar L. 2006. "Revisiting elementary quantum mechanics with the BenDaniel-Duke boundary condition." *Am J Phys* 74 (5):412.

Souza, V. S., J. D. Scholten, D. E. Weibel, D. Eberhardt, D. L. Baptista, S. R. Teixeira, and J. Dupont. 2016. "Hybrid tantalum oxide nanoparticles from the hydrolysis of imidazolium tantalate ionic liquids: efficient catalysts for hydrogen generation from ethanol/water solutions." *J Mater Chem A* 4 (19):7469–75. doi: 10.1039/C6TA02114J.

Spencer, P., Q. Ye, J. Park, E. M. Topp, A. Misra, O. Marangos, Y. Wang, B. S. Bohaty, V. Singh, F. Sene, J. Eslick, K. Camarda, and J. L. Katz. 2010. "Adhesive/dentin interface: the weak link in the composite restoration." *Ann Biomed Eng* 38 (6):1989–2003. doi: 10.1007/s10439-010-9969-6.

Sun, J., A. M. Forster, P. M. Johnson, N. Eidelman, G. Quinn, G. Schumacher, X. Zhang, and W. L. Wu. 2011. "Improving performance of dental resins by adding titanium dioxide nanoparticles." *Dent Mater* 27 (10):972–82. doi: 10.1016/j.dental.2011.06.003.

Sun, J., E. J. Petersen, S. S. Watson, C. M. Sims, A. Kassman, S. Frukhtbeyn, D. Skrtic, M. T. Ok, D. S. Jacobs, V. Reipa, Q. Ye, and B. C. Nelson. 2017. "Biophysical characterization of functionalized titania nanoparticles and their application in dental adhesives." *Acta Biomater* 53:585–97. doi: 10.1016/j. actbio.2017.01.084.

Sun, J., S. S. Watson, D. A. Allsopp, D. Stanley, and D. Skrtic. 2016. "Tuning photocatalytic activities of TiO_2 nanoparticles using dimethacrylate resins." *Dent
Mater* 32 (3):363–72. doi: 10.1016/j.dental.2015.11.021.

Sunnegardh-Gronberg, K., J. W. van Dijken, U. Funegard, A. Lindberg, and M.
Nilsson. 2009. "Selection of dental materials and longevity of replaced restorations in Public Dental Health clinics in northern Sweden." *J Dent* 37 (9):-
673–8. doi: 10.1016/j.jdent.2009.04.010.

Tavassoli Hojati, S., H. Alaghemand, F. Hamze, F. Ahmadian Babaki, R. Rajab-Nia,
M. B. Rezvani, M. Kaviani, and M. Atai. 2013. "Antibacterial, physical and
mechanical properties of flowable resin composites containing zinc oxide
nanoparticles." *Dent Mater* 29 (5):495–505. doi: 10.1016/j.dental.2013.03.011.

Tay, F. R., and D. H. Pashley. 2009. "Biomimetic remineralization of resin-bonded
acid-etched dentin." *J Dent Res* 88 (8):719–24. doi: 10.1177/0022034509341826.

Tay, F. R., K. M. Moulding, and D. H. Pashley. 1999. "Distribution of nanofillers
from a simplified-step adhesive in acid-conditioned dentin." *J Adhes Dent* 1
(2):103–17.

Tezvergil-Mutluay, A., K. A. Agee, A. Mazzoni, R. M. Carvalho, M. Carrilho, I. L.
Tersariol, F. D. Nascimento, S. Imazato, L. Tjaderhane, L. Breschi, F. R. Tay,
and D. H. Pashley. 2015. "Can quaternary ammonium methacrylates inhibit
matrix MMPs and cathepsins?" *Dent Mater* 31 (2):e25–32. doi: 10.1016/j.
dental.2014.10.006.

Van Landuyt, K. L., J. Snauwaert, J. De Munck, M. Peumans, Y. Yoshida, A.
Poitevin, E. Coutinho, K. Suzuki, P. Lambrechts, and B. Van Meerbeek. 2007.
"Systematic review of the chemical composition of contemporary dental adhe-
sives." *Biomaterials* 28 (26):3757–85. doi: 10.1016/j.biomaterials.2007.04.044.

van Tonder, A., A. M. Joubert, and A. D. Cromarty. 2015. "Limitations of the
3-(4,5-dimethylthiazol-2-yl)-2,5-diphenyl-2H-tetrazolium bromide (MTT)
assay when compared to three commonly used cell enumeration assays."
BMC Res Notes 8:47. doi: 10.1186/s13104-015-1000-8.

WHO. 2012. Oral health fact sheet. http://www.who.int/mediacentre/factsheets
/fs318/en/.

Zhang, Y., Y. Liu, C. Li, X. Chen, and Q. Wang. 2014. "Controlled synthesis of Ag_2S
quantum dots and experimental determination of the exciton Bohr radius."
J Phys Chem C 118 (9):4918–23. doi: 10.1021/jp501266d.

Index

Note: **Bold** page numbers refer to tables and *italic* page numbers refer to figures.

Printed and bound by CPI Group (UK) Ltd, Croydon, CR0 4YY

24/10/2024

01778308-0010